RICE UNIVERSITY

SEMICENTENNIAL PUBLICATIONS

Delayed Implantation

Delayed Implantation

1963

PUBLISHED FOR
WILLIAM MARSH RICE UNIVERSITY
BY
THE UNIVERSITY OF CHICAGO PRESS

Library of Congress Catalog Card Number: 63-18851

THE UNIVERSITY OF CHICAGO PRESS, CHICAGO & LONDON
The University of Toronto Press, Toronto 5, Canada

Published 1963. Composed and printed by THE UNIVERSITY OF CHICAGO PRESS, *Chicago, Illinois, U.S.A.*

Preface

THE CELEBRATION of Rice University's semicentennial year provided an opportunity to assemble a group of biologists with a common interest in delayed implantation in mammals. This opportunity occurred at a particularly appropriate time. Interest in delayed implantation has been stimulated by reports from Australia indicating that the phenomenon of delayed implantation, which had barely been suspected in marsupials a decade ago, is probably a common reproductive pattern in the macropods. Furthermore, the use of experimentally induced delay of implantation in rodents has been serving recently as a method for studying blastocyst-endometrial relationships. In addition, the techniques of biochemistry and of electron microscopy have only lately begun to be applied to the study of the blastocyst and its environment. It therefore seemed appropriate to assemble a group of individuals from several different countries who had different approaches to the study of delayed implantation and, in so doing, to encourage the exchange of information between investigators at a time of increasing interest in delayed implantation.

Under the joint sponsorship of Rice University and the National Science Foundation, a group of approximately sixty speakers and participants from six nations assembled at Rice University from January 23 through 26, 1963. The sessions that they attended ranged in subject from surveys of delay in marsupials and mustelids through laboratory studies of induced delay of implantation to studies of implantation per se. The material presented at the symposium and discussion of the papers constitutes the contents of this volume.

I wish to thank the members of the advisory committee for their early enthusiasm for the project, their efforts in making the symposium possible, and their role in the sessions. Many thanks should also go to the contributors to this volume, who gave freely of their thoughts and time, and to the other participants in the symposium whose interest in the material presented formed an essential part of the give-and-take of the symposium.

ALLEN C. ENDERS

Contents

CARL G. HARTMAN

Introductory Address

AS IS WELL KNOWN, the idea of delayed implantation goes back three hundred years to that master of keen observation, William Harvey (1651), who turned his deer-hunting trips with King Charles to scientific purposes. Two hundred years later, in 1854, the phenomenon interested the great embryologist Theodore Bischoff, and in 1900 the biologist Retzius. If I remember correctly, Keibel's paper in 1902 noted that the inhibited deer embryo was not completely quiescent, for the embryo had many cells in mitosis, a subject that I am looking forward to hearing Dr. Baevsky discuss tomorrow.

With the discovery by Lataste in 1887 and Duval in 1892 of delayed implantation in the lactating rat, an experimental animal was found suitable for experimentation on the possible cause, or causes, of delayed implantation. Daniel in 1910 and both King and Kirkham in 1913 corroborated previous workers but were not active in running down the physiological causes of the phenomenon. It was not until the 1930's, and especially the 1940's, that the endocrine approach was inaugurated. This delay in researches in this direction was due to the fact that the sex hormones were not then known. In the 1920's we were still in the "soup" stage of sex endocrine studies. The isolation and identification of these hormones by Doisy and Edgar Allen, Corner and Willard Allen, Hisaw, Evans, and others belong to the 1930's. So we may say that the 1940's and the 1950's have seen a renewed activity in efforts to elucidate the physiological factors concerned in the phenomenon of delayed nidation and its possible adaptive significance.

I had the opportunity of following several studies along this line in the 1930's myself. Dr. Kaisa Turpeinen of Helsinki worked with Evans and Simpson in the Institute of Experimental Biology in Berkeley on experiments using their purified LH (pardon, ICSH) preparations, with

DR. CARL G. HARTMAN is professor of zoölogy and physiology, emeritus, The University of Illinois; research director, emeritus, Ortho Research Foundation; and research consultant, Margaret Sanger Research Bureau.

the thought that the hormones might stimulate the ovary to secrete additional progesterone, thereby hastening the implantation of the embryo. This, however, remained refractory. Dr. Turpeinen then came to the Carnegie Laboratory in Baltimore, where she was given the facilities to apply progesterone to the experimental animals, again with negative results. Next, Drs. Seegar-Jones and Delfs of the Department of Obstetrics of the Johns Hopkins Hospital had better success using estrogens, as also did Weichert later.

The published papers on this subject have been reviewed by a number of writers, of whom I might mention Amoroso and Marshall in Volume I, Part 2, of Marshall's *Physiology of Reproduction* of 1960, with a summary table on pages 738–39; Blandau in Volume II of the 1962 edition of *Sex and Internal Secretions*, published by Williams and Wilkins Company; and Sir Solly Zuckerman in his two-volume work on the ovary published by Academic Press in 1962.

I might add one more item, my own negative findings on the armadillo on which students and I experimented at the University of Illinois. Our failure to get positive results, in retrospect, makes me feel that this work would better have been left to Texans to solve on Texas armadillos in Texas in the first place.

It is fitting that this conference should be held at a university, for universities, through their organized intelligence, control the future. Universities are not afraid of ideas, though their boards of trustees sometimes seem to be. The three hundred years (with sizable gaps) of study in the area we are here considering emphasizes the fact that there is never a completely new idea—all ideas have pedigrees. Dr. Porter, founder of the *American Journal of Physiology*, said, "No man knows the father of his idea," and Professor Whitehead put it this way: "Everything of importance has been said before by somebody who did not discover it." However, I like to think of research as being like opening a door only to find many doors beyond—closed. I am anticipating that some of these doors will be opened in these two days at Rice University; I know for certain that they will for me.

G. B. SHARMAN

Delayed Implantation in Marsupials

THAT DELAYED implantation occurred in at least one marsupial might have been inferred from the report of Carson (1912) about a zoo female of the red kangaroo (*Megaleia rufa*), which was found to have a young in the pouch that must have been born many months after the death of its male parent. Carson apparently assumed that a double fertilization occurred at a single mating, for he suggested that one egg might have developed in one of the two uteri while the other developed more slowly or lay dormant in the alternate uterus "during the months necessary to account for the delay in birth." Jones (1923, 1944), although aware of Carson's work, suggested that cases of delayed birth in red kangaroos and other marsupials could be explained in terms of storage of viable spermatozoa in the female reproductive tract. Sharman (1955*b*, 1955*c*) showed that in at least two species of marsupials birth occurred after the prolonged storage of a quiescent blastocyst stage in the reproductive tract of the lactating female, and later work has shown that several other marsupial species have a similar type of delayed implantation (Hughes, 1962*a*; Ride and Tyndale-Biscoe, 1962).

DELAYED IMPLANTATION IN THE RED KANGAROO (*Megaleia rufa* DESM.)

The female red kangaroo is polyestrous and monovular (Sharman and Pilton, 1963). The average length of the estrous cycle, as determined by the vaginal smear technique, was 34.81 days, and the average length of pregnancy was 33.17 days. Postpartum estrus occurred about 2 days after parturition and the entry of the young to the pouch (Fig. 1). The intervals between mating and postpartum estrus averaged 35.53 days, and, although this interval is slightly longer than the length of the

G. B. SHARMAN is principal research officer, Commonwealth Scientific and Industrial Research Organization, Division of Wildlife Research, Canberra, A.C.T., Australia.

estrous cycle, it is by no means significantly different from it (Table 1). Postpartum mating was not followed by birth while the young occupied the pouch, but, if the young was removed from the pouch, lactation ceased and birth occurred, in the absence of intervening mating, about 31 days after removal. If the young were retained until they emerged from the pouch at the age of about 236 days, their mothers produced a second young immediately afterward if they had mated at

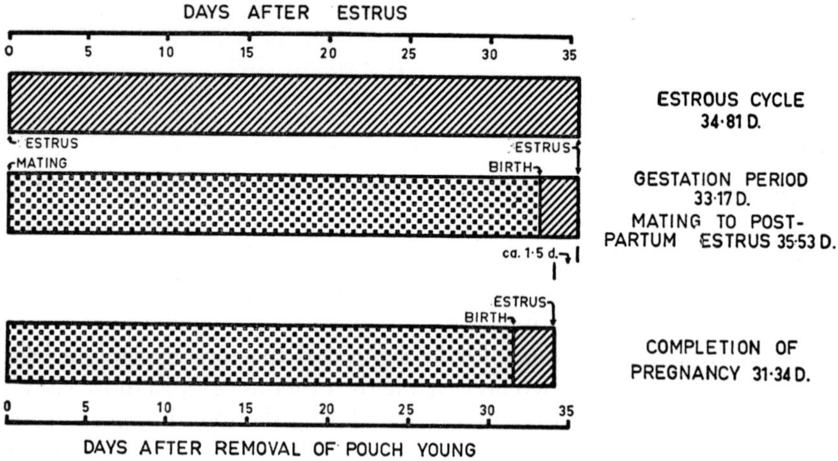

FIG. 1.—Lengths of estrous cycle, gestation period, interval between mating and postpartum mating, and interval between removal of pouch young and birth of young derived from the quiescent blastocyst in the red kangaroo (*Megaleia rufa*). Diagonal hatching indicates absence of embryonic stage; dots indicate presence of embryonic stage.

TABLE 1

REPRODUCTION IN *Megaleia rufa*

Period	Days (Mean ± S.E.)	Reproductive State
Estrus to estrus (estrous cycle)......	{34.81±0.63(16) {35.53±0.52(17)	Non-pregnant Pregnant
Mating to birth (gestation period)...	33.17±0.16(14)	Pregnant
Removal of pouch young to estrus...	{34.67±0.34(3) {34.00±0.89(8)	No blastocyst present Delayed blastocyst completing development
Removal of pouch young to birth (completion of pregnancy)........	31.34±0.35(8)	Delayed blastocyst completing development
Birth to emergence from pouch......	{235.75±2.56(4) {236.50±2.66(10)	No blastocyst present Blastocyst present

Periods inclosed in braces not significantly different.

postpartum estrus. Meanwhile, suckling of the first young, out of the pouch, continued (Pl. I, *1*, *2*). Births that followed the premature removal of young from the pouch, or that followed the normal emergence of young, were also followed by postpartum estrus (Fig. 1). This occurred 34 days after removal of the pouch young, that is, at about the same time after removal as estrus recurred in females that had not had a postpartum mating (Table 1).

Females that had young in the pouch and had mated at postpartum estrus were "pregnant" in the sense that they carried a blastocyst stage of about 0.25-mm. diameter in one or the other uterus (Pl. II, *3*). Blastocysts in the uterus of females with early young in the pouch did not differ in size from those in the uterus of females with advanced young in the pouch, and cell division did not occur in any of 35 blastocysts from females with young aged 7–90 days in the pouch. The precise stage at which the blastocyst began to enlarge in females carrying their pouch young to term varied from female to female, but two females with young aged 213 and 220 days (calculated from measurements) had developing embryos 3 and 5 mm. in diameter in the uterus.

These observations indicate that the red kangaroo has lactation-controlled, delayed implantation. Postpartum mating results in fertilization, but the stimulus of the suckling young in the pouch in some way retards embryonic development, which is completed if the suckling young is lost or removed from the pouch. The relationship between completion of pregnancy and lactation is not simple, since, when the young were retained and suckled in the pouch until they emerged in the normal course of events, embryonic development of the delayed stage was resumed during lactation. There were no differences in the periods of suckling in the pouch between females not carrying delayed blastocysts and those carrying blastocysts that subsequently completed development (Table 1). A remarkable feature is the ability of the female red kangaroo to carry a quiescent but viable embryonic stage of only 0.25-mm. diameter (including the shell membrane) in the uterus for more than 200 days.

Occurrence and Evolution of Delayed Implantation in Marsupials

In all polyestrous marsupials so far studied, with one possible exception (*Macropus canguru*), the gestation periods are shorter than the length of one estrous cycle (Table 2). This contrasts with the condition in polyestrous eutherian mammals, in which pregnancy exceeds the time normally occupied by at least several estrous cycles (Sharman, 1959). Delayed implantation is a feature of reproduction in those marsupials in which the gestation period is nearly equal in length to, but just shorter than, one estrous cycle. It does not occur in such marsupials as *Didelphis* or *Perameles*, in which the estrous cycle is about twice as long as the gestation period (Table 2), and it is known to occur in only one of the five living superfamilies of marsupials recognized by Simpson (1945)—the Phalangeroidea. Within this group it is confined, with one known exception, to the family Macropodidae (kangaroo-like marsupials). The comparatively long gestation period and rudimentary condition at birth of the carnivorous marsupials *Dasyuroides* (Mack, 1961) and *Antechinus* (Marlow, 1961) suggest that development may be discontinuous during pregnancy, but, if delayed implantation does occur, it is mediated by factors other than suckling of young in the pouch.

TABLE 2

OCCURRENCE OF LACTATION-CONTROLLED DELAYED IMPLANTATION IN MARSUPIALS

Family	Without Delayed Implantation	Lengths of Pregnancy and Estrous Cycle (D)				With Delayed Implantation
Didelphidae	*Didelphis virginiana**	13	29			None known
Dasyuridae	*Antechinus flavipes*†	31	monestrus			
Peramelidae	*Perameles nasuta*‡	12	26			
Phalangeridae	*Trichosurus vulpecula*§	17	26			
				?	?	*Dramicia concinna*‖
Macropodidae	*Macropus canguru*#	? variable	34			
				27	28	*Setonix brachyurus***
				33	35	*Megaleia rufa*††
				38	42	*Potorous tridactylus*‡‡
						Also *Protemnodon eugenii*,§§ *P. irma*,‖ ‖ *Thylogale thetis*,## *T. billardierii*,## *Macropus robustus*,*** *Lagostrophus fasciatus*,‖ ‖ *Bettongia cuniculus*,††† *B. lesueuri*‖ ‖

* Hartman (1923); Reynolds (1952).

† Marlow (1961).

‡ Hughes (1962*b*).

§ Pilton and Sharman (1962).

‖ Bowley (1939) showed that a lactating female produced a litter after long separation from males.

\# Gestation period, *ca.* 30 days; estrous cycle, 34 days (Phyllis E. Pilton, personal communication); gestation period 34–35 days (my data), 38–39 days (Owen 1839–47); no evidence of delayed implantation during suckling of early pouch young (Pilton, 1961).

** Sharman (1955*b*).

†† Sharman and Pilton (1963).

‡‡ Hughes (1962*a*).

§§ Sharman (1955*c*).

‖ ‖ Ride and Tyndale-Biscoe (1962).

\## Sharman (unpublished).

*** Ealey (this symposium).

††† Flynn (1930) showed that postpartum estrus and fertilization occurred in this species.

PLATE I

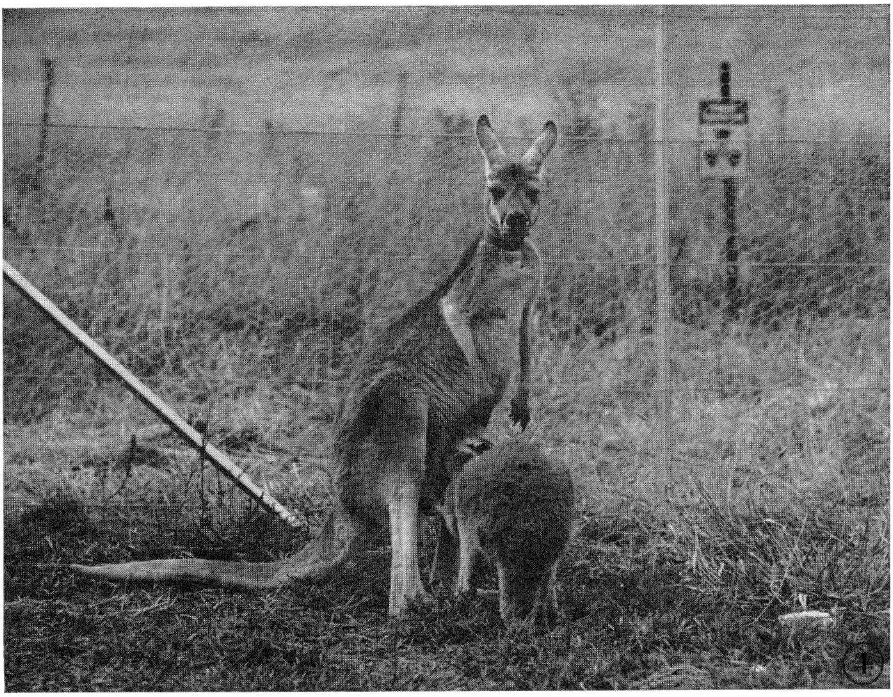

1, Female red kangaroo, with newborn young in the pouch, suckling a 232-day-old young that has just left the pouch.

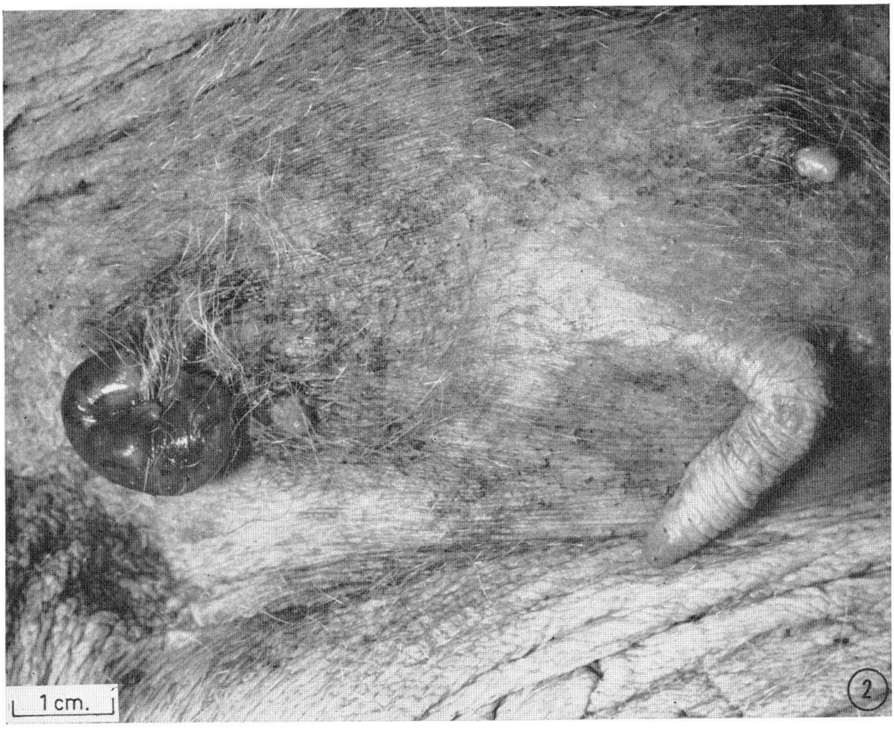

2, Newborn young in the pouch of female shown in *1*. The young is attached to a teat on the upper left; teats at lower left and upper right not lactating; teat at lower right enlarged and producing milk on which the young out of the pouch is being fed.

PLATE II

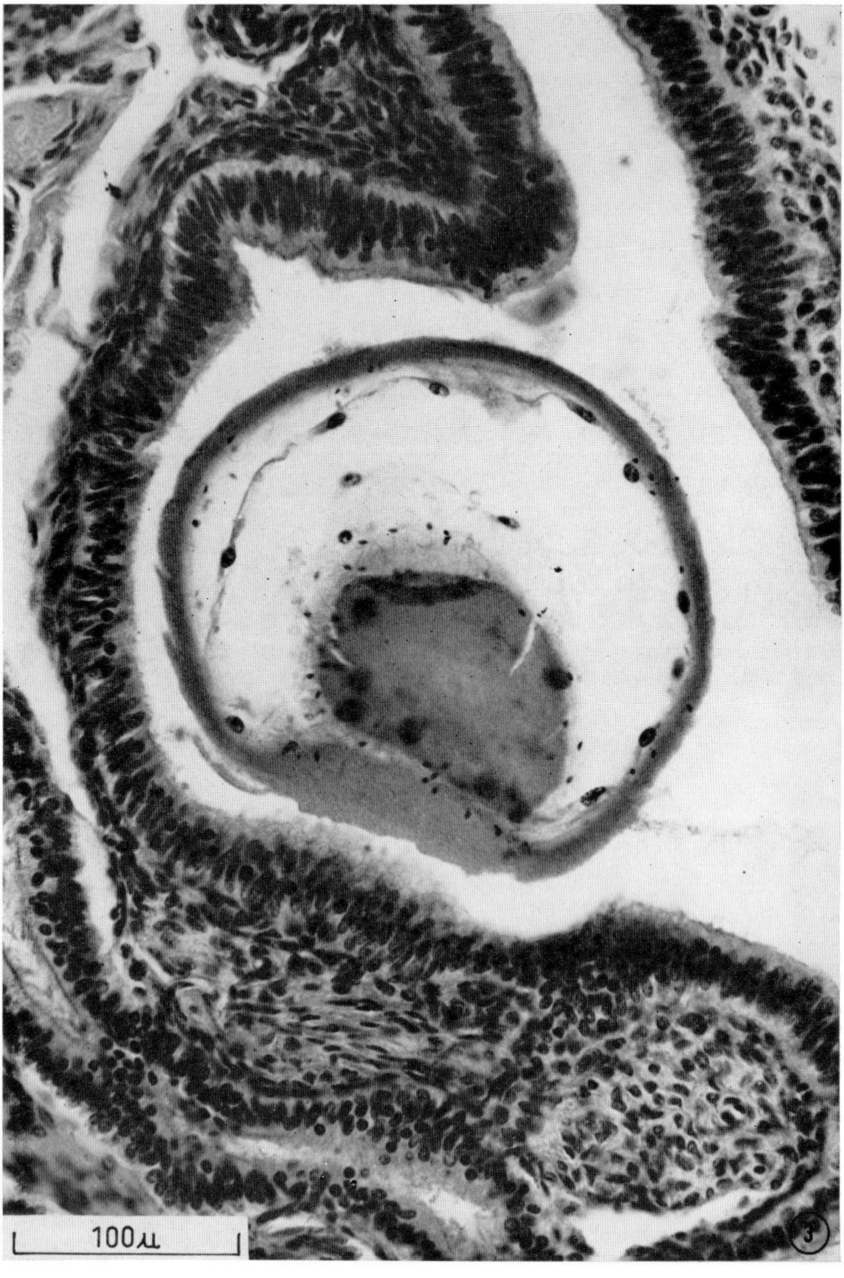

3, Blastocyst in the sectioned uterus of a red kangaroo female with 50-day-old young in the pouch. The blastocyst is seen partly in section (*above*) and partly in surface view (*below*). Blastocyst surrounded by shell membrane in which sperm heads (*black dots*) are imbedded.

In the macropod marsupial *Setonix* the histological and other changes that occur in the reproductive system during the first 27 days of the 28-day estrous cycle are exactly comparable with those occurring during pregnancy except that pregnant females possess a developing embryo in one uterus (Sharman, 1955*a*, 1955*b*). Proestrous changes are already initiated in ovary, uterus, and vagina at the time of parturition. Similar conditions probably prevail in the red kangaroo (*Megaleia*) and in *Potorous* (Fig. 2).

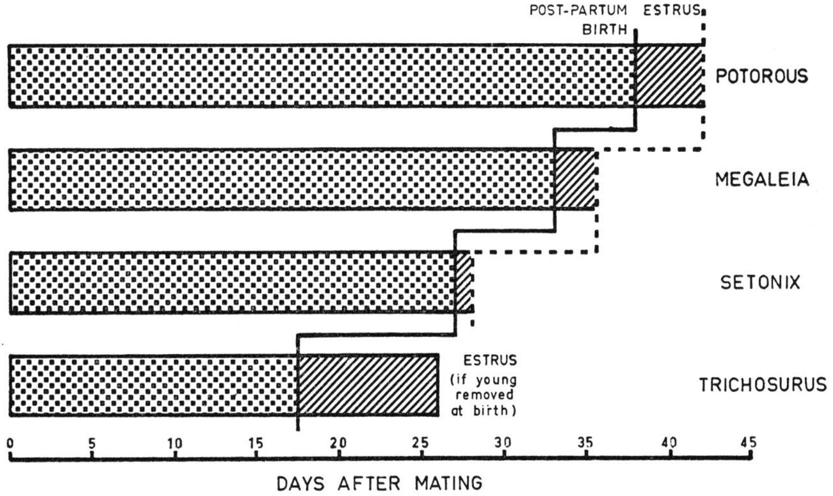

FIG. 2.—Lengths of gestation period and estrous cycle in three marsupials having delayed implantation (*Potorous*, *Megaleia*, and *Setonix*) and in one marsupial that does not have delayed implantation (*Trichosurus*). Diagonal hatching indicates absence of embryonic stage; dots indicate presence of embryonic stage. Note that the estrous cycle is slightly longer than the gestation period in species having delayed implantation and comparatively much longer in the species without delayed implantation.

Fertilization and the subsequent occurrence of pregnancy do not in any way delay postpartum estrus, which happens at the time estrus would occur if pregnancy had not taken place (Fig. 1). In the brush opossum (*Trichosurus*) the changes in the reproductive system during the 17.5-day pregnancy are comparable with those that take place during the first 17–18 days of the estrous cycle (Pilton and Sharman, 1962). Prelactational changes occur in non-mated females following cyclic ovulation, and lactation may be initiated in non-pregnant females, at 16–19 days after estrus, simply by placing a newborn young, which attaches to a teat, in the pouch (Sharman, 1962). Postpartum estrus and ovulation did not occur in *Trichosurus* unless the neonatus is removed at birth. Estrus then recurs at the time expected if the female had not been pregnant (Pilton and Sharman, 1962) (Fig. 2). In *Didelphis* the changes during the short pregnancy are similar to those in the early part of the estrous cycle, and pregnancy does not interrupt the estrous cycle if the young are removed at birth (Hartman, 1923). In the same species a single young is apparently unable to exert sufficient suckling stimulus to maintain lactation and prevent the recurrence of estrus (Reynolds, 1952). These observations suggest that the stimulus of lactation is important in withholding ovulation in marsupials, and it is likely that postpartum estrus occurs in macropods because the onset of lactation is sufficiently delayed, by the comparatively long pregnancy, to allow preovulatory changes to be initiated in the ovary.

It is tempting to postulate that delayed implantation has evolved in the macropod marsupials, the most advanced members of the order, because of an evolutionary trend toward longer gestation periods that have come to occupy almost the entire estrous cycle (Sharman, 1959). Looked at in this way, the evolution of delayed implantation seems almost inevitable, and it might have evolved independently in several lines in which pregnancy was prolonged sufficiently to allow proestrous changes to be initiated before the onset of lactation.

However, postpartum estrus and fertilization are known to occur occasionally in *Trichosurus* (Tyndale-Biscoe, 1955; Pilton and Sharman, 1962), and in the cases studied the embryo derived from the postpartum mating underwent normal development, so two young, separated in age by the period between two fertilizations, came to occupy the pouch. Delayed implantation therefore appears to involve more than the occurrence of postpartum ovulation and fertilization; the mechanism responsible also requires that the corpus luteum, formed at postpartum ovulation, enters an arrested phase (see later) and that the embryo ceases development at the same time.

Delayed implantation does not occur in *Trichosurus*, *Pseudocheirus*, or, as far as is known, any of the family Phalangeridae except the diminutive *Dromicia concinna* (=*Cercaërtus concinnus*) (Table 2). Relevant females of this species have not been examined, so quiescent blastocysts have not been found and the occurrence of postpartum ovulation has not been reported, but Bowley's (1939) results are consistent with the occurrence of delayed implantation, although that author suggested that delayed fertilization was responsible. *Dromicia* is unique among marsupials with delayed implantation in that the female is polyovular, and presumably several quiescent blastocysts are present at one time in the uteri of lactating females. The occurrence of delayed implantation in *Dromicia*, which by all the usual criteria is considered a primitive phalangerid marsupial, and in both subfamilies of the Macropodidae, indicates that the phenomenon is of considerable antiquity in the Phalangeroidea.

The occurrence of delayed implantation has been confirmed in the macropod marsupials *Setonix*, *Megaleia*, *Potorous*, *Macropus robustus*, and *Protemnodon eugenii*. In seven other species (Table 2) such results as have been obtained are consistent with the occurrence of delayed implantation. The only macropod marsupial known that does not appear to have delayed implantation, at least as a general rule, is *Macropus canguru* (the great gray kangaroo). Pilton (1961) did not find corpora lutea of lactation, which accompany quiescent blastocysts in species having delayed implantation, in the ovaries of relevant females.

Several workers have examined large numbers of macropod marsupials to determine the percentage of females carrying delayed blastocysts. In this Wildlife Research division, 100 reproductive systems, collected in inland Eastern Australia from female red kanagroos with young in the pouch, were examined and all had a corpus luteum of lactation in one or other ovary. Fifty of the relevant uteri were serially sectioned, and delayed blastocysts occurred in 35. These results indicate that, although postpartum ovulation was invariable, 30 per cent of females failed to mate at postpartum estrus or there was a considerable loss of quiescent blastocysts from the uteri during lactation. On the other hand, A. E. Newsome (personal communication) found that a high percentage of female red kangaroos in arid inland Australia did not have a corpus luteum of lactation and had not, therefore, had a postpartum ovulation. About half a total sample of 298 female *Setonix*, suckling young in the pouch, were not carrying delayed blastocysts (C. H. Tyndale-Biscoe, personal communication), and 17 of 40 females of this species, from which pouch young were removed, produced another offspring, derived from the delayed blastocyst, 25 or 26 days after removal of the pouch young (Shield and Woolley, 1960). In the domestic colony of red kangaroos used for experimental purposes postpartum estrus failed to occur once in 50 cases. Forty-three females were placed with males at postpartum estrus, and only one failed to mate. Twenty-seven of the 42 postpartum matings have been tested to this date, and 26 of these resulted in the production of young after delayed periods of between 24 and about 220 days.

The Control of Delayed Implantation in Marsupials

In all marsupials having delayed implantation that have been thoroughly studied, the corpus luteum formed at postpartum ovulation (corpus luteum of lactation) has a period of arrested development during the quiescent period of the embryo. In *Setonix* the corpus luteum of lactation begins to increase in size after removal of the suckling young from the pouch, and the blastocyst begins to enlarge almost immediately (Sharman, 1955*b*). In the red kangaroo, corpora lutea of lactation were uniformly small in size in 100 females suckling young up to 190 days, and, in the examination of several hundred reproductive tracts of lactating females with young less than 190 days old in the pouch, no ovary was found in which the corpus luteum of lactation protruded noticeably from the surface. On the other hand corpora lutea associated with post-blastocyst stages, whether these were of normal pregnancy or of blastocysts that had resumed development after a delayed period, often exceeded the rest of the ovarian tissue in size. The almost immediate response of the corpora lutea to the removal of the suckling stimulus suggests that suckling prevents completion of corpus luteum development and that, in the absence of a developed corpus luteum, embryonic development is arrested.

Enders (1961), in his comparative study of the endometrium of delayed implantation in three orders of mammals, concluded that the uterine environment of the blastocysts during delayed implantation was as diverse as the mechanisms that produce delay. Delayed implantation in marsupials has something in common with delayed implantation in rodents in that in both orders delay occurs during lactation. In rodents, as in marsupials, the life of the corpus luteum of lactation is prolonged during delayed implantation, and Brambell and Rowlands (1936) showed that implantation after a period of delay in the bank vole was accompanied by renewed growth of the corpus luteum. However, in the rat and mouse the corpus luteum is apparently functional during the delayed period (Courrier and Baclesse, 1955, cited by Amoroso and Finn, 1962), and the uterine decidual reaction may be evoked (Krehbiel, 1941). This is in contrast to the condition in marsupials in which no luteal changes occur in the uterus during delayed implantation and the endometrial condition approaches that of anestrus. Further comparisons are made between marsupials and various eutherian mammals having delayed implantation in another paper (Tyndale-Biscoe) in this symposium.

In the red kangaroo, resumption of development by the delayed blastocyst occurs when young less than 200 days old are removed from the pouch and also when young more than 200 days old continue suckling and occupy the pouch for most of the time. In the latter case resumption of embryonic development does not occur in response to the removal of the suckling stimulus or to the imminent cessation of lactation, since the young continues to suckle for at least a further 4 months. Assuming that, once development is renewed, it occurs at the same rate in females suckling advanced young as it does in those from which early young are removed, it is possible to calculate the time of resumption of development by backdating from the time at which birth is observed. This in no way correlates with the time at which the young first temporarily emerges.

In one female red kangaroo, which was fertilized at a single mating just after a young had emerged from the pouch, the gestation period was over 40 days, which is very different from the gestation period in two other females suckling a single young out of the pouch and from the average gestation period in non-lactating females. (Table 3). The possibility that young suckling outside the pouch might induce delayed development in further red kangaroo blastocysts was tested by giving an extra young to females that already had one young suckling outside the pouch. Both young used the same teat alternately. The gestation period, while suckling two young out of the pouch, was not noticeably prolonged in any of those females (Table 3). The pouch young were removed from five females that had been mated at postpartum estrus and that had two young suckling from outside the pouch. In these the

TABLE 3

INFLUENCE OF SUCKLING YOUNG, OUT OF POUCH, ON EMBRYONIC DEVELOPMENT OF *Megaleia rufa*

Period	No. Days	Condition
Gestation period	33.17±0.16*	Non-lactating
	31.8–33.8, 33.7, 40.0–41.2	Suckling 1 young
	32.0–32.7, 33.2, 33.6–34.6	Suckling 2 young
Completion of pregnancy	31.34±0.35*	Non-lactating
	31.1, 31.5	Suckling 1 young
	31, 35, 38, 43, 54	Suckling 2 young

* From Table 1.

intervals between removal of pouch young and birth of another young, derived from the quiescent blastocyst, were 54, 43, 38, 35, and 31 days compared with intervals of 31 days in two females suckling a single large young out of the pouch and a mean of 31.34 days for non-lactating females from which a pouch young was removed (Table 3). In two of the five foster-mothers the blastocyst apparently resumed development after removal of one, or both, of the young suckling outside the pouch (Fig. 3).

CONCLUSIONS

It is concluded from the experiments reported above that the primary stimulus concerned in inhibition and resumption of development by marsupial blastocyst is tactile and not directly related to the presence of a young in the pouch, to the amount of milk actually secreted, or to a fall in milk yield. The following is a summary of the reasoning on which this conclusion is based.

1. *Presence of Young in Pouch.* Resumption of development by the

quiescent blastocyst occurs in females carrying advanced young in the pouch, and the young derived from the blastocyst is born, in some cases, less than a day after complete emergence of the earlier occupant of the pouch. This seems to rule out presence of young in the pouch as an inhibiting factor on the blastocyst.

2. *Amount of Milk Secreted.* Development of the blastocyst ceases shortly after fertilization when the embryo consists of a single layer of cells and when a young weighing no more than a few grams is suckled in the pouch. Development is resumed when the young weighs about

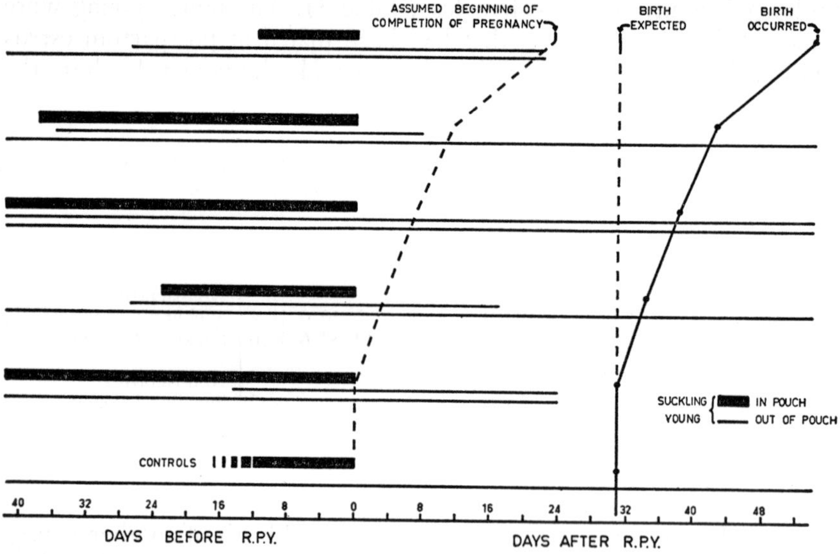

FIG. 3.—Intervals between removal of pouch young and birth in lactating red kangaroos. Controls suckling one or no young out of pouch; experimental animals suckling two young out of pouch; *R.P.Y.* = removal of pouch young.

2 kg. and is growing rapidly and when it is reasonable to assume that the amount of milk actually secreted vastly exceeds that produced when delay is induced. However, the early young in the pouch does not release the teat and cannot reattach if removed before the age of about 40 days (Sharman and Pilton, 1963), whereas the advanced young frequently releases the teat, protrudes its head from the pouch or leaves the pouch entirely.

3. *Fall in Milk Yield.* When the pouch young were removed from females suckling two other young outside the pouch, which must have been accompanied by a fall in milk yield, the blastocyst resumed development immediately in only one of five females. That these females received more mammary stimulation than did females suckling a single

young out of the pouch is indicated by the observations reported in Table 4. The most reasonable interpretation is that the tactile stimulus exerted by the suckling young in the pouch is responsible for inducing

TABLE 4

PERIODS OF SUCKLING: FEMALE *Megaleia rufa* WITH 1 AND 2 YOUNG OUT OF POUCH

No. of Suckling Young	No. of Hours Obs.	Minutes of Suckling		
		Own Young	Foster-Young	24-Hr. Period
1	96	203	....	50.75
2	48	133	59	96.0

the quiescent phase in the marsupial blastocyst and that the same stimulus is responsible for maintaining the quiescent phase irrespective of the presence of a pouch young and fluctuations in the milk yield.

Acknowledgments

I am indebted to the chief of the C.S.I.R.O. Division of Wildlife Research, Mr. H. J. Frith, for allowing me to quote his unpublished data on breeding in wild populations of the red kangaroo. The help of Mr. John Libke (animal maintenance), Mr. Frank Knight, and Mr. James Merchant (technical assistance) is gratefully acknowledged. Mr. J. H. Calaby read the manuscript and made numerous helpful suggestions. The photographs for Plates I and II were taken by Mr. Ederic Slater.

References

Amoroso, E. C., and C. A. Finn. 1962. Ovarian activity during gestation, ovum transport and implantation. In S. Zuckerman (ed.), The Ovary, Vol. 1. London: Academic Press.

Bowley, E. A. 1939. Delayed fertilization in *Dromicia*. J. Mammal., **20**:499.

Brambell, F. W. R., and I. W. Rowlands. 1936. Reproduction in the bank vole (*Evotomys glareolus* Schreber). Phil. Trans. Roy. Soc. London, **226**: 71–97.

Carson, R. D. 1912. Retarded development in a red kangaroo. Proc. Zool. Soc. Lond., **1912**:234–35.

Enders, A. C. 1961. Comparative studies on the endometrium of delayed implantation. Anat. Rec., **139**:483–97.

Flynn, T. T. 1930. The uterine cycle of pregnancy and psuedo-pregnancy as it is in the diprotodont marsupial *Bettongia cuniculus* with notes on other reproductive phenomena in this marsupial. Proc. Linn. Soc. N.S.W., **55**: 506–31.

Hartman, C. G. 1923. The oestrous cycle of the opossum. Am. J. Anat., **32**:353–421.

HUGHES, R. L. 1962*a*. Reproduction in the macropod marsupial *Potorus tridactylus* (Kerr). Aust. J. Zool., **10**:193–244.

———. 1962*b*. Role of the corpus luteum in marsupial reproduction. Nature, **194**:809–91.

JONES, F. WOOD. 1923. The Mammals of South Australia. Part 1. Adelaide: Government Printer.

———. 1944. Some curiosities of mammalian reproduction. Part 2. Concerning the life of the sperm. J. Obstet. Gynaec. Brit. Emp., **51**:533–64.

KREHBIEL, R. H. 1941. The effects of lactation on the implantation of ova of a concurrent pregnancy in the rat. Anat. Rec., **81**:381–92.

MACK, G. 1961. Mammals from South-western Queensland. Mem. Queens. Mus., **13**:213–28.

MARLOW, B. J. 1961. Reproductive behaviour of the marsupial mouse, *Antechinus flavipes* (Waterhouse) (Marsupialia) and the development of the pouch young. Aust. J. Zool., **9**:203–18.

OWEN, R. 1839–47. Marsupialia. In R. B. TODD (ed.), The Cyclopaedia of Anatomy and Physiology. London: Longman, Brown, Green, Longmans and Roberts.

PILTON, P. E. 1961. Reproduction in the great grey kangaroo. Nature, **189**: 948–85.

PILTON, P. E., and G. B. SHARMAN. 1962. Reproduction in the marsupial *Trichosurus vulpecula*. J. Endocrin., **25**:119–36.

REYNOLDS, H. C. 1952. Studies on reproduction in the opossum (*Didelphis virginiana*). Univ. Calif. Pub. Zool., **52**:223–83.

RIDE, W. D. L., and C. H. TYNDALE-BISCOE. 1962. Mammals. Fauna Bull. W. Aust. 2. (In press.)

SHARMAN, G. B. 1955*a*. Studies on marsupial reproduction. 2. The oestrous cycle of *Setonix brachyurus*. Aust. J. Zool., **3**:44–55.

———. 1955*b*. Studies on marsupial reproduction. 3. Normal and delayed pregnancy in *Setonix brachyurus*. *Ibid*., pp. 56–70.

———. 1955*c*. Studies on marsupial reproduction. 4. Delayed birth in *Protemnodon eugenii*. *Ibid*., pp. 156–61.

———. 1959. Evolution of marsupials. Aust. J. Sci., **22**:40–45.

———. 1962. The initiation and maintenance of lactation in the marsupial *Trichosurus vulpecula*. J. Endocrin., **25**:375–85.

SHARMAN, G. B., and P. E. PILTON. 1963. The life history and reproduction of the red kangaroo (*Megaleia rufa*). Proc. Zool. Soc. London., Vol. **141**. (In press.)

SHIELD, J. W., and P. WOOLLEY. 1960. Gestation time for delayed birth in the quokka. Nature, **188**:163–64.

SIMPSON, G. G. 1945. Principles of classification and a classification of mammals. Bull. Amer. Mus. Nat. Hist., **85**:1–350.

TYNDALE-BISCOE, C. H. 1955. Observations on reproduction and ecology of the brush-tailed possum, *Trichosurus vulpecula* Kerr (Marsupialia), in New Zealand. Aust. J. Zool., **3**:162–84.

Discussion was deferred until after Dr. Tyndale-Biscoe's paper.

C. H. TYNDALE-BISCOE

The Role of the Corpus Luteum in the Delayed Implantation of Marsupials

SUCCESSFUL IMPLANTATION in eutherian mammals depends upon a close synchronization between the postestrous stage of the embryo and the endometrium (Austin, 1961) and also upon a precise balance of gonadal hormones (Shelesnyak, 1960). In species that have delayed implantation, embryonic development is arrested immediately prior to implantation. It has probably evolved independently several times as an adaptation by the blastocyst to a uterine environment inimical to successful implantation and the continuance of growth and development that follows therefrom.

In macropod marsupials the embryo is arrested at the unilaminar blastocyst stage, as in eutheria, but, unlike in them, implantation does not take place immediately after the resumption of development. Indeed, implantation is not associated with the phenomenon at all, and it should more correctly be termed "embryonic diapause."

In the quokka, *Setonix brachyurus*, blastocysts have been transferred synchronously to other animals six days after the end of the delay period and have developed normally thereafter (Tyndale-Biscoe, 1963*b*). In this species and in two other macropod marsupials, *Protemnodon rufogrisea* and *Potorous tridactylus*, breakdown of the shell membrane and close apposition of the trophoblast to the uterine epithelium does not occur until late pregnancy (Sharman, 1961). Before this stage the vesicle can be rolled out of the opened uterus undamaged.

Although the adaptation in marsupials has not, therefore, resulted from a need to await suitable conditions for implantation, embryonic diapause, as in eutheria, is associated with an endocrine and uterine environment different from that of normal gestation, and subsequent growth and development are dependent on the appearance of a secretory or luteal endometrium. Marsupials thus afford the opportunity to ex-

C. H. TYNDALE-BISCOE is lecturer, Department of Zoölogy, Australian National University, Canberra, A.C.T., Australia.

amine the endocrine mechanism of embryonic diapause without the additional complexity of imminent implantation.

The present results on the relationship among the ovaries, uterus, and embryo before and after removal of the pouch young are mainly derived from observations and preliminary experiments in *Setonix brachyurus*. Removal of the pouch young is followed by resumption of ovarian activity in both pregnant and non-pregnant animals and, apart from the enlargement resulting from the developing embryo, no histological or physiological differences are apparent between the two states, since blastocysts transferred to non-pregnant animals develop normally (Tyndale-Biscoe, 1963*b*). This resumption of ovarian activity and the features associated with it constitute the delayed cycle of reproduction.

The animals used in this work and the surgical and other procedures used to obtain the material have been described (Tyndale-Biscoe, 1963*a*). Blastocysts and ova were flushed from the uteri in saline or in a mixture of Krebs-Ringer bicarbonate and quokka serum if they were to be transferred. Uteri and ovaries were sectioned at 10μ and stained with Harris' hematoxylin and eosin. From ovaries, every twenty-fifth section was mounted in series, and the three diameters of graafian follicles and corpora lutea were measured after mounting. One was obtained by multiplying the number of sections in which the structure appeared by 0.25 mm., and the other two were the greatest and the least diameter of the largest section of the structure. Estimates of the total number of luteal cells in each corpus luteum were obtained with the use of a Zeiss ($\times 10$) projection-screen head. A part of the section of the corpus luteum, on which the two diameters were measured, was projected onto the ground-glass screen at a magnification of $\times 630$, which gave a sample field 0.01 mm. thick with an 0.11-mm. radius. All the luteal-cell nuclei observed in each of four random fields were counted, and the mean was obtained. Preliminary counts of more fields (20) in alternate sections through each of several corpora lutea gave estimates that were not significantly different from these. The total number of cells was then calculated by (vol. corpus luteum)/(vol. sample field) $\times$ mean number nuclei in four sample fields.

Hormones and drugs used were estradiol diproprionate (Ovocyclin, Ciba) in oil; serum gonadotrophin (Gestyl, Organon) in water; an acetone-dried powder of horse anterior pituitaries (AP118B), similar to that described by Rowlands and Williams (1941), prepared as a saline suspension; and reserpine (Serpasil, Ciba) in aqueous solution.

The Delayed Cycle in *Setonix*

In lactating quokkas follicular growth and development are arrested and the single corpus luteum of postpartum ovulation remains small, similar-sized glands being found in animals that had been lactating for 7 or for 100 days (Fig. 1). Growth of the corpus luteum resumes during the first 4 days after removal of the pouch young and continues until day 19; thereafter it continuously diminishes in size (Fig. 1).

Histologically, this growth is due to both hypertrophy and hyperplasia of luteal cells and not to hypertrophy alone, as in the normal cycle

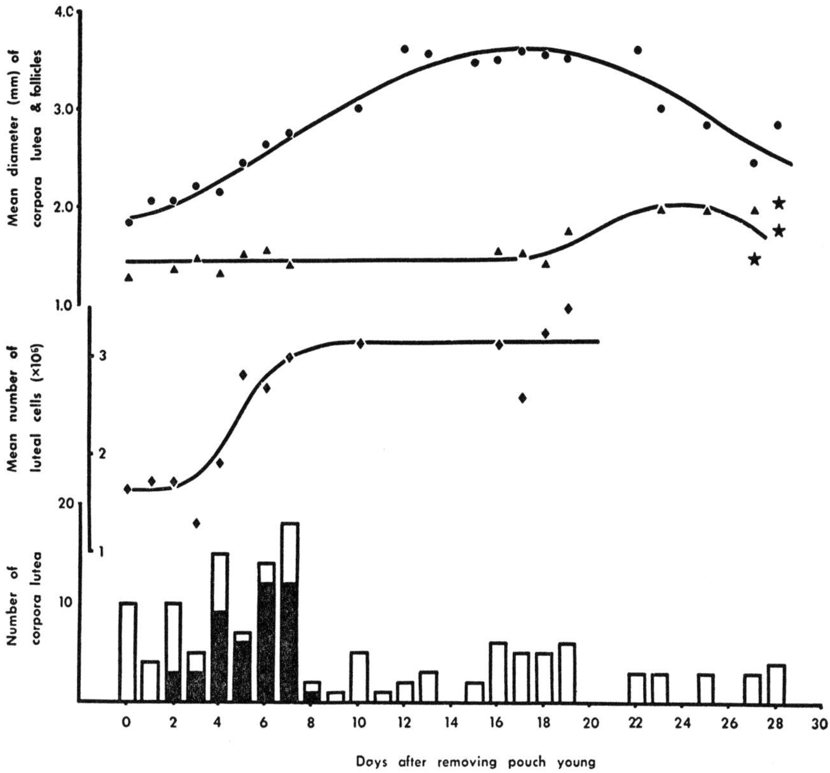

FIG. 1.—Synopsis of changes in ovaries and corpus luteum during delayed cycle of reproduction that follows removal of pouch young. ● = Mean diameter of corpora lutea. Fitted regression line, weighted for number of observations and daily variance. ▲ = Mean diameter of largest graafian follicle. ◆ = Mean number of luteal cells per corpus luteum. ■ = Number of animals in which the luteal cells of the corpus luteum were undergoing mitosis among all those examined. ✶ = Day of ovulation in three animals.

uninterrupted by lactation (Sharman, 1955*a*). The contribution of hyperplasia has been assessed by estimating the total number of luteal cells in each corpus luteum, and the means of these estimates for each day after removal of the pouch young show an increase from about 1.5 million cells during days 0–3 to about 3 million cells during days 7–19 (Fig. 1). An analysis of variance of the estimates for day 2 and day 7 shows that the difference between these days is significant at the 1 per cent level (26 d.f., VR = 11.87).

This period of hyperplasia coincides with the only period during the delayed reproductive cycle when mitoses have been observed in luteal cells. No mitoses were seen in the corpora lutea of lactating animals, but over 60 per cent of the animals examined between days 2 and 8 showed mitoses in the corpora lutea (Fig. 1), and in some they were numerous (Pl. I, *2*). It is unusual, in most mammals examined, for any hyperplasia to occur in the cells derived from the membrana granulosa during corpus luteum growth (Brambell, 1956), although mitoses are common in derivatives of the theca interna during initial development. In *Setonix* this initial stage occurs before lactation inhibition, and, even if some theca interna elements contribute to the luteal tissue, as Sharman (1955*a*) has suggested, the extent of mitotic activity observed between days 3 and 7 after removal of the pouch young clearly indicates that membrana granulosa cells are contributing largely to the hyperplasia. Since hyperplasia has not been observed in the normal cycle later than the third day after estrus, its occurrence in the delayed cycle may be associated with the long period that may elapse between formation of the corpus luteum and its secretory activity. Bassett (1949) has shown that hyperplasia contributes to the second period of corpus luteum growth in the pregnant rat 12–15 days after estrus.

Decrease in size of the corpus luteum after day 19 is accompanied by degenerative changes in the luteal cells, especially their nuclei, and an increase in connective tissue (Pl. I, *4*). Coincident with this, one follicle begins to grow, and mitoses are common in the cells of the membrana granulosa and theca folliculi from day 19 to day 27. Ovulation occurs 26–27 days after removal of the pouch young (Fig. 1). No ovulation had occurred by day 23 in seventeen animals with enlarged follicles; one had ovulated by day 27, and two by day 28. Ovulation thus occurs 8–9 days after the corpus luteum has begun to decline, which is similar to the sequence in the normal cycle (Sharman, 1955*a*).

During lactation the uteri approach the condition of seasonal anestrus. The diameter during anestrus is 3–5 mm., during lactation 5–7 mm., and the endometrial glands are longer and more coiled than in anestrus. They are lined by low columnar cells with relatively large oval nuclei (Pl. II, *5*). Following removal of the pouch young, the histological changes follow the same sequence as in the normal estrous cycle (Sharman, 1955*a*), but the timing coincides with the different development of the corpus luteum. The luteal phase, characterized by enlarged glands composed of tall columnar cells with chromophobic cytoplasm and small basally situated nuclei (Pl. II, *6*), first appears in some animals on day 6, and from days 8 to 22 the endometria of all animals were luteal.

Proestrous changes begin on day 23 (Pl. II, 7). Leucocytic infiltration of stroma and gland lumina in the late pregnant or parturient uterus was observed to be much heavier than that in the non-pregnant uterus and is probably associated with absorption of the fetal membranes, some of which remain in the uterus at parturition (Pl. II, *8*). Spermatozoa, from postpartum copulation, have been seen in the glands and lumen of non-pregnant uteri (Pl. II, *9*) but not of parturient uteri, even in the same animal.

In *Setonix* there is no growth or development of the unilaminar blastocyst during the period of delay as there is in the badger (Canivenc, 1957;

TABLE 1

DIMENSIONS OF OVA AND BLASTOCYSTS FROM MACROPOD MARSUPIALS DURING LACTATION AND AFTER REMOVAL OF POUCH YOUNG

	Megaleia rufa		*Macropus robustus*		*Setonix brachyurus*		VR
	N	$\bar{x}$ and s.e.	N	$\bar{x}$ and s.e.	N	$\bar{x}$ and s.e.	
From lactating animals							
Ova							
Shell diam.	5	0.316±0.012	15	0.308±0.012	10	0.242±0.015	...
Inner mass	...	.134± .018	...	.109± .030	...	...	3.549 (not significant)
Blastocysts							
Shell diam.	10	.312± .008	10	.317± .012	21	.262± .003	...
Trophoblast	...	0.246±0.008	...	0.212±0.011	...	...	1.268 (not significant)
After removal of pouch young							
Blastocysts, day 4, shell diam.	...	...	...	...	11	.268± .003	9.06 (significant)
Blastocysts, day 6, shell diam.	...	...	...	...	18	0.281±0.006	...

Neal and Harrison, 1958) and the roe deer (Hamlett, 1935). Retention in the uterus is evidently passive, since, in the animals that do not become fertilized at postpartum ovulation, the ovum is often retained for equally long periods in the uterus (Table 1). Thus 10 pregnant females were separated from males three weeks before parturition, and an ovum was recovered from the uterus of each animal 22–52 days after postpartum ovulation.

The mean diameter of the shell membrane of these ova was not significantly different from viable blastocysts recovered from pregnant, lactating animals (Table 1), but the ova could be readily distinguished by the absence of the spherical trophoblast within the shell and the presence of cellular debris in its stead. Similarly, in an examination of flushings from the uteri of lactating females of the hill kangaroo (*Macropus robustus*) and the plains kangaroo (*Megaleia rufa*), both unfertilized ova and blastocysts were recovered from females carrying young of all ages. In these also the mean diameters of the shell membrane were the same, and blastocysts were distinguished by the greater diameter and appearance of the trophoblast (Table 1). Hartman (1919) illustrated unfertilized ova of similar appearance, from *Didelphis*, that had been retained in the uterus throughout the gestation of the fertilized ova of the same ovulation. This resistance of the marsupial shell membrane, even of unfertilized eggs, may be a factor in the preservation of quiescent blastocysts.

The quiescent condition of the uterus during lactation might be thought to be a contributory factor in the passive retention of ova and blastocysts. However, in one quokka that was separated from males during two successive estrous cycles and was mated at the third estrus two ova and one blastocyst were recovered from the uteri, indicating that ova can be retained through all phases of the estrous cycle.

Significant enlargement of the outer diameter of the blastocyst occurs between day 4 and day 6 after removal of the pouch young, but not earlier (Table 1). Thereafter, the diameter of the embryonic vesicle enlarges very rapidly to a diameter of 13–14 mm. by day 16 (Fig. 2), this phase of rapid growth coinciding with the luteal phase in the uterus. Three embryos that were recovered on day 16 were at the 17-somite stage, so most of the earlier growth was expansion of the vesicle, and organogenesis must occur during the last ten days of gestation. Breakdown of the shell membrane and the establishment of close apposition of the vascular omphalopleur to the endometrium occurs about day 20 (Sharman, 1961).

The duration of four pregnancies accurately timed from removal of the pouch young to birth ranged from 24 days and 8 hours to 25 days and 7 hours (Table 2), which lie within the period reported by Shield and Woolley (1960). However, a fifth animal had not given birth after 27 days and 19 hours, although the fetus was alive and successfully suckled for a week in the pouch of another animal. This fetus was heavier than any other of the newborn young, which suggests that it was postmature. The neonatal weight is no greater than that of one neonatus born to an animal captured during the first pregnancy of the season (Table 2).

In normal pregnancy, uninterrupted by lactation, birth occurs 27 days after estrus and postpartum ovulation two days later (Sharman, 1955*b*), whereas in delayed pregnancy birth occurs about 25 days, and postpartum ovulation about 27 days, after removal of the pouch young. Since reproductive processes are arrested at the stage reached four days after estrus, birth and postpartum ovulation occur about two days later than expected if activity resumed immediately after removal of the pouch young. This conclusion is supported by the results of ovariectomy during the delayed cycle (Tyndale-Biscoe, 1963*a*). Removal of both ovaries during the first two days after removal of the pouch young prevented all development of the blastocyst and the endometrium for as long as

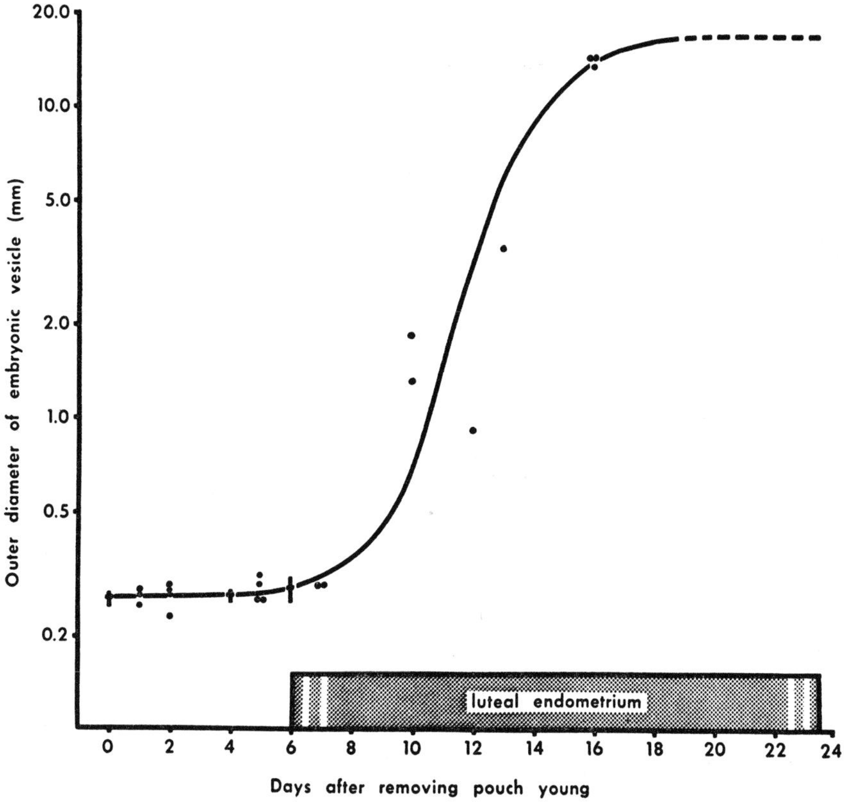

FIG. 2.—Growth of embryonic vesicle after removal of pouch young and correlation with occurrence of luteal phase in the endometrium. For days 0, 4, and 6 the means and standard deviations, derived from Table 1, are plotted; for other days individual observations are plotted.

28 days, whereas removal any time later than day 2 did not prevent the resumption of embryonic development or the appearance of the luteal condition in the endometrium. Similar results were obtained if only the one ovary bearing the corpus luteum was removed or if progesterone was given for the first seven days after bilateral ovariectomy performed when the pouch young was removed. It is thus evident that secretions of the corpus luteum are essential both for resumption of

embryonic development and for the appearance of the luteal endometrium, on which the subsequent nourishment of the embryo depends.

These may, however, be two separate functions of the corpus luteum. The luteal phase does not develop in the uterus until day 6 at the earliest, whereas the blastocyst has resumed development by day 3 and measurable growth occurs during days 4–6, so it appears to be stimulated directly by secretions of the corpus luteum before any changes have occurred in the uterus.

TABLE 2

LENGTH OF GESTATION AFTER REMOVAL OF POUCH YOUNG: NEONATAL MEASUREMENTS IN *Setonix*

	Animal No.	Prior Lactation (Days)	Interval from RPY to Birth		Neonatal Weight (gm.)	Crown-Rump Length (Mm.)
			Days	Hours		
Normal gestation......	0885	....	....	....	0.310	....
Delayed gestation......	0973	28	24	8± 2	0.390	14.5
	1466	67	24	12± 1	.322	14.2
	0822	65	24	22	.370	14.5
	0133	79	25	7	.321	13.5
(In uterus at autopsy)..	2916	80	>27	19	[0.413]	[14.3]
From Shield and Woolley (1960)...........	3♀♀	....	24	12±12	....	....
	14♀♀	....	25	12±12	....	....
0.5 mg/day reserpine injected on days 1–5 after RPY..........	1256	38	30	11±10	0.350	14.5

In the rat and mouse most evidence indicates that progesterone inhibits blastocyst growth (Whitten, 1957; Canivenc and Laffargue, 1956; Cochrane and Meyer, 1957) and estrogen precipitates implantation (Shelesnyak, 1960). Nevertheless, progesterone stimulates expansion of the rabbit blastocyst (Pincus, 1937), and, indeed, the early development of the rabbit and *Setonix* is more similar in this respect than either is to the rat or mouse.

The Mechanism of Lactation Inhibition

Sharman (1955*b*) suggested that secretions of the corpus luteum during lactation might be sufficient to inhibit follicular growth and possibly also to contribute to the maintenance of lactation, while being insufficient to induce endometrial and embryonic development. However, postpartum ovulation is not invariable in *Setonix* or in *Megaleia*

PLATE I

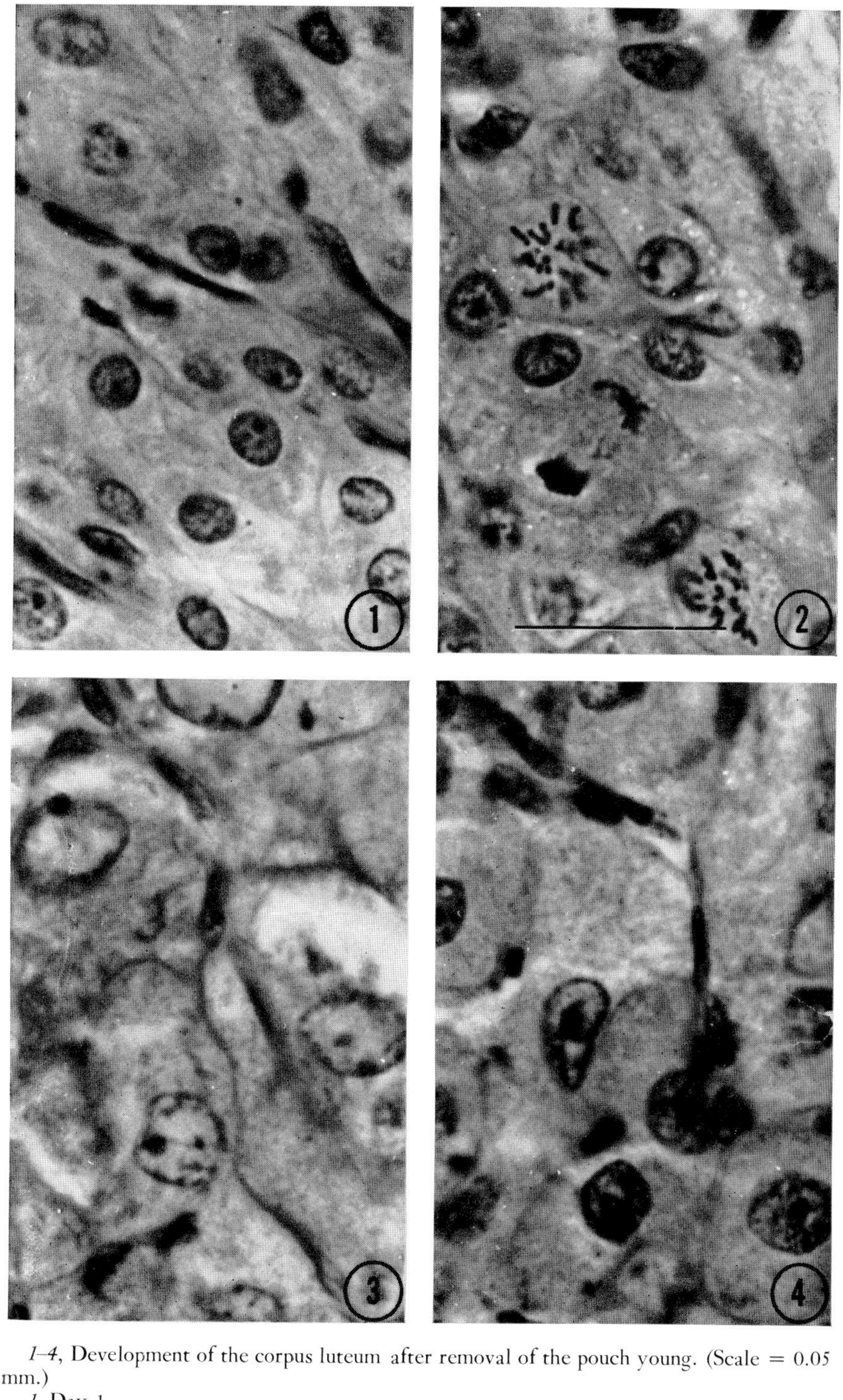

1–4, Development of the corpus luteum after removal of the pouch young. (Scale = 0.05 mm.)

1, Day 1.

2, Day 4. Note mitoses in luteal cell nuclei.

3, Day 17, corpus luteum at full size.

4, Day 23, degenerative changes apparent in the nuclei. This animal has an enlarged follicle on the other ovary and the uteri were proestrous (see Pl. II, *7*).

PLATE II

5–9, The condition of the uterus successive days after removing the pouch young. (Scale = 0.1 mm.)

5, Day 1, typical of lactation.

6, Day 12, fully luteal condition, characterized by basally situated nuclei and chromophobic cytoplasm, especially in the outer glands.

7, Day 23, proestrous condition, associated with an enlarged follicle. Note mitoses in epithelia of lumen and glands.

8, Day 26, postpartum uterus. Numerous leucocytes in the stroma and glands and indistinct luminal epithelium.

9, Day 26, non-pregnant uterus of same animal as in *8*. Note absence of leucocytes from lumen and glands, well-formed luminal epithelium, and presence of spermatozoa in lumen and glands.

PLATE II

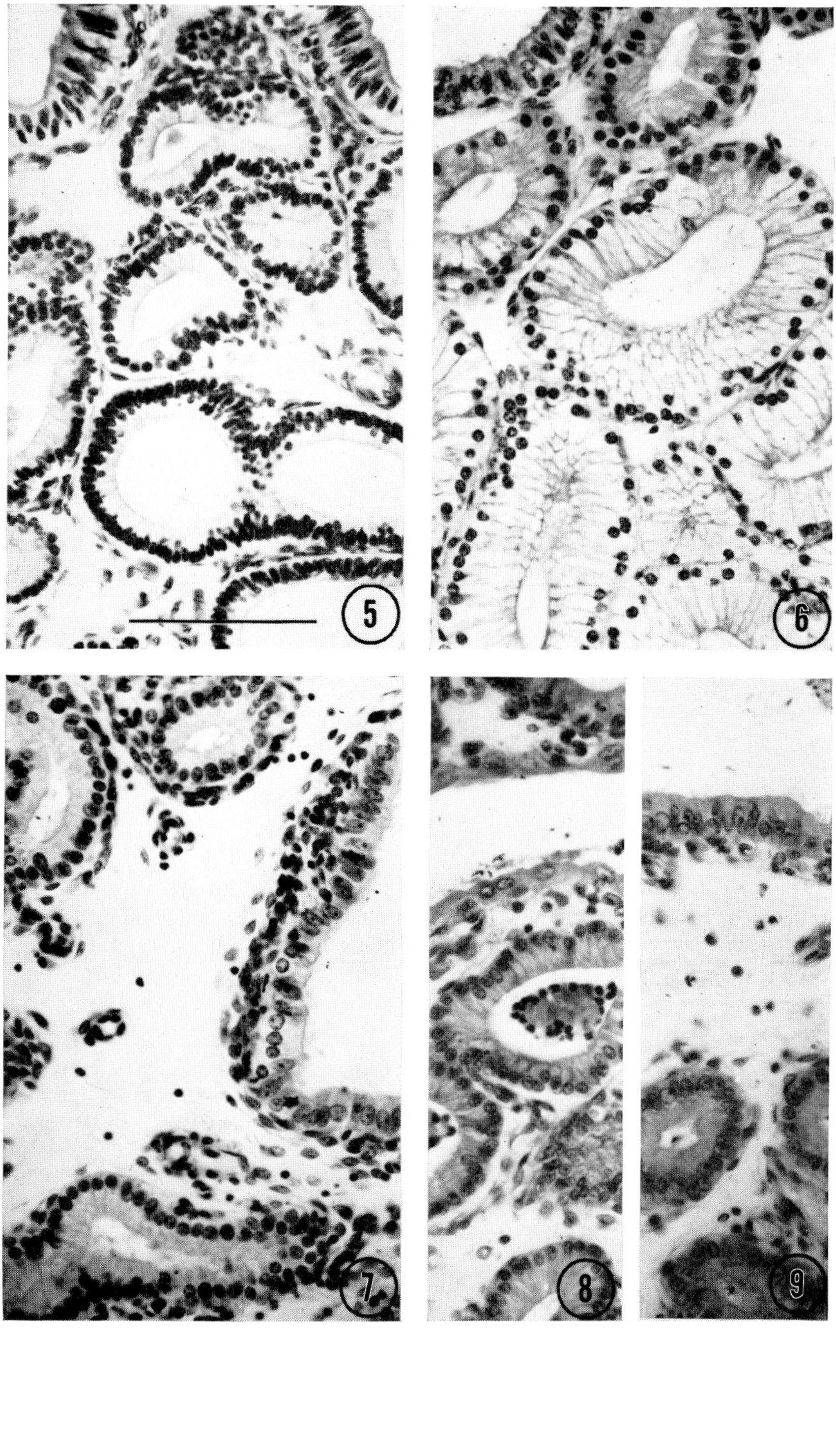

(Sharman, 1963). Eleven of 298 lactating quokkas examined did not have a corpus luteum of postpartum ovulation and failed to undergo the delayed cycle after removal of the pouch young. No evidence of follicular growth during lactation was found in these animals or in one animal from which the ovary bearing the corpus luteum was removed during continuing lactation. Three of the 11 animals, however, each had an enlarged follicle 18 and 23 days after removal of the pouch young.

All twelve animals were suckling normal pouch young, and two other animals bilaterally ovariectomized during lactation also continued to suckle their young normally.

At autopsy of the three ovariectomized animals a quiescent blastocyst of normal appearance was recovered from each one, indicating that neither resorption nor further development of the embryos followed these procedures. This contrasts with the results of Buchanan, Enders, and Talmage (1956) on the armadillo, in which removal of the ovary bearing the single corpus luteum during delayed implantation caused resorption of the blastocyst, whereas bilateral ovariectomy induced premature implantation.

The corpus luteum, during lactation, is thus without significant influence on either the maintenance of lactation or the retention of the blastocyst, and follicular growth and ovulation are inhibited independently of its presence. In *Didelphis* (Hartman, 1923) and also in *Trichosurus* (Pilton and Sharman, 1962), ovulation is inhibited during lactation, and in these species corpora lutea are not formed after parturition.

In *Setonix*, when the corpus luteum is removed within two days of removal of the pouch young, ovulation occurs prematurely from the remaining ovary (Tyndale-Biscoe, 1963*a*), whereas if the operation is performed later than day 2, ovulation occurs at about the usual time (Fig. 1). Thus, removal of the pouch young enables the ovaries to resume activity, provided that the corpus luteum is absent after day 2, because after this day the corpus luteum itself exercises an inhibition on follicular growth. From this it appears that both the corpus luteum and the ovaries are released from restraint by removal of the pouch young.

The inhibition of both the ovaries and the corpus luteum during lactation suggests that secretion of gonadotrophins from the anterior pituitary is reduced during this period. Furthermore, the quiescent condition of the corpus luteum suggests that prolactin, which has been assayed from the pituitary of another macropod marsupial (Purves and Sirett, 1959) and is presumably present in *Setonix* during lactation, is not luteotrophic in this species, which thus resembles the rabbit and the monkey (Cowie and Folley, 1955).

The delayed implantation that occurs during lactation in rats and mice is likewise associated with low levels of gonadotrophins (Whitten, 1955; Greenwald, 1958) and a high concentration of prolactin. Because of the luteotrophic activity of prolactin in these species (Evans, Simpson, Lyons, and Turpeinen, 1941), however, the corpora lutea are active and the endometrium progestational. Implantation can be induced by injecting serum gonadotrophin (Whitten, 1955) or very small doses of estrogen (Krehbiel, 1941; Weichart, 1942).

Preliminary attempts to induce resumption of reproductive activity in *Setonix* using either serum gonadotrophin or estrogen were unsuccessful. Three lactating quokkas, given a single injection of 200 i.u. serum gonadotrophin, showed no enlargement of the corpus luteum or development of the uteri 17 days later, but none of them was pregnant. Two other lactating quokkas, given a single injection of 5 μg. estrogen each, showed no development of the corpus luteum, uterus, or blastocyst 25 days later.

These results, though inconclusive, are not unexpected, since it is clear that these hormones injected into lactating rats or mice are effective in precipitating implantation only in a progestational environment, whereas in *Setonix* the uterus is quiescent during lactation.

In order to test the conclusion that a general reduction in pituitary gonadotrophin levels is responsible for delayed implantation in *Setonix*, five lactating quokkas were injected with an extract of horse anterior pituitary having both FSH and LH activity (Rowlands and Williams, 1941). Injections of 1 mg/day were given for 4 days, and the animals were examined 15 days after the first injection. All five were still suckling pouch young, and in two of them the corpus luteum was enlarged to the size normal for the middle of the cycle, and the uteri were enlarged and fully luteal. Only one contained a blastocyst, and it had not resumed development. In each of the other three, which were not pregnant, several follicles were enlarged and luteinized, but in none was the corpus luteum of postpartum ovulation enlarged, although in two of these animals also the uteri were luteal. These results support the view that the corpus luteum is inhibited during lactation by a lack of gonadotrophin secretion and that reproductive activity is not necessarily incompatible with lactation.

Observations on one wild and eight captive animals also support this view. During the examination of several thousand lactating quokkas by members of the University of Western Australia, one animal was observed to have two young in the pouch, whose ages, estimated from pes and tail length (Shield and Woolley, 1961), were 41 days and 15 days, respectively. Allowing for errors in estimation, the difference in age is clearly the duration of the second cycle, which was not delayed at all. Similar cases of two young occupying the same pouch and differing in age by the length of one estrous cycle have also been recorded for *Megaleia rufa* (Jones, 1944; Sharman and Pilton, 1963).

In eight captive quokkas, growth of the corpus luteum and the blastocyst resumed during lactation. There was no correlation with the duration of lactation already undergone, but in all cases the estimated date when development had resumed coincided with the date of capture on Rottnest Island and transport to the mainland. Stress has been shown to extend the period of delayed implantation in rats (Mayer, 1959) and has been suggested as the cause of certain cases of exceedingly long gestation in captive badgers (Neal and Harrison, 1958), but in *Setonix* stress appears to have had an opposite effect in these few animals.

If delayed implantation in *Setonix* is due to reduced levels of pituitary gonadotrophin during lactation, it should be possible to prolong the inhibition after removing the pouch young by inhibiting gonadotrophin secretion. In rats reserpine provokes the secretion of prolactin, indicated by mammary-gland development (Meites, Nicoll, and Talwalker, 1959) and the maintenance of corpora lutea in a secretory state (Psychoyos, 1958), but appears to inhibit gonadotrophin secretion (Kehl, Audibert, Gage, and Armager, 1956). These results resemble the condition in the lactating rat, and reserpine given to rats during the first eight days of pregnancy induced delayed implantation as in lactation (Mayer, Meunier, and Thevenot-Duluc, 1960).

In a single experiment with *Setonix* the pouch young were removed from four animals, and sufficient reserpine was injected daily for the next five days to maintain the animals in a state of torpor. One animal died on day 6, and the pouches of the other three were examined daily from day 23 to day 34 for new offspring. Only one of these was pregnant, and it gave birth on day 31, six days later than animals not treated with reserpine (Table 2). This young one was the normal neonatal size; it became attached to a teat and continued to grow and develop until removed 38 days later. The reserpine appeared to have delayed the resumption of embryonic development for a further six days after removal of the pouch young.

These observations in *Setonix* indicate a similarity between the mechanism of delayed implantation in this species and the rat and mouse. The stimulus of suckling is the proximate factor in the rat and mouse (Brambell, 1937), and Sharman (1963) has shown that it is almost certainly the proximate factor inducing delay in macropod marsupials. In both orders delayed implantation is probably associated with reduced secretion of gonadotrophin, but in the rat and mouse the effect of this in the ovaries, and indirectly in the uterus, is obscured by the luteotrophic effect of prolactin upon the corpora lutea, which does not occur in macropod marsupials. This results in the most interesting difference between the two orders: whereas the rodent blastocyst is stimulated to further development by estrogen, the marsupial blastocyst is stimulated by progesterone.

Acknowledgments

This work was undertaken during the tenure of a studentship from the Commonwealth Scientific and Industrial Research Organisation, Austrialia, and was supported by a grant from the University of Western Australia and a special grant from the C.S.I.R.O. to Professor H. Waring for marsupial research.

Grateful acknowledgment is made to Dr. C. R. Austin, formerly of the National Institute of Medical Research, London, for providing the extract of horse anterior pituitary; to Mr. C. A. P. Boundy, Division of Mathematical Statistics, C.S.I.R.O., for advice and assistance with the statistics; and to Dr. J. W. Shield for permitting use of his observations on a quokka bearing two young in the pouch.

Finally, I am much indebted to Professor Waring for his interest and advice and to Dr. G. B. Sharman for many fruitful discussions.

References

Austin, C. R. 1961. The Mammalian Egg. Oxford: Blackwell.

Bassett, D. L. 1949. The lutein cell population and mitotic activity in the corpus luteum of pregnancy in the albino rat. Anat. Rec., **103**:597–610.

Brambell, F. W. R. 1937. The influence of lactation on the implantation of the mammalian embryo. Am. J. Obstet. & Gynec., **33**:942.

———. 1956. Ovarian Changes. In A. S. Parkes (ed.), Marshall's Physiology of Reproduction, Vol. 1, Part 1. 3d ed. London: Longmans, Green & Co.

Buchanan, G. D., A. C. Enders, and R. V. Talmage. 1956. Implantation in armadillos ovariectomized during the period of delayed implantation. J. Endocrin., **14**:121–28.

Canivenc, R. 1957. Étude de la nidation différée du blaireau européen (*Meles meles*). Ann. Endocrin., **18**:716–36.

Canivenc, R., and M. Laffargue. 1956. Survie prolongée d'œufs fécondés non implantés, dans l'utérus des rattes castrées et injectées de progesterone. C.R. Acad. Sci., **242**:2857–60.

Cochrane, R. L., and R. K. Meyer. 1957. Delayed nidation in the rat induced by progesterone. Proc. Soc. Exp. Biol., **96**:155–59.

Cowie, A. T., and S. J. Folley. 1955. Physiology of the gonadotrophins and the lactogenic hormone. In G. Pincus and K. V. Thimann (eds.), The Hormones. Vol. 3. New York: Academic Press.

Evans, H. M., M. E. Simpson, W. R. Lyons, and K. Turpeinen. 1941. Anterior pituitary hormones which favour the production of traumatic uterine placentomata. Endocrinology, **28**:933–45.

GREENWALD, G. S. 1958. A histological study of the reproductive tract of the lactating mouse. J. Endocrin., **17**:17–23.

HAMLETT, G. W. D. 1935. Delayed implantation and discontinuous development in mammals. Quart. Rev. Biol., **10**:432–47.

HARTMAN, C. G. 1919. Studies in the development of the opossum, *Didelphis virginiana*. J. Morph., **32**:1–144.

———. 1923. The estrous cycle in the opossum. Am. J. Anat., **32**:353–421.

JONES, F. W. 1944. Some curiosities of mammalian reproduction. 2. Concerning the life of the sperm. J. Obstet. Gynaec. Brit. Emp., **51**:533–64.

KEHL, R., A. AUDIBERT, C. GAGE, and J. ARMAGER. 1956. Influence expérimentale de la réserpine sur l'activité hypophyso-génitale. C.R. Soc. Biol., **150**: 981–83.

KREHBIEL, R. H. 1941. The effects of theelin on delayed implantation in the pregnant lactating rat. Anat. Rec., **81**:381–92.

MAYER, G. 1959. Recent studies on hormonal control of delayed implantation and super-implantation in the rat. Mem. Soc. Endocrin., **6**:76–83.

MAYER, G., J.-M. MEUNIER, and A. J. THEVENOT-DULUC. 1960. Prolongation de la grossesse pars retards de nidation obtenus chez la ratte par administration de réserpine. Ann. Endocrin., **21**:1–13.

MEITES, J., C. S. NICOLL, and P. K. TALWALKER. 1959. The effects of reserpine and serotonin on milk secretion and mammary growth in the rat. Proc. Soc. Exp. Biol., **101**:653–65.

NEAL, E. G., and R. J. HARRISON. 1958. Reproduction in the European badger (*Meles meles* L.). Trans. Zool. Soc. London, **29**:67–120.

PILTON, P. E., and G. B. SHARMAN. 1962. Reproduction in the marsupial *Trichosurus vulpecula*. J. Endocrin., **25**:119–36.

PINCUS, G. 1937. The metabolism of ovarian hormones, especially in relation to the growth of the fertilized ovum. Cold Spring Harbor Symp. Quant. Biol., **5**:44–55.

PSYCHOYOS, A. 1958. Considérations sur les rapports de la chlorpromazine et de la lutéotrophine hypophysaire. C.R. Soc. Biol., **152**:918–20.

PURVES, H. D., and N. E. SIRETT. 1959. A study of the hormone contents of the rostral and caudal zones of the pars anterior of the wallaby pituitary. Aust. J. Exp. Biol., **37**:271–78.

ROWLANDS, I. W., and P. C. WILLIAMS. 1941. Comparative activity of the gonadotrophin in horse pituitary glands and in pregnant mare's serum. J. Endocrin., **2**:380–94.

SHARMAN, G. B. 1955*a*. Studies on marsupial reproduction. 2. The oestrous cycle of *Setonix brachyurus*. Aust. J. Zool., **3**:44–55.

———. 1955*b*. Studies on marsupial reproduction. 3. Normal and delayed pregnancy in *Setonix brachyurus*. *Ibid*., pp. 56–70.

———. 1959. Marsupial reproduction. In Biogeography and Ecology in Australia. Monogr. Biol., **8**:332–68.

———. 1961. The embryonic membranes and placentation in five genera of diprotodont marsupials. Proc. Zool. Soc. London, **137**:197–200.

SHARMAN, G. B., and P. E. PILTON. 1963. The life history and reproduction of the red kangaroo (*Megaleia rufa*). Proc. Zool. Soc. London. (In press.)

SHELESNYAK, M. C. 1960. Nidation of the fertilised ovum. Endeavour, **19**: 81–86.

SHIELD, J. W., and P. WOOLLEY. 1960. Gestation time for delayed birth in the quokka. Nature, **188**:163.

———. 1961. Age estimation by measurement of pouch young of the quokka (*Setonix brachyurus*). Aust. J. Zool., **9**:14–23.

TYNDALE-BISCOE, C. H. 1963*a*. The effects of ovariectomy in the marsupial, *Setonix brachyurus*. J. Reprod. & Fertil. (In press.)

———. 1963*b*. Blastocyst transfer in the marsupial, *Setonix brachyurus*. *Ibid.* (In press.)

WEICHERT, C. K. 1942. The experimental control of prolonged pregnancy in the lactating rat by means of oestrogen. Anat. Rec., **83**:1–18.

WHITTEN, W. K. 1955. Endocrine studies on delayed implantation in lactating mice. J. Endocrin., **13**:1–6.

———. 1957. The effect of progesterone on the development of mouse eggs *in vitro*. *Ibid.*, **16**:80–85.

DISCUSSION (*Chairman:* A. C. ENDERS)

A. ENDERS: In the illustration the blastocyst seemed to be in a slight crypt.

SHARMAN: In the slide it is in a crypt, but this is not invariably the case.

GREENWALD: Selye produced a pseudopregnancy in the rat by applying turpentine to the mammae, which released LTH. Have you applied turpentine or any irritant to the teats to see whether this would take the place of the suckling stimulus of two young outside the pouch in delaying implantation?

SHARMAN: I have never attempted that method.

HARTMAN: It is easy to demonstrate a reflex stimulation of the uterine musculature upon stimulation of the nipple. Women are cognizant of this when the baby is put to the breast.

In 1931 Drs. A. C. Ivy, Arthur Koff, and I (1931, Am. J. Obstet. & Gynecol., **22**:388–99) at the Carnegie Laboratory in Baltimore, made a motion picture of the contractions of the monkey uterus upon light faradic stimulation of the nipple. For the first time we saw the waves of contraction in a primate uterus; these began at the uterotubal junctions as the pacemakers.

As to the coagulum seen in the lumen of the uterine glands, constituting evidence of secretion, Dr. George Bartelmez (1937, Physiol. Rev., **17**:28–72) contended that there is also active secretion in the proliferative phase of the cycle but that the myometrial activity in this phase is such as to squeeze out of the glands the coagulable products of secretion.

The "depression" produced by the ovum in the soft and yielding uterine mucosa (especially marked in the opossum) reminds me of the paper on opossum ova by Spurgeon and Brooks (1916, Anat. Rec., Vol. **10**), which appeared simultaneously with my paper on 415 living opossum eggs and vesicles (1916, J. Morph., **27**:1–83). The former authors had only degenerating unfertilized ova, which, with their tough shell membranes, made deep depressions in the fluffy mucosa.

NELSON: Dr. Hartman mentioned a nervous connection between the nipple and the uterus. I am sure that he had in mind the release of oxytocin incident to the suckling stimulus and the effect of such oxytocin upon the uterus.

MANN: May I ask the speaker what effect hypophysectomy has on delayed implantation in these animals?

TYNDALE-BISCOE: We have never attempted this experiment.

AMOROSO: Is there a delay of implantation with the first pregnancy?

SHARMAN: No, because there are no suckling young in the pouch.

GLASSER: Have you attempted to put a foster young with the female in order to cause a delay in the first pregnancy?

SHARMAN: I have put two outside the pouch to try to delay initial development, but this was not achieved. Delay was extended by two young suckling outside the pouch after removal of the young from inside the pouch.

MAYER: I should like to ask Dr. Tyndale-Biscoe whether there is some information on the nature of the luteotrophic factor in marsupials. It does not seem to be prolactin, a hormone that acts as a luteotrophic factor in rats; it does not seem to be estrogen, a hormone that maintains the functional life of corpora lutea in hypophysectomized rabbits (see Robson). What, then, can be the luteotrophic factor in marsupials? Does LH stimulate the function of the corpus luteum?

TYNDALE-BISCOE: The powder I used was extract of horse pituitary. I tried injecting prolactin into lactating animals, but it had no effect upon the corpus luteum or the embryo.

MAYER: Can you get results with a hypophyseal graft?

TYNDALE-BISCOE: No grafting has been attempted.

WIMSATT: I was interested in Dr. Sharman's statement—when he showed slides of two different-sized young attached to two different-sized teats—that the "quality" of the milk was different in each case. This seems remarkable. Could you, Dr. Sharman, provide us with some further details?

SHARMAN: I have not analyzed the milk, but the early milk is clear, low in solids and fats. Later in suckling it is thick and high in solids and fats. They are definitely different. So it is likely that the female produces milk of two different sorts simultaneously. Bolliger showed that this was indeed the case, but his analyses were done on single mammary glands of animals suckling young of different ages, not on two mammary glands from the same female.

HARTMAN: I was amazed to learn that the marsupial liver is able to change progesterone to pregnanediol, since I believed this function to be confined to the higher primates (chimpanzee and man). Certainly the rhesus monkey, whose secretory endometrium is indistinguishable from that of the human, does not excrete a molecule of pregnanediol, either in the secretory phase of the menstrual cycle or in pregnancy (Marker and Hartman, 1940, J. Biol. Chem., **133**:529–37).

SHARMAN: Pregnanediol is excreted in the urine of the marsupial *Trichosurus*. No difference between the levels excreted by pregnant and non-pregnant females at the same time after estrus was demonstrated.

BIGGERS: Can you tell us something about the rate of regression of the mammary gland after a joey finally stops suckling?

SHARMAN: It depends on the age of young. I have removed larger ones, and it was quite a while afterward.

BIGGERS: Your pictures show that the teat suckled intermittently by a joey that has left the pouch is very large indeed and that a newborn could not possibly become attached to it. Do conditions arise, therefore, in which a gland is unavailable to a newborn animal?

SHARMAN: Yes, a teat that has recently been used would be too large for a newborn young to take into its mouth.

DEANESLY: Spermatozoa were shown in the uterine glands. Under what conditions were they found?

TYNDALE-BISCOE: They were in the non-pregnant uterus of a pregnant animal. Spermatozoa were found only in the uterus without embryos.

A. ENDERS: You have said that blastocysts resume development before any changes appear in the endometrium. Do you think that the stimulus acts directly on the blastocyst rather than on the uterus?

TYNDALE-BISCOE: The blastocyst may be stimulated by secretions of the corpus luteum directly, since the blastocyst resumes development before changes appear in the endometrium.

DAVIES: After one week of hypophysectomy in the rabbit, LH will restore the interstitial cells of the ovary, but apparently they do not function. Following the addition of prolactin, effects are dramatic on the interstitial cells—estrogenic effects appear to predominate.

TYNDALE-BISCOE: In the animals in which the one ovary bearing a corpus was removed during the first two days after removal of pouch young, no development of embryo or development of endometrium occurred. However, proestrous changes occur in the endometrium at day 12 rather than day 23 owing to the premature growth of a follicle in the remaining ovary.

CLEWE: Where within the uterus is the blastocyst found?

SHARMAN: I think I can answer that. An assistant of mine has serially sectioned 50 uteri. The blastocysts are invariably in the lower third of the uterus.

BUCHANAN: In ovariectomy experiments, when ovariectomy was performed within two days after removal of the pouch young, was there no development?

TYNDALE-BISCOE: Autopsy was done 28 days after removal of the ovaries on day 2. The blastocysts were the same size as normal delayed blastocysts in lactating females; there was no shrinkage.

BUCHANAN: When they are ovariectomized later, does development proceed?

TYNDALE-BISCOE: If the ovaries are removed later than day 2 but earlier than day 7, the blastocyst resumes development but does not go to term. If they are removed after more than 7 days, the blastocyst goes to term.

BUCHANAN: Did this animal undergo parturition?

TYNDALE-BISCOE: It was killed two days after expected parturition.

ORSINI: You mentioned that the arrested blastocyst is near the cervical end of the uterus. Where is the implantation site?

SHARMAN: When the blastocyst starts to develop, it does so from this position, but the forward extrusion of tissues, mainly extraembryonic, fills and expands the uterus.

ORSINI: When does it lose the zona pellucida?

SHARMAN: The shell membrane persists throughout delay. In the brush opossum (*Trichosurus*) the shell membrane separates the embryonic membranes from the uterus until the fourteenth day of the 17-day gestation period. It persists longer in the quokka (*Setonix*).

SHELESNYAK: We have observed biochemical changes in decidual transformation in rats well before morphological evidence is evident. When the uteri of rats were cut in three equal sections—ovarian third, middle third, and cervical third—and weighed, we noted that within 24 hours after the decidual inducing stimulus was administered the distal (cervical) third was from 25 to 35 per cent heavier than one-third of the total weight of that horn.

LUTWAK-MANN: I should like to ask two entirely different questions relating to what you have been describing to us. First, has anyone attempted as yet to culture either blastocysts of the marsupials or the very young neonates in the pouch? Second, could one collect the milk from the marsupials (for chemical and other studies) by means of a milking machine, such as is currently used, for example, in virological studies in mice?

TYNDALE-BISCOE: I tried to milk quokkas but got very little with 3 milkings per day, and no milk could be expressed after day 4. I am trying to culture blastocysts now, but, since the species I am working with is monovular, I am attempting to induce superovulation in order to get more eggs.

E. H. M. EALEY

The Ecological Significance of Delayed Implantation in a Population of the Hill Kangaroo (Macropus robustus)

THAT DELAYED IMPLANTATION occurred in the euro, *Macropus robustus*, was first shown in 1957 when blastocysts were blown from the uteri of females carrying pouch young, using the method described by Sharman (1955). Six female euros then had their pouch young removed and were isolated from males. These females were killed after varying periods of time, and one was found to be pregnant 13 days after its pouch young had been removed. These results were later confirmed by Sadleir and Shield (1960*a*), who showed that the period from removal of young to the birth of young from a quiescent blastocyst was between 34 and 36 days. Sadleir (1962) found in wild populations that blastocysts occurred in the uteri of 50–100 per cent of female euros carrying pouch young. Even in drought conditions such as occurred in August, 1959, he recorded that three of a sample of five adult females contained blastocysts.

The phenomenon of delayed implantation is obviously an advantage to animals that hibernate and seals that come ashore only once a year. It is a feature of reproduction in those marsupials in which the gestation period is just shorter than the length of one estrous cycle.

In these, proestrous changes are initiated in ovary and uterus before the onset of lactation, and there is no lactational inhibition of the post-partum ovulation. Delayed implantation may have evolved separately in several lines of marsupials in which the gestation period was extended to almost equal the length of one estrous cycle (Sharman, this symposium). However, one would not expect the blastocysts to be main-

DR. E. H. M. EALEY is senior lecturer in the Department of Zoölogy and Comparative Physiology, Monash University, Clayton, Victoria, Australia.

tained in the uterus for as long as the pouch life of the young from the previous ovulation (as may occur) if delayed implantation were not of some use to the species. Since such a high proportion of individuals in the populations of macropods mentioned carried quiescent blastocysts, it is reasonable to suppose that this phenomenon confers some benefit on these species.

Sharman (this symposium) has shown that if the pouch young is removed from a female red kangaroo that is *not* carrying a quiescent blastocyst, the female does not come into estrus until about 34 days later, that is, nearly the length of time occupied by one estrous cycle. If a blastocyst is carried, this completes development 31 days after removal of the pouch young, that is, 2 days less than the normal gestation period of 33 days. Accepting Sadleir and Shield's figures of about 35 days for the interval between removal of pouch young and birth in the euro, on the analogy of the red kangaroo it is likely that the gestation period is about 37 days and that females not carrying a blastocyst cannot be fertilized again until about 37 days after loss or removal of pouch young.

Therefore, in the case of a female *not* carrying a blastocyst, 74 days must elapse between the loss of the pouch young and the birth of the next, compared with only 35 days for a female carrying a quiescent blastocyst. In a population where significant pouch mortality occurred, this saving of time between loss of pouch young and production of another one could be an advantage under certain circumstances.

Evidence of a high natural mortality among euro pouch young in the study population will be given. The ecological significance of delayed implantation in the euro will be discussed against a background of the breeding pattern that occurred in the study area and in relation to seasonal changes in the nutritional status of the population.

Environment

The study area was situated in the northwest of Western Australia, just north of the Tropic of Capricorn. It was approximately one hundred miles from the sea. Relative humidity was low and usually below 30 per cent. The average daily maximum temperature during summer may be as high as 42° C., while the daily maximum may occasionally reach 49° C.

Rainfall between the months of November and April (summer) averages 7.1 inches, the average for the rest of the year being 2.8 inches. Geographically, the locality falls in the transition from a climate D A'w to E A'd in the Thornthwaite classification (Keast, 1959), that is, between semiarid, tropical steppe with rainfall deficient in winter and arid tropical desert with rainfall deficient in all seasons. Natural waters are widely scattered pools in watercourses that nearly always dry up in summer.

The principal vegetation consists of *Triodea spp.* and low trees (*Acacia spp.*). The dominant food grass is *Triodea pungens.* The protein content of three typical food plants for the period July, 1957, to March, 1958, is set out in Figure 1 and related to rainfall.

Variations in Nutritional Status of the Population

In demonstrating that timing is important in euro breeding, one should know at what time of the year the female euro is in the best condition to meet the greatest demands of her young. It can be seen

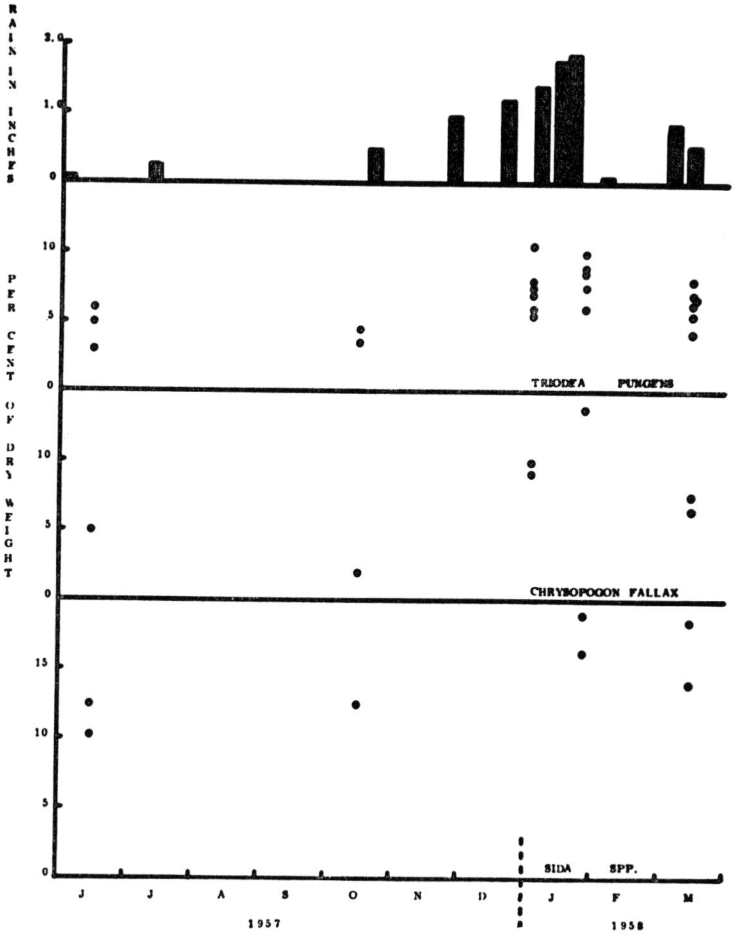

Fig. 1.—Seasonal changes in the protein content of three kinds of food plants eaten by the euro.

from Figure 1 that even in a good year most of the summer rain may have fallen by the end of January. The protein content of the food plants is highest about that time and is reduced by March.

However, the nutritional state of the euro population, as indicated by hemoglobin concentration of the blood (Fig. 2), is highest in April–May. It can be seen from Figures 3 and 6 that the pouch life of a euro is seven to eight months, so females with young born in the previous September and October would be able to supply sufficient milk when

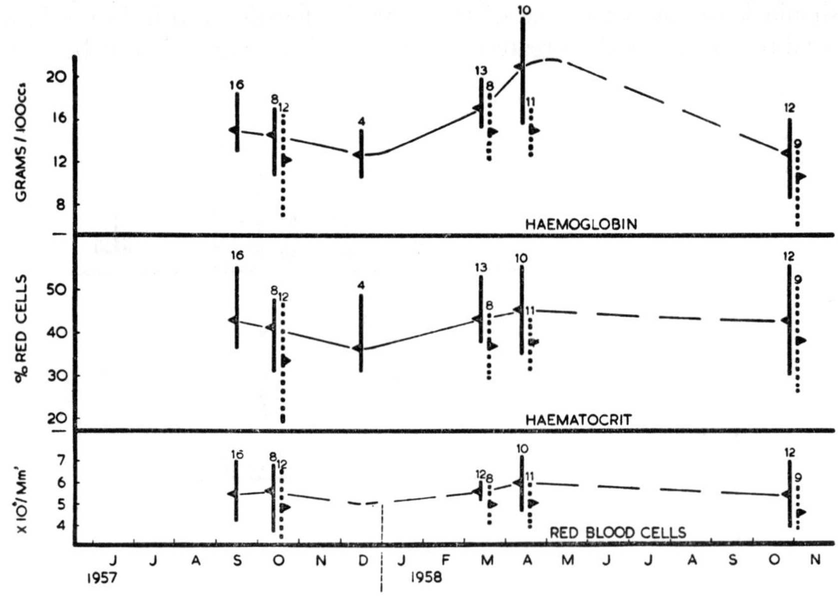

FIG. 2.—Seasonal changes in some constituents of the blood of wild euros. Means and ranges are given. Means are joined by thin lines. Broken vertical lines indicate values for euros on a study where only low protein forage was available.

their young are making the greatest demands in April–May, as it is then that the parent's level of nutrition is highest. The later they are born, the worse are their chances of survival unless winter rain falls.

EVIDENCE OF CHANGES IN REPRODUCTIVE ACTIVITY OF FEMALES

Preliminary investigations indicated that euros could breed at any time of the year and suggested that breeding could sometimes be opportunistic. However, evidence will be given below of a seasonal increase in breeding occurring in early summer (September to November) well before any summer rain fell.

Large samples were collected at about six monthly intervals. So that each sample could be obtained as quickly as possible, procedures were streamlined and some operations omitted from the program. For instance, reproductive organs were collected only from adult females *without* pouch young, the rest being classed as in "lactation anestrus" and their pouch young measured. The age of pouch young was determined by means of a curve constructed by Sadleir (1962).

EVIDENCE FROM SAMPLES

The best way of presenting the evidence for seasonal changes in reproductive activity is to describe the composition of the samples. The following descriptions of the samples of females shot should be read with reference to Figures 4 and 5.

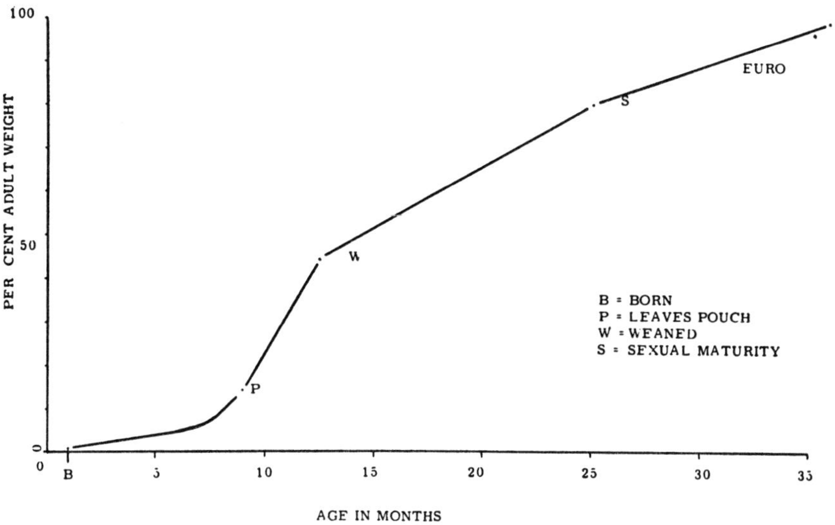

FIG. 3.—Growth rate of euro expressed as percentage of adult body weight

Sample Shot June 21–23, 1957 (130 Females). Although this sample was taken in midwinter when conditions were mild, many animals were thin and apparently starving. The previous summer rains were late in falling and were inadequate. This would account for the poor conditions of the animals sampled. Of the adults, 14 per cent were either anestrous or approaching this condition. Only 10 per cent were reproductively active, and 70 per cent carried pouch young. Of the latter, the incidence of very young animals (30 per cent) was comparatively high. This figure suggests that some of the larger pouch young may have died of malnutrition and that quiescent blastocysts had then developed.

Sample Shot in February, 1958 (177 Females). There were no anestrous females in this sample, and those that were not in the cyclic condition or pregnant had pouch young. Many of the pouch young were newborn and so must have completed their uterine development after the rain had fallen. However, a considerable number had been conceived *before* rain fell, when animals were in a semistarved condition. Figure 5 shows an increase in births during the months of October, November, and December, 1957.

Unfortunately, only reproductive organs of adult females without pouch young were collected. Some of these had only one obvious corpus

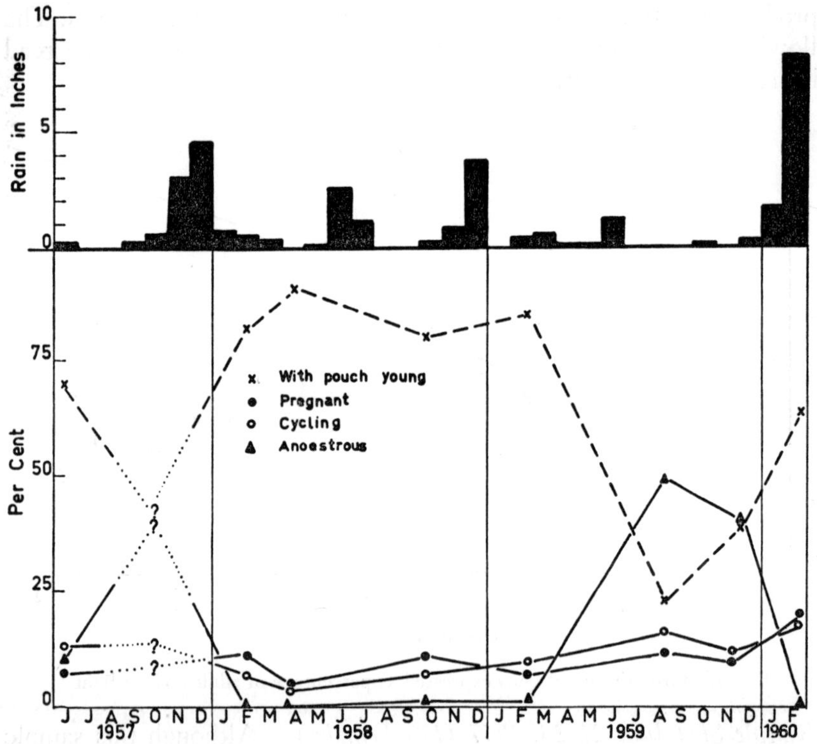

FIG. 4.—Changes in different reproductive classes of adult females in relation to rainfall

luteum, indicating that they were reproductively active for the first time in some months. They had, therefore, been in anestrus before the rain fell. Other females had several corpora lutea, which indicated that they had become reproductively active before the rain fell but had either not been fertilized or, if they had, the young had not survived.

Sample Shot in April, 1958 (100 Females). This sample confirmed that breeding activity increased *before* the summer rain and showed that a peak of births had also occurred in February. By this time, almost all females had pouch young. Very few were cyclic, and none were anestrous.

Sample Shot in October, 1958 (200 Females). Before this sample was taken, useful winter rain had fallen. The high survival rate of the young born in February–March, 1958, may have been related to this rain. Evidence of the high survival rate can be seen in Table 1, which shows that 44.3 per cent of the adult females had unoccupied lactating nipples, that is, 44.3 per cent had survived to leave the pouch and were suckling

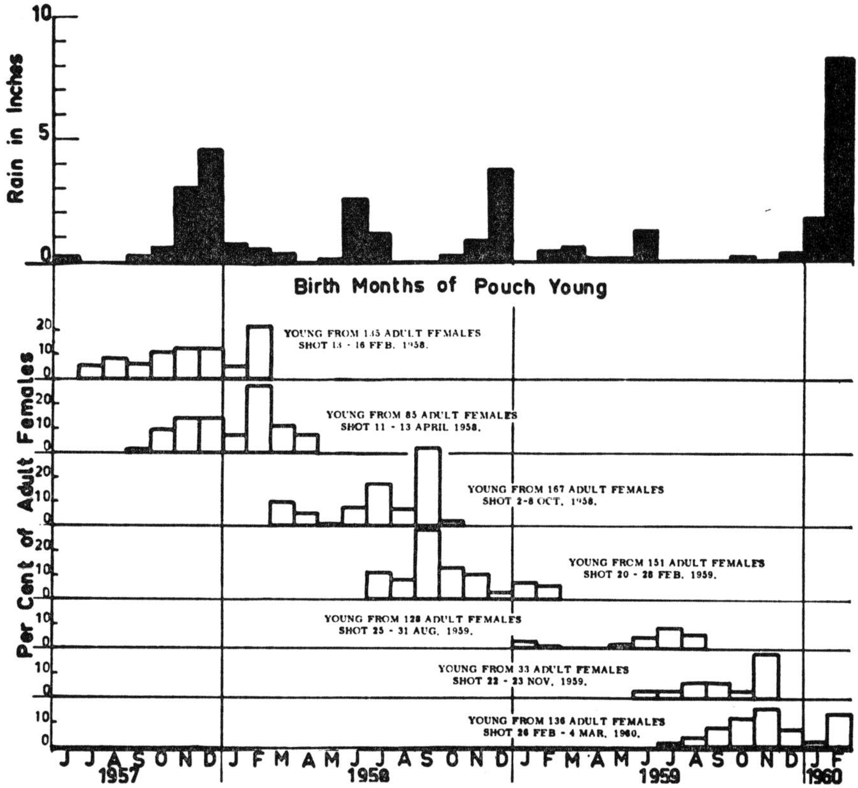

FIG. 5.—Percentage of pouch young born each month. Expressed as percentage of the adult females in each sample and compared with rainfall.

from outside. As they left the pouch, they were apparently replaced by other newborn young. Figure 5 shows the incidence of newborn young to be high in October.

Many of these newborn young probably came from quiescent blastocysts that were fertilized a month after the peak in births that occurred in February. On numerous occasions, females with seven- to eight-month-old pouch young were also found to contain uterine fetuses. These could not have come from recent fertilizations because the female would have been in lactation anestrus. Sadleir and Shield (1960*b*) have shown with a captive euro that a delayed blastocyst could implant while the first young was still in the pouch. This resulted in replacement of the first pouch young by a newborn one as soon as the first left the pouch. This allows females to take advantage of a run of favorable seasons such as this by the immediate production of a new fetus without the delay of an estrous cycle after the first young leaves the pouch.

The general situation in October was virtually the same as that revealed by the last two samples, in which there were no anestrous females, but some were cyclic or pregnant, and many had pouch young.

TABLE 1

FEMALE EUROS SHOT FOR BREEDING STUDY

Reproductive State	June 23, 1957	February 13–16, 1958	April 11–13, 1958	October 2–8, 1958	February 20–28, 1959	August 25–31, 1959	November 22–23, 1959	February 26–March 4, 1960
	Number of Females Shot							
Immature	30	42	15	33	49	72	17	63
Mature	100	135	85	167	151	128	33	136
Total females shot	130	177	100	200	200	200	50	200
	Classes of Mature Females Expressed as Per Cent of Total Adult Females							
Anestrous	14	0	0	2.4	0.8	48.3	39.4	0
Cycling	10	4.4	3.5	3	5.4	9.3	6	10.9
Postestrous or pregnant	3	2.2	1.2	4.2	3.9	7	6.1	6.6
Definitely pregnant	8	11.1	4.7	10.8	7	11.7	9	19.1
Total with no pouch young	35	17.8	9.4	20.4	17	76.6	60.5	36.8
With young in pouch	71	82.2	90.5	79.6	85.4	23.4	39.4	64
With young at foot (enlarged unoccupied nipples)	24	27.3	18.8	44.3	47.3	55.1	18.1	23.5

This was very different from the situation in the previous October, or even in the winter of 1957, when a number of females were anestrous.

Sample Shot in February, 1959 (200 Females). The summer rains were late in falling this season and, when they came, were insufficient to produce adequate plant growth. In any case, there could not have been much breeding activity after this rain because most of the females already had pouch young, and, since they were in lactation anestrus, they were simply not available. After the previous good season, most of the pouch young had survived the comparatively hard summer, and 47.3 per cent of the adult females had unoccupied, enlarged nipples, indicating that many young had survived to leave the pouch and were now at foot.

Sample Shot in Late August, 1959 (200 Females). There was a dry winter in 1959, and, since this followed scanty summer rains, the district was in a state of drought according to the standards of the local residents. Many euros were very thin, although the summer had not even started. Only 23.4 per cent carried pouch young, and 48.3 per cent were classed as anestrous on the macroscopic appearance of their reproductive tracts. However, microscopic examination showed numerous mitoses in over 30 per cent of these. The presence of mitoses in the uteri of an otherwise apparently anestrous female is considered to indicate that uterine growth was taking place prior to an estrous cycle. The absence of corpora lutea in the ovaries of these animals indicated that they had been sexually inactive for some time. It is of interest that so many were emerging from anestrus without the stimulus of rain or improved pasture conditions.

Although only 23.4 per cent were carrying pouch young, 55.1 per cent had successfully reared pouch young, which were now suckling from outside the pouch.

Sample Shot in November, 1959 (50 Females). All these were in a state of semistarvation. Some were in such bad condition they that were barely able to hop away when approached. Of the 34 adults, 40 per cent were anestrous and, although no rain had fallen since the previous sample, the number carrying young in their pouches had increased to 40 per cent. In other words, some animals were in fact emerging from anestrus and producing young, and many of these had been recently born.

Sample Shot in February–March, 1960 (200 Females). This sample was taken after heavy rain had fallen. All adult females had come out of anestrus and were either in a cyclic condition, pregnant, or among the 64 per cent with pouch young. Unfortunately, only the reproductive tracts of the 25 per cent without pouch young were preserved. Of these, 5.5 per cent had one recent but degenerating corpus luteum and 0.5 per cent had two. These animals had either not been fertilized during the summer or, if they had, the young had not survived, and many had probably been replaced by a young from a quiescent blastocyst.

Mortality among Pouch Young

Direct Evidence of Mortality

Local sheep farmers and aboriginals report that, when harassed by a dingo or an eagle, a euro ejects its young, which is then devoured by the predator. These reports were confirmed when the remains of five young euros were found in the nest of a wedge-tailed eagle (*Aquila audax*); all had hind feet measuring less than 148 mm. in length, indicating that all were less than five months old and normally would not have left the pouch at that stage.

On several occasions during the dry time of the year (October to December), a female euro that had a pouch young when she was originally captured and marked had lost it by the time she was recaptured several weeks later. On other occasions, emaciated young were found dead in the pouch, suggesting that the milk supply was failing. As the mother would no doubt soon eject the dead and putrifying pouch young, the chances of finding one dead are not good. It is likely, therefore, that death of pouch young through malnutrition is the commonest type of mortality.

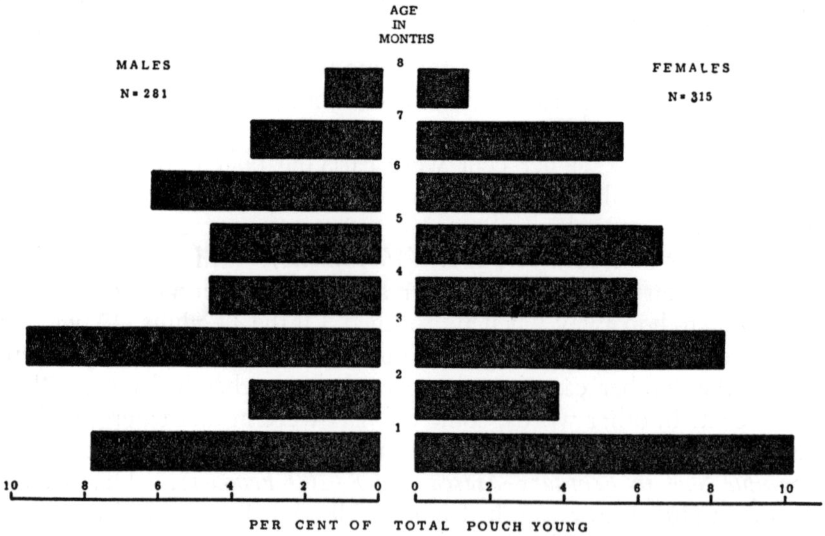

FIG. 6.—Age pyramid for euro pouch young, constructed from all pouch young taken from females shot in study area.

MORTALITY WITHIN INDIVIDUAL COHORTS OF POUCH YOUNG

It can be seen in Figures 3 and 6 that young leave the pouch between 7 and 8 months after birth. Therefore, when two different samples have been taken less than 7 months apart, pouch young calculated by hind-foot measurement as having been born during a certain period will be represented in each sample. Table 2 gives details of three separate cohorts that have each been sampled twice. It can be seen that in each case there were fewer young in the second sample.

Although a sample of 200 females was shot on each occasion, the number of pouch young calculated to have been born in each month was not considered adequate to estimate mortality accurately. Therefore, the percentage mortality shown can be only an indication that mortality occurred. Table 2 shows young calculated to have been born during July, August, and September, 1958, which were sampled in October, 1958, and February, 1959. Between the taking of those samples a mortality of about 18.5 per cent occurred. Young born in February, 1959, showed a mortality of the order of 80 per cent between February, 1959, and August, 1959. There is evidence that a high mortality did in fact occur among pouch young born about that time. The sample of 128 adult females shot in August, 1959, did not include any pouch young born in March or April of that year. This was despite the fact that Sadleir (personal communication) found newborn young during this period. This high mortality is not unexpected, since drought conditions then prevailed. Results from samples shot in August, 1959, and February, 1960, showed a mortality of about 33 per cent among young born in August, 1959.

TABLE 2

MORTALITY AMONG POUCH YOUNG

Birth Months of Pouch Young	Dates Samples Were Taken		Per Cent* Carrying Young		Difference	Mortality (Per Cent)
	First Sample	Second Sample	First Sample	Second Sample		
September, 1958 August, 1958 July, 1958	October, 1958	February, 1959	52.9	43.1	9.8	18.5
February, 1959	February, 1959	August, 1959	4	0.8	3.2	80
August, 1959	August, 1959	February, 1960	5.5	3.7	1.8	32.7

* The number of females carrying the cohort of pouch young born during the particular period in question is expressed as a percentage of the adult portion of each sample of females.

EVIDENCE OF MORTALITY FROM COMBINED SAMPLES OF POUCH YOUNG

The hind-foot measurements from a total of 596 pouch young that were taken from all females shot on the study area were combined to construct the age pyramid shown in Figure 6.

Since most young leave the pouch during the eighth month after birth, only the results from birth to the age of seven months can be used. It can be seen that comparatively few two-month-old pouch young were sampled. The apparent anomaly can be explained by the fact that there was a considerable difference in the number of young born from month to month (see Fig. 5) and by the coincidence of peaks or dips that occurred when samples were combined. *Despite* the deficiency of two-month-old young, it is nevertheless possible to demonstrate that considerable mortality occurred during the seven months of pouch life. The sample was composed of 281 males and 315 females. Since it was not possible to demonstrate a different mortality rate for each sex, the sexes were combined for the assessment of mortality among pouch young. The combined results of all pouch young aged three months and under composed 43.1 per cent of the total pouch young. Those aged four to seven months composed only 31.3 per cent. It is not probable that this difference occurred by chance, so it indicates a considerable mortality. Because of the great variability in the breeding patterns, more samples collected over a longer period than 2½ years would be necessary to assess over-all mortality rate among pouch young in this area.

Discussion

It has been suggested (Waring, 1956; Sharman, 1959) that the quiescent blastocyst was important in replacing pouch young that were lost accidentally or were thrown out by the parent during flight. Others have pointed out the advantage of this mechanism if males and females were separated for long periods, but in the euro this does not occur, and Sadleir (1962) has shown that there is no significant change in male fertility throughout the year. Sadleir (1962) suggests that the role of the blastocyst is to extend the period of time during which females can produce young during times of seasonal stress. This would certainly be the case and would be an advantage if rain fell in time to prevent the replacing pouch young from dying of starvation. This was probably happening in mid-1959 until, finally, when rain did not eventuate, most animals ceased ovulating and went into anestrus.

Most of the foregoing suggestions concerning the importance of the blastocyst are, indeed, valid. However, the data presented indicate that delayed implantation is ecologically important in connection with timing of pouch-young development and seasonal conditions. It can be seen from Figures 4 and 5 and Table 1 that, unless most of the females already had pouch young (e.g., in September and October, 1958), there was a general increase in breeding activity before the advent of the summer rains. This was shown by the increase in the number of pouch young during the periods from October to December, 1957, and September to November, 1959. This latter increase was foreshadowed by the number of animals in early proestrus that were recorded in the sample shot in August, 1959. It is important that as many as possible pouch young start their careers in early summer so that they can benefit from the good nutritional condition of their mothers (see Fig. 2) in the following April and May. Conditions during the period September to December can be very severe, and a high pouch mortality is likely to occur. The quick replacement of dead pouch young by means of delayed blastocysts must be a definite advantage because the replacing pouch young would have commenced development by the time rain finally fell.

If the summer rains should be scanty, plant growth would not be as prolific and females would not reach such a high level of nutrition. The length of time over which they could produce adequate milk to insure survival of the now enlarged pouch young would then be more critical. Scanty summer rain and no winter rain are normal in the desert to the northeast of the study area, so for the euros that exist there it is likely that timing of breeding would be very important.

On the other hand, if there is adequate summer rain followed by good winter rain, there will be a high survival among pouch young. As they leave the pouch, their places are taken by newborn young from the delayed blastocysts. The time needed to go through an estrous period is saved, and full advantage can be taken of the extended good season.

In all years there was a *decrease* in the number of births recorded in December and/or January. This did not coincide with an increase in the number of anestrous females or a decrease in the number of cyclic females that were, in fact, in a condition to become pregnant. The number of recent corpora lutea found in the ovaries of females shot in February supported the theory that there had been no decrease in fertility in the females. However, the presence of these corpora lutea indicated that either (*a*) fertility among the males was reduced during the hottest part of the year or (*b*), if the females had been fertilized, the fetuses of early pouch young had died. As Sadleir (1962) has shown, there is no significant change in fertility among males, therefore (*b*) must apply. Perhaps a combination of such factors as malnutrition, extremely high temperatures, and dehydration caused this mortality among pouch young. Whatever the causes, it is likely that many of the pouch young that died were replaced by young from quiescent blastocysts. These were born around February. Young born then would leave the pouch before the severe summer weather had commenced. If winter rain fell, they would have a good chance of survival.

The foregoing arguments suggest that timing in regard to the birth of young can be important for their subsequent survival and that the availability of a quiescent blastocyst is of use in this. However, the saving of time between one birth and the next when euros are continuously breeding during good seasons may be even more important because it would allow a higher "intrinsic rate of natural increase" (Birch, 1948; Cole, 1954). For example, a female producing one young every eight months could produce five young in a little over three years. On the other hand, if she produced one every nine months, she could produce only four young in the same period.

It cannot be said that postpartum ovulation evolved because of the advantages outlined above, since opossums (*Trichosurus*) quickly come into estrus only 8 days after loss of pouch young, so have another young

25 days after loss. Both opossums and gray kangaroos (*Macropus canguru*) may mate while carrying advanced young in the pouch, so the young that emerges from the pouch is replaced immediately by a newborn that has *not* been carried for months as an unimplanted blastocyst (Sharman, this conference).

Postpartum ovulation may be merely an unavoidable by-product in marsupials that have a gestation period shorter than the estrous cycle. Once this has evolved, the advantages of maintaining a quiescent blastocyst for a long period would cause this character to be fixed by natural selection.

Summary

A seasonal variation in the nutritional state of the euro population has been demonstrated. An increase in reproductive activity occurs at such a time that the young are becoming large when the parents are best able to supply adequate milk. However, this reproductive activity occurs before the main rain has fallen, and there is considerable mortality among the young. Many of the young that die can be replaced by others from quiescent blastocysts. Time is saved, and the replacing young have a better chance of obtaining enough milk for survival when they are larger than if they had been born about a month later, as they would have been if the mothers had gone through another estrous cycle and been fertilized.

When there is a prolonged good season, the mechanism of delayed implantation insures that the maximum number of pouch young are produced in the shortest time.

References

Asdell, S. A. 1946. Pattern of Mammalian Reproduction. Ithaca, N.Y.: Comstock Pub. Co.

Birch, L. C. 1948. The intrinsic rate of natural increase of an insect population. J. Am. Ecol., **17**:15–26.

Cole, L. C. 1954. The population consequences of life history phenomena. Quart. Rev. Biol., **29**:103–37.

Ealey, E. H. M. n.d. Biology of the euro, *Macropus robustus*. Ph.D. thesis, Library of University of Western Australia, 1962.

Keast, A. 1959. The Australian environment. Biogeography and Ecology in Australia, pp. 15–35. (Monog. Biol., VIII.)

Sadleir, R. H. n.d. Fertility studies of macropods with special reference to the euro, *Macropus robustus* Gould, and the marloo, *M. rufus* Desmarest, in the arid northwest of Western Australia. Ph.D. thesis, Library of University of Western Australia, 1962.

Sadleir, R. H., and J. W. Shield. 1960*a*. Delayed birth in marsupial macropods—the euro, the tamar and the marloo. Nature, **185**:335.

———. 1960*b*. Delayed birth in a hill-kangaroo, the euro (*Macropus robustus*). Proc. Zool. Soc. London, **135**:642–43.

SHARMAN, G. B. 1954. Reproduction in marsupials. Nature, **173**:302.
———. 1955. Studies on marsupial reproduction. II. The estrous cycle of *Setonix brachyurus*. Aust. J. Zool., **3**:44–55.
———. 1959. Evolution of marsupials. Aust. J. Sci., **22**:40–45.
WARING, H. 1956. Marsupial studies in Western Australia. Aust. J. Sci., **18**: 66–73.

DISCUSSION (*Chairman:* R. J. HARRISON)

EALEY: Before someone asks the question, "Why has the species evolved a shorter pouch life if the saving of 35 days is so important?" I will answer it now. The euro has a slower rate of growth and development than has the sheep in the same area. Therefore, its energy requirements are always less and the chances of survival of young in times of starvation are always greater. This may explain why euros can breed in this area and sheep cannot. For this reason, I do not think that there would be selection for a shorter pouch life and faster development.

HARRISON: Can you tell me, to enlighten my ignorance, something about the fossil record of the kangaroo? Have the climatic conditions of the country changed over a long period of time?

EALEY: There has been increasing aridity over many years. The country is much more arid than it was. There once was a generally more dense vegetation. The present plant associations, dominated by eucalypts, are comparatively recent.

ALDEN: Am I correct in understanding your data, and your interpretation of it, that the animal anticipates increased rainfall and produces young, which would then be able to take advantage of increased rainfall, even though the health of the mothers is impaired by adverse environmental conditions?

EALEY: Yes, that is correct—this sort of pattern is known to occur in some other marsupials and placentals as well as birds. In some passerine birds it is controlled by changing length of day. In sheep, shortening day length is important.

BIGGERS: In times of drought, is the mammary secretion reduced so that the growth of the joey is retarded? If so, does this result in the joey's residing in the pouch longer than in times of greater rainfall, thereby extending the period of delayed implantation?

EALEY: We made successive measurements of pouch young carried by marked females. During one drought we found that the growth rates of a few were slightly retarded. I cannot say whether these pouch young left the pouch after the usual period as stunted animals or whether their pouch life was extended. If the latter occurred, it is possible that the time of delayed implantation may also have been extended.

BUCHANAN: Did you say that, even though conditions are bad, they come into breeding condition? When weather conditions are bad and proestrous changes appear, do fewer come into estrus? With populations in poor condition, do fewer animals come into estrus at all?

EALEY: Yes, by the end of the bad season, 60–70 per cent had young, so most of them must have come into estrus and conceived *before* rain fell.

BUCHANAN: Even when an animal is in bad condition, can it breed and carry young?

EALEY: Yes, it can breed, but pouch mortality is no doubt high until rain falls.

DEMPSEY: I am fascinated with the use you made of indices of nutritional status. Do you have information as to the nutritional status of females as compared to males? What drain of nutrition in females is caused by carrying pouch young, as measured by the index?

EALEY: The samples were just not big enough. We could handle blood analysis of only 10–20 animals at one time. There was no difference between male and female values.

DEMPSEY: In view of the specialization of these animals to survive in a bad environment, do they build up more females in the population?

EALEY: No difference in mortality rate between male and female pouch young could be demonstrated. There is a difference in sex ratio in favor of females.

TYNDALE-BISCOE: We once shot a euro that had a pouch young, very emaciated, and a blastocyst of 0.9 mm., compared with 0.3 mm. for the delayed blastocyst. In dry conditions the pouch young may continue to grow until it becomes a serious drain on the mother. When it dies, the delayed blastocyst resumes development, is born, and continues to grow to the same stage. This process could continue until favorable conditions of rainfall enable the mother to nourish the pouch young through to weaning. If this were so, the occurrence of delayed implantation would give the animal carrying a blastocyst an advantage over the animal that did not carry one.

HARRISON: The European badger can delay for over two years, and we have a suspicion that in captivity it may delay for even longer.

GLASSER: Relative to fecundity, what is the nutritional factor that is rate-limiting—the total number of calories consumed or the number of calories consumed as protein?

EALEY: There is always an excess of calories in the form of indigestible cellulose. This is converted by the ruminal flora into fatty acids, which can be used by the euro. The bacterial population requires a minimum level of crude protein to convert cellulose. Therefore, the protein level in the vegetation is a limiting factor.

WILLIAM A. WIMSATT

Delayed Implantation in the Ursidae, with Particular Reference to the Black Bear (Ursus americanus *Pallas*)

KNOWLEDGE OF THE reproductive biology of bears understandably is fragmentary and inconclusive. Most information has been obtained from observations of captive animals in zoölogical gardens, supplemented by scattered and fortuitous observations on wild bears and hunters' kills. The bulk of it concerns the European brown bear (*Ursus arctos*), the polar bear (*Thalarctos maritimus*), and the American black bear (*Ursus americanus*), but there exists a smattering of isolated observations relating to other species. Virtually all that is positively known are the seasons of breeding and parturition, the approximate duration of gestation, and the facts that the young are born in a relatively immature state and that sexual maturity is not achieved before the second or third year of life (and perhaps later in some species). Further, it has long been suspected that embryonic development may be characterized by a period of delay in implantation, such as occurs in various other carnivores, but positive proof has thus far been lacking. Since the older literature on reproduction in bears has been adequately summarized by Hamlett (1935) and Asdell (1946), I shall not review it here. With the exception of a recent study by Rausch (1961), nothing significant on the subject seems to have been published since the time of Asdell's review. While Rausch's study was primarily concerned with problems of dentition and growth in the Alaskan black bear, he nevertheless presents some valuable observations on the reproductive biology of this species in Alaska.

Since I shall be mainly concerned here with the black bear and additions to our knowledge of its reproductive biology, it is desirable to

DR. WILLIAM A. WIMSATT is professor and chairman of the Department of Zoölogy, Cornell University, Ithaca, New York.

summarize what has been learned concerning reproduction in this species prior to the present study. The data have been gleaned from Baker (1912), the reviews of Hamlett (1935) and Asdell (1946) and the recent study of Rausch (1961). Estrus and breeding occur in early summer, usually in the latter half of June or early July, and seemingly are independent of regional origin or captivity status. The duration of estrus is unknown, but Rausch (1961) has stated that it may be comparatively short. Parturition occurs in midwinter, usually in late January or early February, providing an elapsed time between ovulation and the birth of the young of approximately 7–8 months (about 220 days).

The preovulatory follicle is large; a mature one in a bear killed by Rausch in late June measured 9 × 12 mm. Corpora lutea endure throughout pregnancy, but after parturition they involute rapidly, and within 4–5 months are reduced to corpora albicantia scarcely a millimeter in diameter (Rausch, 1961).

The age at which female black bears become sexually mature is not precisely known, and, as Rausch suggests, it may vary with latitude and individual growth rates. Successful first breedings in captive females of known age have been reported at $3\frac{1}{2}$ years (Baker, 1912; R. J. Hock, cited by Rausch, 1961) and $6\frac{1}{3}$ years (Rausch, 1961).

It is commonly held that female black bears produce young only in alternate years. This notion is substantiated by observations of Rausch (1961) on two wild bears killed in late June and early July, each of which had borne three cubs some months earlier. Neither had ovulated, although killed at a time when this should have occurred, and the ovaries contained no maturing large follicles. On the other hand, Baker (1912) indicates that estrus may be induced each year at the normal time in captive black bears if the cubs of the year are taken from their mothers in May. This observation implies the existence of a mechanism that inhibits estrus during the prolonged lactational period (the latter overspans the time when estrus would normally occur) and could account for the alternate-year breeding cycle of adult females.

In the black bear normally two or three young are produced each pregnancy, but the number of ova released at ovulation may be as many as four, and in captive bears litters of four have been recorded (Baker, 1912).

It appears from earlier observations that all bears about which anything is known have essentially similar breeding cycles and pregnancy sequences. In addition to the black bear, these include the European brown bear, polar bear, and grizzly bear. It has generally been assumed that in all of them pregnancy is characterized by a period of developmental arrest of the embryos prior to implantation, resulting in a delay in the attachment of the blastocysts to the endometrium. This belief has been based on evidence that is indirect, but compelling, nevertheless. Fundamentally, the conclusion rests on the long interval that passes between breeding and parturition in conjunction with the failure to find macroscopically visible embryos before the last few weeks of gestation and the relatively undeveloped state of the young at birth (9–12 oz.; Baker, 1912). Since the possibility of an ovulatory delay, as occurs in hibernating bats, can be effectively ruled out, delayed implantation, already known to occur in other carnivores, appeared to provide the most logical explanation of the observed facts. Final proof, which involves successful recovery of unimplanted blastocysts from the uterus at sufficiently long intervals after the presumed time of ovulation to foster confidence that their development is indeed arrested, had not been successfully accomplished.

This proof has finally been obtained in the material that forms the basis of this report. The observations to be presented will provide a description of free blastocysts recovered from the uterus many weeks after ovulation had occurred. In addition, there will be described for the first time in a bear pertinent histological and cytological characteristics of the corpora lutea and endometrium during the delay and early postimplantation periods, as well as observations on the distribution of total lipids, which are a prominent feature of the endometrial tissues during pregnancy in the bear. The carrying-out of most other histochemical tests was precluded by the nature of fixation of the material, all of which was preserved in 10 per cent neutral formalin.

In general, my observations substantiate earlier concepts of the probable nature of the pregnancy cycle in bears and give conclusive support to the long-held belief that pregnancy in bears, as with certain other carnivores, is characterized by a period of deferred implantation of the blastocysts that endures for several months. It follows that the rapid postimplantation development of the embryos is accomplished wholly in the last 6–8 weeks of the prolonged gestation period. The pregnancy cycle in the black bear will thus be shown to resemble in all major respects the cycles of other carnivores already known to display a prolonged period of embryonic arrest prior to implantation.

Material and Methods

The material on which this report is based is summarized in Table 1, which indicates the age,[1] weights, reproductive status, and dates of autopsy of the individual specimens. The bulk of the material was ob-

[1] Accurate aging of wild-caught bears is difficult, for reliable criteria of age have not yet been firmly established. It is quite possible that some of the estimated ages herein provided are erroneous. For present purposes, in the case of obviously adult bears, the absolute age is not important. It is important, however, in the presumed yearling and two-and-one-

TABLE 1

SUMMARY OF MATERIAL

No.	Date	Weight (Lb.)	Age (Yr.)	Ovarian Analysis
S- 68....	Late May	?	1½	4 Large follicles, 7 mm.
A-100....	6/11	99	1½	2 Large follicles, 1 atretic
A-102....	6/14	180	4½	3 Corpora lutea
A-101....	6/14	68	1½	Small atretic follicles
A-126....	6/17	34	1½	Primary follicles only
A-103....	6/18	109	1½	1 Large follicle, 7 mm., atretic
A-38a*...	6/20	?	2½	3 Corpora lutea
A-107....	6/22	40	1½	Primary follicles only
A-104....	6/22	152	2½–4½	2 Large follicles, atretic
A-105*...	6/22	175	4½+	2 Corpora lutea
A- 27....	6/23	?	4½+	2 Corpora lutea
A-108....	6/23	?	2½–3½	3 Large follicles, atretic
A-109....	6/24	150	4½+	3 Corpora lutea
A- 39....	6/29	146	2½	Medium follicles, atretic
A-110....	7/1	98	2½	Small follicles, atretic
A-111....	7/2	47	1½	Primary follicles only
A- 28....	7/9	176	1½–2½	Small follicles, atretic
A-127....	7/9	129	5½+	3 Large follicles, atretic
A-112....	7/9	123	4½+	3 Large follicles, atretic
A- 40....	7/10	170	7½	2 Corpora lutea
A-113....	7/10	101	2½	2 Corpora lutea
A-128....	7/11	110	4½–5½	3 Large follicles, atretic
A- 32....	7/12	?	1½	Medium follicle, atretic
A- 33....	7/13	195	4½+	5 Corpora lutea
A-129....	7/15	112	2½–3½	2 Large follicles, atretic
A-130....	7/17	112	3½	2 Large follicles, atretic
A- 34....	7/18	?	4½+	Small follicles, atretic
A- 35....	7/18	50	Cub	Primary follicles only
A- 42....	7/23	105	2½	3 Corpora lutea
A-114....	7/24	141	3½	Small follicles, atretic
A-131....	7/25	125	2½–4½	3 Corpora lutea
A- 43....	7/30	171	6½	3 Corpora lutea
A- 44....	8/5	155	8½	2 Corpora lutea
A-132....	8/5	110	2½–4½	2 Corpora lutea
A-115....	8/9	179	4½+	2 Corpora lutea
A-133....	8/11	130	6½	3 Corpora lutea
A-134....	8/13	119	4½	2 Corpora lutea
A- 36....	8/15	146	6½–7½	3 Corpora lutea
A-135....	8/18	110	7½–8½	Small follicles, atretic
A-118*...	8/22	140	3½	4 Corpora lutea
A- 45....	8/24	162	3½	3 Corpora lutea
A-117....	8/24	130	2½–4½	1 Corpus atreticum
A-119....	8/25	108	2½	Primary follicles only
A- 38....	8/18	?	3½–4½	Medium and small follicles, atretic
A-136....	8/26	143	8½	3 Corpora lutea
A-120....	8/27	27	Cub	Primary follicles only
A-121*...	8/27	204	2½–3½	4 Corpora lutea
A-122....	8/28	187	4½+	Small follicles, atretic
A-137....	8/28	134	2½–4½	2 Corpora lutea
A-123....	8/29	160+	3½	2 Corpora lutea
A-124*...	8/30	317	4½	3 Corpora lutea
A-138....	9/2	80	2½	1 Corpus luteum
A-125....	9/6	171	4½+	Small follicles, atretic
29....	11/23	?	?	3 Corpora lutea
A- 25†...	12/12	?	8½	2 Corpora lutea
A- 22†...	12/12	?	6½	2 Corpora lutea

* = Blastocysts recovered.
† = Pregnant (i.e., postimplantation).

tained from bears live-trapped from the wild in a four-county area of the Adirondack Forest Preserve in northern New York and in Allegheny County in the western part of the state. Trapping was carried out over a three-year period, but only during the summer months, between late May and early September. Several hundred bears were caught, of which 53 females of various estimated ages were killed for a study of the reproductive and other organs.

The reproductive organs were preserved in toto in 10 per cent neutral formalin, in most instances after the uterine horns had been slit open for most of their length along the antimesometrial border. Washing out the uterine lumen for the purpose of recovering any blastocysts that might be present unfortunately was attempted on only a few of these bears, but free vesicles were obtained from 7 animals, 2 killed in late June and 5 in the latter half of August. All were preserved in 10 per cent neutral formalin.

In addition to these wild-caught bears, the material includes two entire reproductive tracts of known-age females killed at the Watertown, New York, Zoo on December 12, 1956; the tracts were preserved without dissection in 10 per cent formalin. Each contained two embryonic swellings (Pl. I), one in each cornu, but they present different stages in the postimplantation development. One uterus contained embryos of approximately 20 somite pairs (7–8 mm.), the other, embryos in the advanced limb-bud stage (15+ mm.). A final specimen, represented in this material by a group of serial sections of the uterine cornua generously provided by Dr. Harland W. Mossman (No. 29 in Table 1), was from a bear shot in Price County, Wisconsin, on November 23, 1958. The tract, which contained no embryonic swellings, was preserved in Baker's formal-calcium and subsequently cleared in methyl salicylate for the purpose of determining the location of any free vesicles that might be present. Three of these were found, and the portions of the uterus containing them were excised, imbedded in paraffin, and sectioned serially. The ovaries of this specimen were not available for study, but their contents are indicated in Table 1.

The histological procedures utilized with the material were fairly routine. Blocks of the uterus and slices of the ovaries at the desired levels were imbedded in paraffin and sectioned at 5–8 μ. These were mounted on slides and stained with Harris' hematoxylin and eosin, the Masson trichrome procedure (with the substitution of aniline blue for

---

half-year-old age classes, for these provide the basis of my conclusions relative to the time of attainment of sexual maturity (cf. n. 2). Until the actual ages of these bears are established (and an effort is being made at the research laboratory of the N.Y.S. Conservation Department to establish better criteria for doing so), these conclusions must be regarded as strictly tentative.

the usual light green), the PAS procedure followed by counterstaining in hematoxylin, and the Mallory azan procedure.

Great difficulty was experienced with the free blastocysts owing to the extreme fragility of the zona pellucida. Several were destroyed in vain attempts to secure sections from paraffin-, agar-, and celloidin-imbedded blastocysts. Satisfactory results were finally obtained by imbedding the blastocysts in gelatin (which collapsed the zona, but not completely) and sectioning them at 10 μ in a Harris-type histological cryostat at −20° C. The sections were mounted on slides without fixative and were stained just before they completely dried out. The stains employed were hematoxylin and eosin, the PAS procedure, Hale's dialyzed iron, and Alcian blue (a modification of the method of Pearse [1960]).

Finally, small segments of selected uteri and ovarian slices were imbedded in gelatin and sectioned at 10 μ in the histological cryostat. The free sections, after having been washed, were stained directly in a solution of Sudan black B (Gurr) in 70 per cent alcohol for 5–8 minutes; they were then briefly rinsed in 50 per cent alcohol, floated onto slides in water, and mounted in glycerine jelly. Similar sections were variously extracted in absolute acetone, hot pyridine, or a methyl alcohol–ether mixture (1:1) overnight before being stained in Sudan black. A few sections were mounted directly in glycerine without previous extraction or staining.

Observations

GROSS MORPHOLOGY OF THE FEMALE REPRODUCTIVE ORGANS

The reproductive tract (Pl. I, *1A*) is of the typical carnivore type, consisting of a bicornuate uterus, with moderately elongated cornua. The latter meet in a relatively short common chamber or corpus uteri, which communicates with the cervix. The dimensions of the cornua in adults are similar to those presented by Rausch (1961) in the Alaskan black bear, being 100–130 mm. in length and 8–10 mm. in width. In immature bears the tract is smaller, the diameter of the cornua seldom exceeding 2 or 3 mm. The oviduct is relatively short and terminates in an ovarial bursa, which communicates with the peritoneal cavity through a prominent ostium. The ovaries are variable in size and shape, but typically are somewhat flattened oval bodies, which in adults may have a greatest diameter of 20–28 mm. They are appreciably smaller in immature bears. Ovaries containing large follicles or corpora lutea appear less flattened and often show rounded prominences or bulges at the sites of these structures. However, pediculated corpora, such as described by Wright and Rausch (1955) in the wolverine, were not observed.

THE OVARIAN CYCLE

The bears here studied are divisible into four groups in accordance with the condition of their ovaries: (1) immatures,[2] 10, (2) adults with large[3] but non-viable follicles, 11, (3) adults with corpora lutea, 29, and (4) adults with neither large follicles nor corpora lutea, 6. The simultaneous occurrence of large follicles *and* corpora lutea was never observed. The chronology of these ovarian states in the adult bears is indicated in Table 2, which reflects the functional history of the ovary

TABLE 2

ANALYSIS OF OVARIAN CONTENTS IN ADULT BEARS ACCORDING TO MONTH OF SACRIFICE

Date	No. Bears	Large Follicles Present	Corpora Lutea	Atretic Large Follicles Present	Lack Follicles or Corpora Lutea
May (late)	1	1*	.....	.....	.....
June	10	1*	5	4	.....
July	14	.....	6	5	3
August	17	.....	13	2	2
September	2	.....	1	.....	1
October	.....	.....	No material	.....	.....
November	1	.....	1	.....	.....
December	3	.....	3	.....	.....
Totals	48	2	29	11	6

* Yearling bears; cf. n. 2 of text.

[2] The "immature" category is a somewhat ambiguous one in that it includes both cubs and yearling (1½ years) bears. Five yearlings killed in June and July contained neither large follicles nor corpora lutea in their ovaries and were adjudged to be sexually immature. On the other hand, three yearlings, one killed in May and the other two in June, contained in the ovaries graafian follicles larger than 6½ mm. in diameter. These were still normal and developing in the May specimen, one of two was atretic in the June 11 specimen, and the single follicle of the June 18 specimen was likewise atretic. A corpus luteum was not found, however, in any yearling bear. Since corpora lutea have been found in the two-and-one-half-year-olds, it is evident that sexual maturity can be achieved in females by the third summer, but the occurrence of large follicles in the ovaries of some yearlings raises the possibility that under favorable circumstances of nutrition and growth it could happen as early as the second summer. It is not without interest that those yearlings which display large follicles seemed to be at the top of their weight class (two weighed 99 and 109 lb., respectively; weight of the third was not available), while those without large follicles were much smaller (68, 34, 40, 47 lb., respectively; the weight of one was unknown).

[3] For the purposes of this report a "large" follicle is one of outstanding size, in comparison with other follicles present, and measuring not less than 5–6 mm. in greatest diameter. Such follicles were observed in a viable condition only in late May and early June and are presumably those which in the normal course of events achieve maturity and rupture. The use of the term "medium" will imply follicles less than 2 mm. Additionally, "primary" follicles are considered to be those in which the ovum is surrounded by only a single layer of granulosal cells; "secondary" follicles possess two or more layers of granulosal cells but lack an antrum; follicles are called "tertiary" when they become vesicular (graafian), regardless of size.

through the most important phases of the reproductive cycle. It is regrettable that adult bears with viable large follicles were not obtained, for all my June adults had either already ovulated or possessed large follicles undergoing atresia. Only yearling specimens were available from late May and early June, and, although two of these had large viable follicles (and hence are included in Table 2), it is not certain that these would have become ovulatory. The uteri of these animals were comparable in size and development, however, to those of adults. Nevertheless, the presence of the viable follicles at this time, in conjunction with the finding of only atretic follicles or corpora lutea in older bears just a few days later, strongly indicates that in New York State bears achieve estrus in late May or the early part of June and probably seldom later than mid-June. Determination of the time of ovulation is obviously important if the occurrence of delayed implantation in these bears is to be established.

A brief histological characterization of the whole ovary in relation to the different functional states just mentioned is desirable before I trace in greater detail the history of the corpus luteum. The ovaries of the immature bears (exclusive of the two yearlings with large follicles already mentioned) have a similar organization and resemble those of Alaskan black bears of equivalent age described by Rausch (1961). Medium or large vesicular follicles are typically absent. In cubs (four to six months of age) only primary and small secondary follicles were found, but in yearlings, in addition to primary and secondary follicles, a few small vesicular follicles up to 2 mm. in greatest diameter were likewise present. Nearly all of these showed evidence of atresia, however, so their growth is inhibited while they are still quite small. Interstitial cells, which are observed in the ovaries of bears of all ages and at all seasons, are especially prominent in the ovaries of immatures. Those of more recent formation are arranged in spherical clusters, mirroring the follicular structure whence they were derived, while those formed earlier are arranged in irregular nests and cords separated by narrow strands of fibrous connective tissue.

In the yearling bear of late May, which possessed large viable follicles (S-68 in Table 1) and, in this respect at least, was presumably comparable to preovulatory adults, primary follicles were not abundant (at least not in the vicinity of the large follicles—the ovary was not sectioned serially) but, where present, tended to be grouped in irregularly dispersed clusters lying just beneath the prominent tunica albuginea. Corpora atretica, 1–2 mm. in greatest diameter, were very numerous, as they are in older bears earlier in the summer, and the stroma of the ovary was filled with nests and cords of interstitial cells derived from atretic follicles of an earlier period. The germinal epithelium was prominent, as it was in all ovaries examined histologically. It consists of columnar cells that rest on the fibrous tunica albuginea without the intervention of a specialized basement membrane.

The ovaries of adult bears with atretic large follicles, or lacking large follicles or corpora lutea, resemble in other respects those of bears with corpora lutea, so the following remarks apply in general to all three conditions. Slight individual variations are noted, but by and large the organization of the ovaries shows no dramatic changes through the summer months. Primary and secondary follicles are not abundant but tend to be arranged in irregular groups beneath the tunica albuginea. Atresia among these small follicles is much in evidence. Growing vesicular follicles are typically absent, and corpora atretica measuring 1 or 2 mm. in greatest diameter may be very numerous or may be few in number; the impression is gained that they are more numerous and prominent earlier in the summer than in later months. The ovarian stroma is characteristically fibrous and always shows numerous strands and nests of interstitial cells distributed throughout the substance of the ovary except within the tunica albuginea. Their appearance seems not to alter appreciably through the summer months. In Sudan black–stained frozen sections the germinal epithelium and the interstitial cells show up prominently, for both are rich in lipid droplets.

The ovaries of the single November specimen (No. 29, Table 1) that had corpora lutea were not available for study, so the preceding description applies only to the ovaries of bears killed between late May and early September. Some minor alterations were noted over the conditions previously described, however, in the ovaries of the two "pregnant" specimens sacrificed in early December (A-25 and A-22, Table 1). The cells of the germinal epithelium are lower, and primordial follicles are virtually absent. Secondary follicles are present but relatively scarce, and nearly all were observed to be in various stages of atresia. There had apparently been some growth of small vesicular follicles up to 1 or 2 mm. in diameter, for there were several of these in each ovary, but in every case they were undergoing atresia, some with the development of prominent thecal cuffs of interstitial cells and some without. A few corpora atretica of comparable size were likewise present. Just when during the fall months this follicular growth was initiated, whether before or after implantation had occurred, could not be determined. Interstitial cells, either singly or in small clusters or cords, were scattered throughout the stroma except in the hilus region, but their aggregations were more widely separated and less conspicuous than in summer-killed animals. Also, for the most part, they were smaller and contained less lipid than in summer animals. Only interstitital cells associated with currently atretic follicles were of larger size and contained more lipid droplets. In general, the ovarian stroma of these "pregnant" bears appeared more densely fibrous than did the stroma in the ovaries of bears killed during the summer months.

CORPORA LUTEA

The following description of the corpora lutea is based on the ovaries of 29 summer-killed animals that bore them and the 2 post-implantation specimens killed in early December. It should be emphasized at once that the corpora of the summer animals show a comparable organization and histological character, subject to slight individual variation, regardless of the time at which they were killed between late June and early September. A dramatic change in histological character was noted only in the two "pregnant" December specimens. The number of corpora observed in individual bears varied from one to five, but two or three was the most common finding. They were usually divided between the two ovaries, but as many as four were encountered in a single ovary.

In summer bears the corpora tend to be smaller in greatest diameter than the preovulatory follicles that gave rise to them—provided that we may assume the 9 × 12-mm. follicle described by Rausch (1961) in an Alaskan black bear killed in late June to be representative of the size ultimately achieved by preovulatory follicles. In the 29 bears here analyzed the corpora lutea varied in greatest diameter from 4 to 8 mm., but most averaged 6 or 7 mm. There was no tendency for smaller corpora to be present in bears killed earlier in the season, for smaller and larger corpora were equally characteristic of bears killed throughout the period from June to September. In general, however, younger corpora were characterized by a relatively larger central "cavity," which was either rounded or slit-like, but even this difference was not consistent, for larger cavities have been observed in some late summer bears. Following the collapse of the follicle at ovulation, the ingrowth of connective tissue into the former follicular antrum is rapid, and, even in a mid-June specimen in which blastocysts were in an early stage of formation, the invasion of connective tissue into the cavities of the forming corpora was virtually complete.

The corpora of summer-killed animals show, in general, a "radial" organization of their histological components. From the theca, sheets and strands of connective tissue pass vertically inward, converging on the connective-tissue-filled central area. These strands contain numerous small arterioles, easily distinguished by their heavy coats, and similar vessels are observed in the central mass of connective tissue. The lutein cells are sandwiched between these parallel septa in thick columns. These are further subdivided into smaller, often spherical, aggregations by delicate connective tissue strands that are continuous with the primary septa. If care is taken, capillaries may be observed within these finer septa, but a rich vascularization is not ordinarily seen.

The lutein cells are of moderate size, averaging 20–40 μ in diameter, and possess rounded, polygonal, or angular profiles. Mitotic figures, which are reasonably numerous in the peripheral zone of the corpora, seem to involve thecal and septal elements rather than the primary lutein cells. The cytoplasm of the lutein cells shows a variable texture. As seen in hematoxylin and eosin preparations, many of the cells are relatively homogeneous or finely granular in appearance. Numerous others reveal a delicate vacuolation, either uniformly distributed or restricted to only a part of the total cytoplasmic area. Less abundantly, still other cells contain one or more larger vacuoles, which may occupy half or more of the total cytoplasmic area. Most of these features are easily seen in Plate II, *2*. In frozen sections stained with Sudan black (Pl. II, *3*) the lutein cells for the most part reveal a uniform bluish-black wash in the cytoplasm. Superimposed upon it are uniformly blackish or grayish droplets of lipid that correspond in size and distribution to the vacuolar apparatus noted in hematoxylin and eosin preparations. Most of the lipid droplets are extracted by lipid solvents, but the background wash in the cytoplasm resists extraction. While some individual variation was noted in the degree of vacuolation of the lutein cells from one corpus luteum to another, large lipid vacuoles seemed to occur more often in lutein cells nearer the primary septa and in the peripheral and central regions of the corpora lutea than in between.

It was not possible to determine with certainty in my material whether all the lutein cells are derived from the granulosa or receive contributions from the thecal interstitial tissue. All about the periphery of the corpora, and wherever connective tissue septa pass inward, one observes numerous nests of insterstitial cells incorporated within the substance of the gland in much the way they are in species in which "thecal lutein cells" contribute to the formation of the corpus luteum. These cells are readily distinguished from the lutein cells of granulosal origin by their frankly smaller size and vacuolated achromatic cytoplasm. Intermediate forms between these and the larger granulosal lutein cells were not positively identified, however. In the functional corpora of the two "pregnant" December specimens these smaller cells are scarcely in evidence, and it might be presumed that they have either undergone regression or have transformed into functional lutein cells, which in my material are indistinguishable for those of granulosal origin.

In the two postimplantation specimens killed in December the corpora lutea have experienced a number of changes over the summer condition just described. First of all, they are much larger, averaging 9–10 mm. in greatest diameter, indicating a two- to four-and-one-half fold increase in volume over the corpora of the summer "delay" period. The radial arrangement of septa and lutein cells so characteristic of summer corpora is scarcely evident, the glands being divided more homogeneously into irregular masses of lutein cells. A central area filled with connective tissue is still prominent, but the periphery of the corpus presents a more regular surface to the adjacent stromal elements. The intercalation of interstitial cells between the peripheral lutein cells and along the connective tissue septa is not apparent. A dramatic change seems to have occurred in the vascular framework. The gland is permeated by an exceedingly rich vascular plexus of a density assuring that most cells are proximate to a capillary vessel. The capillaries, instead of being small and indistinct as in the summer corpora, are at many places widely dilated and appear sinusoidal in character.

The lutein cells, too, have changed markedly over their summer condition. They have now increased greatly in size, averaging 70–90 μ in diameter, or a volumetric increase of nearly thirteen fold. This results from an increase in cytoplasmic mass, for the nuclei have enlarged but little if at all. Over all, as seen in hematoxylin and eosin-stained preparations, the cells have a homogeneous or finely granular texture, but many do show aggregates of small vacuoles, usually confined to a restricted region of the cytoplasm. The largest vacuoles characteristic of summer corpora are virtually absent. Most of these features are shown in Plate II, *4*. In Sudan black–stained frozen sections the cytoplasm reveals a homogeneous black ground coloration that varies in intensity from cell to cell and resists extraction by lipid solvents. The various orders of smallish vacuoles noted in hematoxylin and eosin preparations are represented in frozen sections by sudanophilic droplets of various configurations. The smaller of these, which usually occur in dense aggregates, are stained uniformly black; the slightly larger ones, which occur alone or in loose aggregates, often show a densely sudanophilic outer ring inclosing a central droplet that is Sudan-negative. Most of these droplets are removed by lipid solvents. Some of these features are visible in Plate II, *5*, which depicts a section of corpus luteum from one of the "pregnant" bears stained with Sudan black. Finally, at various places within the central core of connective tissue, loose aggregations of extravascular leucocytes occur; these are especially prominent in frozen sections, owing to the numerous sudanophilic granules and droplets present in their cytoplasm. Leucocytes are not so numerous in the corpora of summer-killed bears.

MICROSCOPIC ORGANIZATION OF THE UTERUS

Since the over-all microscopic organization of the uterus in the black bear does not differ radically from that of other, better-known carnivores, I shall focus mainly on those features which appear most important in supporting the products of fertilization during the "delay" and early postimplantation periods; for all practical purposes this involves only the endometrium. A rigorous histological analysis of the entire uterus has not yet been undertaken, so the following observations pertain only to the cornua and, specifically, to an area encompassing the mesial two-thirds, from which blastocysts have been recovered and in which, in the two December specimens, implantation had occurred.

General Description. The organization of the uterine wall is illustrated in Plate III, *6*. The adventitial coat is thin, consisting only of delicate connective-tissue fibrils and cells. The myometrium is very prominent, even in the immature uterus. Over most of the circumference of the uterus it comprises two well-defined and closely apposed laminae of nearly equal thickness. In the outer layer the muscle fibers are oriented longitudinally, paralleling the axis of the cornu, while the orientation within the inner layer is circular and at right angles to those of the outer layer. Only the inner layer forms a continuous investment for the endometrium; at the mesometrial side the outer layer separates from the inner and passes off into the broad ligament as two distinct muscular laminae lying within its dorsal and ventral surfaces, respectively. Blood vessels entering the uterus within the ligament pass between these two muscular layers. At the mesometrial side the inner, circular layer of muscle is generally thicker than elsewhere about the uterine circumference. Both muscle layers are very compact, and little evidence of interdigitation of fiber bundles between them is seen. The myometrial-endometrial boundary is abrupt, and a "spongy" zone of intercrescent muscle bundles, vessels, and connective tissue, as described by Enders *et al.* (1958) in the armadillo, is not apparent. At the point near the mesometrial side of the uterus where the outer muscle layer diverges from the inner there was seen in some sections an intermediate layer of muscle, which at the mesometrial pole passes into the center of the broad ligament. Where present, its fibers interdigitate extensively with those of the inner circular layer of muscle and less extensively with those of the outer layer. It is possible that this muscle represents anchoring slips of the uterine round ligament.

The major arteries entering the uterus from the broad ligament ramify between the inner and outer coats of the myometrium. These give rise to penetrating branches, little diminished in size, which perforate the circular muscle layer and form a second irregular plexus of large convoluted vessels just within the endometrium. From this plexus smaller branches follow a tortuous course through the basal half of the endometrium, gradually diminish in size, and become less tortuous within the superficial region. The details of the capillary aborizations from the endometrial vessels could not be determined in the thin sections used.

The endometrium as a whole is of variable thickness, for the uterine lining is thrown into a series of longitudinal folds, at least four of which are relatively constant (Pl. III, *6*). Most prominent are two fleshy folds that project into the lumen from the lateral sides midway between the mesometrial and antimesometrial borders of the uterine tube. A lower, more acuminate fold protrudes upward from the mesometrial side, and antimesometrially there is another fold, smaller than the lateral ones, which is sometimes subdivided into two. The endometrium is thickest within the folds and thinnest beneath the luminal "crypts" that separate them. The greatest thickness observed in an immature uterus was 0.5 mm., but in "delay" uteri the endometrium may be as thick as 2 mm. within the large lateral folds.

During the delay period the endometrium is divisible into three regions on the basis of the form and distribution of the glands and the organization of its connective tissues. The deepest layer comprises the narrow zone between the glandular fundi and the inner muscle layer of the myometrium. It is composed of relatively coarse bundles of collagenous fibers and few cells; within it lies the inner vascular plexus described earlier. The intermediate, and broadest, region is that part occupied by the gland crypts, and it extends up to the level of the necks of the glands. Here the collagenous bundles are finer, and the interfibrillar ground substance is relatively prominent. Connective-tissue cells are numerous but are rather widely dispersed. The most superficial region comprises the subluminal tissue, within which lie the neck segments of the uterine glands. The crowding-together of these segments, with an attendant compression of the surrounding connective tissues, sometimes gives this zone a relatively congested appearance, but actually the connective tissue fibrils are more delicate here than in the other two zones.

The surface epithelium in the immature uterus is simple and low columnar, the nuclei occupying nearly the entire height of the cells. At least in the mesial two-thirds of the cornua there are no cilia. In the mature uterus, during the delay period, the epithelium retains its simple character, but the cells are much taller, and their apices are rounded and bulge into the lumen (Pl. IV, 7). The oval nuclei are displaced about one-third of the way up from the cell base, and there is a wide supranuclear zone, the apical half of which is homogeneous and finely granular; that portion just above the nucleus, however, as well as the basal cytoplasm, is markedly vacuolated. This organization is more apparent in August speciments than in those of June. In Masson and azan preparations "terminal bars" are sometimes distinct opposite the bases of the apical blebs. Pseudo-stratification of the epithelium, often seen in the uteri of other mammals, is not prominent during the delay period in the bear.

In the immature uterus the endometrial glands are simple tubular, slightly convoluted structures and are relatively few in number. In the adult uterus they are far more numerous and take origin from the surface epithelium over the entire endometrial surface. They seem to achieve their maximum preimplantation development shortly after ovulation, so their structure remains relatively constant during the prolonged delay period. At this time they are divisible histologically into three parts: a short isthmus; a relatively narrow and straight neck segment, which occupies the shallow superficial zone of the endometrium; and the longer, wider, greatly convoluted, and sometimes branched secretory crypts, which occupy the whole of the broad intermediate zone of the endometrium.

The isthmus portion is represented by a short constricted segment at the point where the gland joins the surface epithelium. The cells are lower here and more crowded than in the neck segment or surface epithelium. The neck segment arises abruptly from the short isthmus and is made up of cells that resemble in most respects the surface epithelial cells, being of similar height and provided with a comparably wide supranuclear zone. The apical band is finely granular, but below and just above the nucleus the cytoplasm is markedly vacuolated (Pl. IV, *7*).

The girth of the neck segment is appreciably greater than that of the isthmus, although not so great as the secretory crypts below. The gland lumen is typically widest in the neck segment, gradually narrows in the upper portions of the secretory crypts, and is usually smallest in the glandular fundi.

The secretory crypts, including the fundi, differ from the neck segments principally in the size and character of the epithelial cells that compose them (Pl. IV, *8*, *9*). While the girth of these portions appreciably exceeds that of the neck segments, the luminal diameter is often much smaller because of the greater height of the gland cells. In a typical crypt, as seen in Masson or hematoxylin and eosin preparations, the cells superficially resemble those in a mucous acinus. They have a tall columnar, sometimes pyramidal, form, being half again as tall as the cells of the neck segments. The rounded nucleus is situated close to the cell base and is overlaid by a supranuclear cytoplasmic zone that is more extensive than that of any of the other epithelial components of the uterus. Characteristically, the cytoplasm below and above the nucleus is markedly vacuolated and achromatic. At the cell apex, however, the cytoplasm is more chromatic and somewhat granular in texture. In favorable sections "terminal bars" are occasionally observed below the rounded free margins of the cells.

In the late May yearling bear, which possessed large viable graafian follicles and in which the uterus was of comparable size and development to that of older bears (S-68, Table 1), the morphology of the surface epithelium and glands differs only slightly from the conditions just described in the "delay" uterus. The surface epithelium is somewhat lower over all, and the supranuclear band of cytoplasm is narrower. Also the cells lack the marked basal vacuolation characteristic of the delay uterus. The glands are numerous but, especially in the cryptal portions, are less highly developed. The organization of the crypts more nearly resembles that of the neck segments, the cells being lower and less vacuolated than in the delay uterus, and the lumina are wider. Histochemical differences, which are more dramatic, will be stressed shortly.

Histochemical Characteristics. Histochemical observations were limited to PAS-positive substances and total lipids as visualized with Sudan black. During the delay period, at least from mid-June to September, no significant variations were observed in the over-all histochemical picture.

Within the endometrial connective tissue diastase-resistant PAS-positive reactions were most prominent in the fibrillar elements, especially those which comprise the basement membranes underlying the various epithelia. Reactivity is most intense within the superficial subluminal zone of the endometrium, where the connective tissues are compressed between the gland neck segments. The relatively scant homogeneous ground substance was everywhere only mildly positive. Sudanophilic lipids were nowhere observed within the endometrial connective tissues, except for small granules within the cytoplasm of an occasional extravascular leucocyte.

Among the epithelial elements PAS-positive materials are largely restricted to the glands, where they are observed both in the neck segments and in the crypts. Within the neck segments a few minute diastase-resistant granules are typically found within a narrow apical zone of the cytoplasm and sometimes just outside the cells at the luminal border (Pl. IV, *10*). A similar picture is observed in the cryptal segments, except here granules may also be observed deeper in the cell between the vacuoles that extend to the subterminal band of cytoplasm. PAS-positive material is also present here and there within the lumina of the glands, but not abundantly, and the great majority of luminal profiles seen in sections are clear. With the exception of a few small granules within the Golgi zone just above the nucleus, PAS-positive substances were not observed in the surface epithelium.

In contrast to the relative paucity of PAS-positive materials within the epithelial elements, lipids are abundant in both surface and glandular epithelia throughout the delay period. Typically, they are most abundant in the glandular neck segments, but nevertheless both the crypts and the surface epithelium are generously endowed (Pl. V, *11, 12*). Other than this quantitative difference, the form and distribution of lipids within the cells were similar in the glandular and surface epithelia. The lipids occur as droplets of variable size, which are most concentrated in the basal cytoplasm beneath the nucleus and in the lower half of the supranuclear zone; generally, the larger droplets are basally situated. Some droplets are invariably observed also in the apical regions of the cells, especially in the neck segments of the glands, but they tend to be smaller than those more deeply situated and are more widely dispersed in the cytoplasm. All these droplets are readily removed by lipid solvents, and birefringence in them could not be demonstrated under the polarizing microscope. The lipid material appears to be retained within the epithelial cells, for sudanophilic substances were not observed in the glandular lumina or in that of the uterine tube.

The histochemical picture just described during the delay period differs radically from that observed in the preovulatory uterus, especially in regard to the epithelial elements. The yearling bear from late May (S-68, Table 1), several times previously mentioned, is believed to be representative of the preovulatory condition. Within it the relative abundance of PAS-positive substances and lipids in the epithelial cells is essentially reversed over the conditions observed in the "delay" uterus. The surface epithelium is again largely deficient in PAS-positive material, but the glandular epithelia are rich in diastase-resistant small granules (Pl. V, *13*). These are largely restricted to a variably wide apical zone of the cytoplasm. The zone occupied by granules tends to be narrower in the neck segments than in the crypts, but the density of the granules is greater in the neck segments. Also, in contrast to the "delay" uterus, the glandular lumina and the lumen of the uterus contain an abundance of PAS-positive material, presumably the secretion product of the glands. The texture of this luminal secretion varies, showing finely granular, flocculent, and homogenous colloid-like configurations.

In the preovulatory uterus lipids are virtually absent from both the surface and the glandular epithelia (Pl. V, *14*). Here and there a few small droplets are seen beneath and just above the nuclei, but the over-all picture stands in marked contrast to the rich lipid endowment of the epithelia in the uterus of the delay period.

The lipid content of the epithelial elements of the uterus was also examined in a December bear in which implantation had recently occurred (A-25, Table 1), and differences from the "delay" condition were noted. Frozen sections were obtained from the uterine tube just mesial to the implantation chamber, and others were obtained from within the chamber. In the uterine tube mesial to the conceptus, lipids are still moderately plentiful in the neck and upper cryptal segments of the glands, but they have disappeared entirely from the lower two-thirds of the crypts and from the surface epithelium (Pl. VI, *15*). Within the implantation chamber the endometrium has been extensively eroded, except at the mesometrial side, where chorionic invasion does not occur. In the eroded areas only the lower third or so of the gland fundi remain. A few of these show a moderate content of lipid droplets (Pl. VI, *16*), but the majority lack lipid altogether. At the mesometrial side, where the endometrium is intact, there is a luxuriant glandular apparatus. Here lipids are again confined to the neck and upper cryptal segments of the glands (as in the uterus mesial to the implantation chamber), the deeper crypts and the surface epithelium being free of fat.

Blastocysts

In all, free blastocysts were recovered from the uteri of seven bears, two killed in the latter half of June and five in late August. The number recovered from individual bears varied from two to four and, with the exception of one specimen, corresponded to the number of corpora lutea in the ovaries. In this specimen, killed on August 22, the ovaries contained four corpora, but only three blastocysts were recovered.

Unfortunately, the blastocysts recovered from the late-June specimens were not available to me, but photographs of one of them were provided and are reproduced in Plate VII, *19*. In comparison with the structure of blastocysts recovered in late August, it is evident that in these June specimens development was still in progress. Cleavage had progressed to the point where there is a clear differentiation of inner cell mass and trophoblast, but the cell mass is still joined to the trophoblast at various points by cellular retinacula. It is also evident, from the size of the inner cell mass relative to the vesicle as a whole, in comparison with this relationship in August specimens, that the developing June blastocysts are appreciably smaller than those recovered later in the summer.

The ten blastocysts recovered from three different bears in late August varied only slightly in size and were all comparably developed, suggesting that a developmental arrest had indeed occurred. These vesicles measured 1.25–1.75 mm. in over-all diameter. With the exception of those recovered from one bear (Pl. VIII, *20A*), all the blastocysts had undergone appreciable shrinkage, showing up as small spherical masses floating about freely within the presumably unshrunken zonal sphere (Pl. VIII, *20B*). The single instance in which shrinkage of the blastocysts within the zona did not occur makes it clear, however, that in life the blastocysts completely occupy the zonal cavity and have a total diameter no less than that of the interior of the zonal sphere.

In the non-shrunken blastocysts it is apparent that the trophoblastic cells are greatly flattened and spread out, for the widely dispersed fine punctae visible in Plate VIII, *20A*, represent the cell nuclei stained with hematoxylin; they are much more crowded together in the shrunken specimens. As observed in intact blastocysts, the inner cell mass consists of a small, sharply circumscribed opaque disk; when viewed from the side, it is seen to be nearly as thick as it is wide, and it presents a hemispherical contour to the blastocyst cavity. The diameter of the disk is approximately 60–80 μ.

The specimen shown in Plate VIII, *20B*, was one of four identically developed blastocysts recovered from a bear killed on August 27. All four showed a condition not seen in those recovered from any of the other bears, a condition that must therefore be regarded as unique, namely, the presence of two inner cell masses. In each, one cell mass is larger than the other, the larger one being about normal size. In three of the blastocysts the larger and smaller cell masses are approximate; in the fourth they are separated by a distance equal to about a quarter of the circumference of the vesicle. This doubling of the inner cell mass could bespeak a monovular twinning, and its occurrence in all four blastocysts recovered from a single bear may well indicate a genetic predisposition toward monovular twinning in this individual.

The zona pellucida in the formalin-preserved blastocysts proved to be a thick, glassy, and resilient membrane, resembling in these respects the zonas of "delay" blastocysts in various mustelids (e.g., the fisher [Eadie and Hamilton, 1958] and the marten [Marshall and Enders, 1942]). It can be torn with fine forceps, however, to effect the relase of the blastocyst within. In such dissections the impression was gained that the zona is composed of several layers. A fine striation paralleling the zonal surface could usually be seen in sections, and, just within the outer surface, elongate refractile clefts oriented in the plane of the aforementioned striations were irregularly distributed, but gross "onion skin" type of concentric organization was not apparent in sections stained with hematoxylin, Masson, PAS, Alcian blue, or Hale's dialyzed iron. The staining reactions of the zona are perhaps of some interest. It is colored a pale blue after hematoxylin, a reddish brown with Masson, a moderately intense bluish with Hale's dialyzed iron, and an intense red with PAS; Alcian blue stains it not at all. The last reaction presumably indicates an absence of acidic polysaccharide complexes within the zona.

Besides the blastocyst, there also exists within the zonal cavity an amorphous semihyaline material that differs in its staining reactions from the zona. The substance remains unstained after hematoxylin, Masson, and Hale's dialyzed iron; is faintly positive with PAS; and stains intensely blue-green with Alcian blue in acid solution. The last two reactions presumably indicate the presence of a highly polymerized polysaccharide complex of some acidity. A similar coagulum was noted by Marshall and Enders (1942) in the zonal cavity of the marten.

The histological organization of the inner cell mass is illustrated in Plate VI, *17*, *18*, from a section stained with hematoxylin and eosin. It is seen to consist of a solid ball of rather large cells and is slightly flattened on top. The cell profiles are rounded or polygonal, and the boundaries are easily distinguished. The nuclei tend to be centrally situated and are surrounded by a copious cytoplasm that is finely vacuolated (foamy) and relatively achromatic. While not completely shown in the plane of focus of the photographs, the cell mass is separated from the zona by a covering of flattened trophoblastic cells continuous with the peripheral trophoblast of the vesicle wall. There is as yet no evidence of the differentiation and spread of presumptive entoderm, so the "delay" vesicle, at least in late summer, is still completely monodermic. Rigorous cell counts have not as yet been carried out, but the inner cell mass illustrated is comprised of no more than 35–50 cells. The trophoblastic nuclei in the lower blastocyst of Plate VIII, *50A*, were counted and number approximately 70. Since about a quarter of the total surface is visible, this would provide, as a rough estimate, approximately 280 cells in the outer trophoblastic wall of the blastocyst, or something over 300 cells in the blastocyst as a whole. Marshall and Enders (1942) report that the inner cell mass of the delay blastocyst in martens contains 300–400 cells, which seems very high. Their Figure 2, purporting to show an inner cell mass, is not very convincing, for to me it resembles an entire blastocyst very much shrunken and collapesd.

It was mentioned earlier that three unimplanted blastocysts were found in the uterus of the November specimen provided by Dr. Mossman. Unfortunately, since these were sectioned in utero, they were completely demolished during the sectioning process and only bits of the zona and a few cell fragments are visible in the sections. Accordingly, nothing of their structure can be made out. On the other hand, at the level of each blastocyst the lumen is expanded in such a way as to form a circular "pocket" approximately 1.5 mm. in diameter (Pl. III, *6*). Each pocket undoubtedly represents the "imprint" of the blastocyst lodged at that point, and, since the blastocysts were still intact when the endometrium was fixed, we may assume that each of these three blastocysts had a diameter of approximately 1.5 mm.

Discussion and Conclusions

It has been shown that, in New York bears, ovulation occurs during the last three weeks of June and probably not thereafter. Unimplanted blastocysts have been recovered in late June, the end of August, and late November. Two pregnant specimens were obtained in mid-December in which, judging from the development of the conceptuses implantation, could not have occurred more than a week or two previously. Hamlett (1935) reported the recovery of a 2-mm. embryo from a bear killed in Pennsylvania on December 2 that obviously could also have implanted only a short time before. Collectively, these observations finally prove what has long been suspected—that embryonic development in the black bear is characterized by a delay in the implantation of the blastocysts and that the quiescent period endures approximately five months, at least at the latitude of New York State. These findings in the black bear enhance the probability that a similar delay period occurs in other species of bears, for their reproductive sequences, as far as they are known, resemble that of the black bear.

What the present observations cannot tell us with certainty is whether embryonic differentiation and expansion of the blastocyst are fully suppressed or merely greatly slowed down during the delay period. The earliest specimens recovered in June were appreciably smaller than those obtained at summer's end, but they were obviously still actively differentiating and probably no more than a few days past ovulation. The late-summer specimens were all collected within a few days of one another and hence do not represent a chronological series. The late-November specimens, which could have provided the answer, were all destroyed in the process of sectioning; I have given reasons for my belief that they were probably of the same size as the late-summer blastocysts, but of course their degree of embryonic differentiation could not be assessed. A final answer must await the recovery and study of free blastocysts from bears killed in the late fall shortly before implantation occurs. Fischer (1900) has indicated that the free blastocysts of the European badger (*Meles*) slowly expand during the delay period, but Hamlett (1932, 1935) found no indication of this in the American badger (*Taxidea*). In most mammals showing discontinuous development embryonic differentiation is arrested before the primary entoderm is formed, and the black bear appears to belong to this group. The European roe deer (*Capreolus*) represents the only known exception to this, for in this species not only entoderm but primary amniotic cavity and the embryonic shield slowly differentiate during the delay period (Keibel, cited by Hamlett, 1935).

It has also been shown that the bear resembles other carnivores with discontinuous development in that the zona pellucida is unusually thick and resistant and that it persists throughout the delay period. This contrasts with the situation in the armadillo, in which, according to Hamlett (1935), the zona disappears in the quiescent period.

Changes in the structure and histochemistry of the endometrium from the preovulatory to the delay and pregnancy conditions have been described. These principally involve the epithelial elements, especially the glands. The latter are developed somewhat better in the delay than in the preovulatory uterus, but thereafter they experience no radical change before implantation. The outstanding histochemical feature of the endometrium during the delay period is the great abundance of lipid in all epithelial components. It is virtually absent, however, in the preovulatory uterus and disappears from the surface epithelium and gland crypts in the early pregnant uterus. On the other hand, diastase-resistant PAS-positive granules are abundant in the glandular epithelium and lumina in the preovulatory uterus but are greatly reduced in the uterus of the delay period. Enders *et al.* (1958) recorded a similar abundance of lipids in the glandular and surface epithelia of the armadillo uterus during delay and noted also a slight diminution following implantation. They likewise succeeded in demonstrating small amounts of glycogen in the glands during the delay period and, at the luminal borders of many of the gland cells, a "thin fringe" of PAS-positive saliva-resistant mucopolysaccharide. Following implantation in the armadillo, great vacuolation of the gland cells associated with an increase in glycogen content was noted. As far as lipids and saliva-resistant PAS-positive substances are concerned (glycogen could not be investigated in my formalin-fixed material), the endometrium of the bear more or less resembles that of the armadillo during the delay period. Histological changes in the uterus before, during, and after the delay period have been described in various carnivores, most notably the mink (Hansson, 1957; Enders, 1952), American badger (Hamlett, 1932), European badger (Neal and Harrison, 1958; Canivenc, 1960) and several pinnipedia (cf. Canivenc, 1960). An equivalent condition has been found in all, that is, an endometrium that shows all the characteristics of the follicular (estrogenic) phase and few, if any, of the luteal (progestational) phase. In general the picture here described in the black bear is similar. The glandular and surface epithelia are more hypertrophied during the delay than during the preovulatory phase, but evidence of secretory activity in the glands is diminished during the delay period in comparison with the preovulatory uterus. Following implantation, however, the endometrium becomes markedly foliate and the glands experience further growth and hypertrophy.

PLATE I

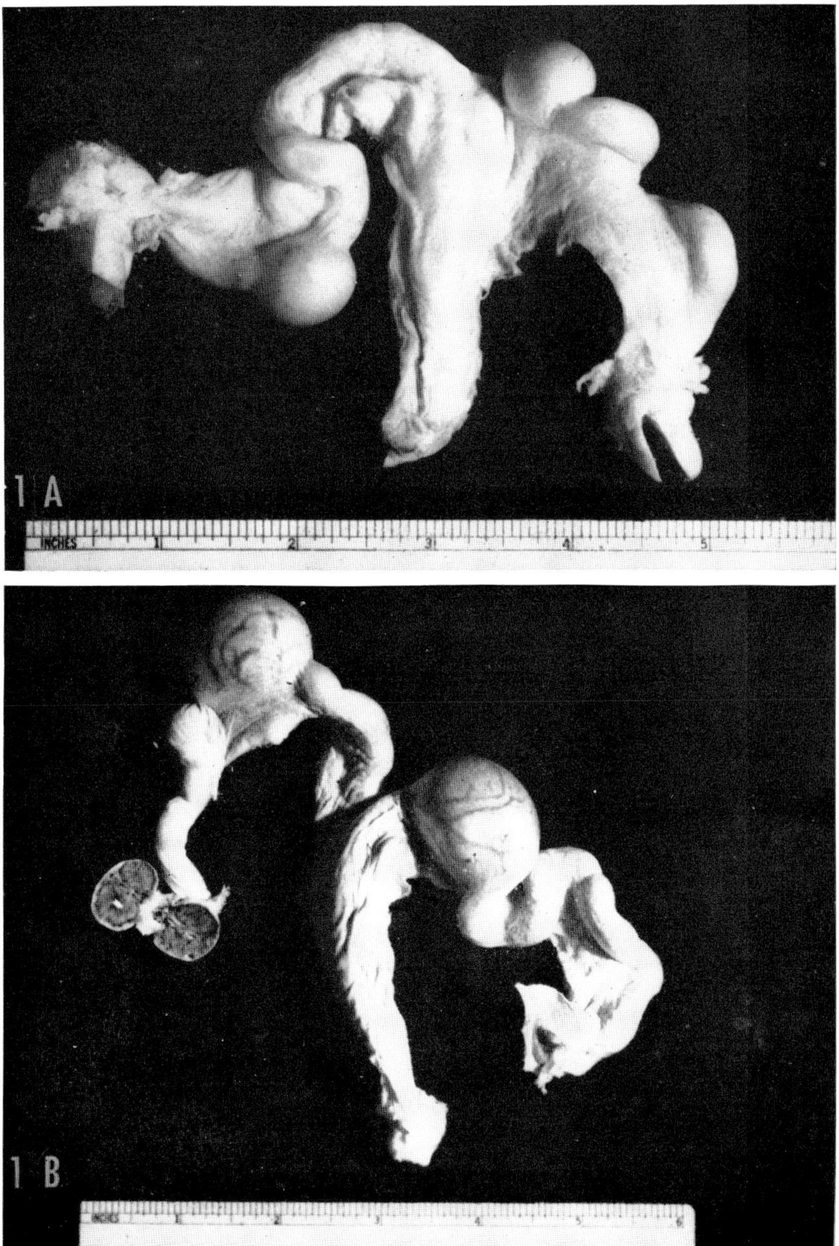

1A, *1B*, Reproductive organs of two "pregnant" bears killed in early December. A single gestation swelling occurs in each cornu of both specimens; they are located about one-third of the way out in the cornua from the corpus uteri.

PLATE II

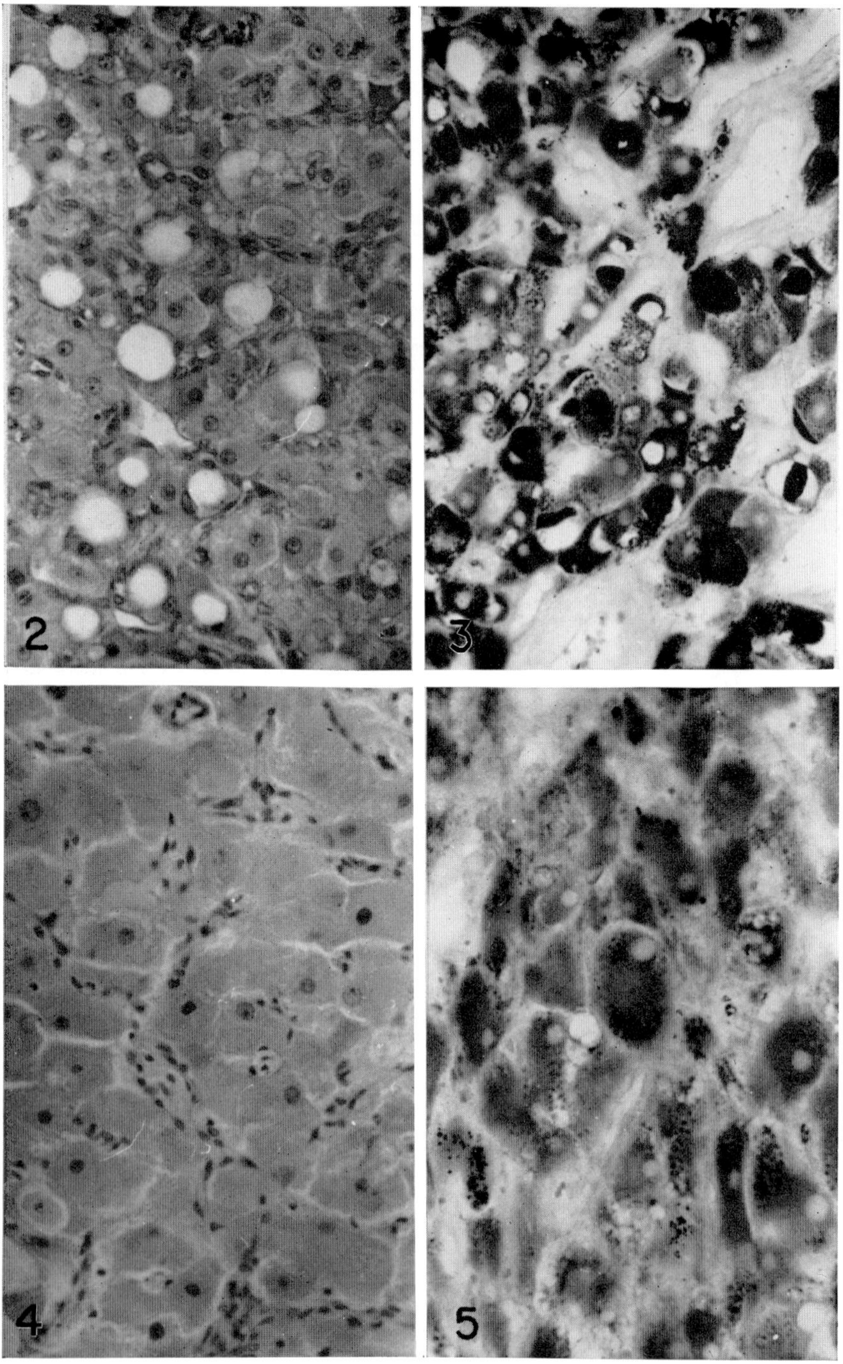

2, Section of corpus luteum from bear with delay blastocysts killed on August 30. Compare with *4*, showing corpus luteum of a "pregnant" December bear. H. & E. ×300.

3, Same corpus luteum as in *2* but stained with Sudan black B. ×300.

4, Corpus luteum of "pregnant" bear killed in early December. Note increase in cell size over "delay" corpora and absence of gross vacuolation. H. & E. ×300.

5, Same corpus luteum as in *4* but stained with Sudan black B. ×300.

PLATE III

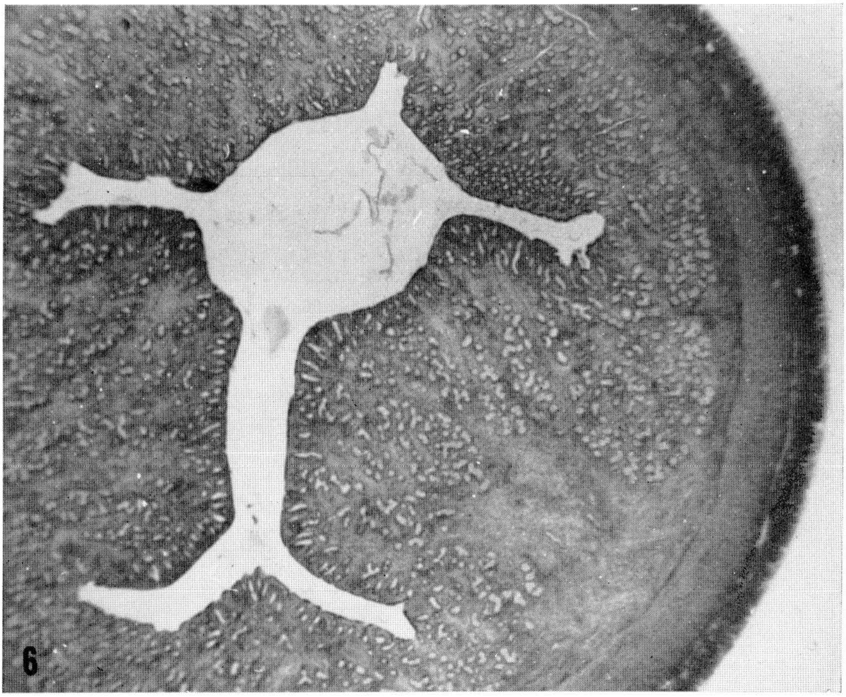

6, Section of uterine wall of bear with delay blastocysts killed in November, showing organization of myometrial and endometrial components. Masson. ×23.

PLATE IV

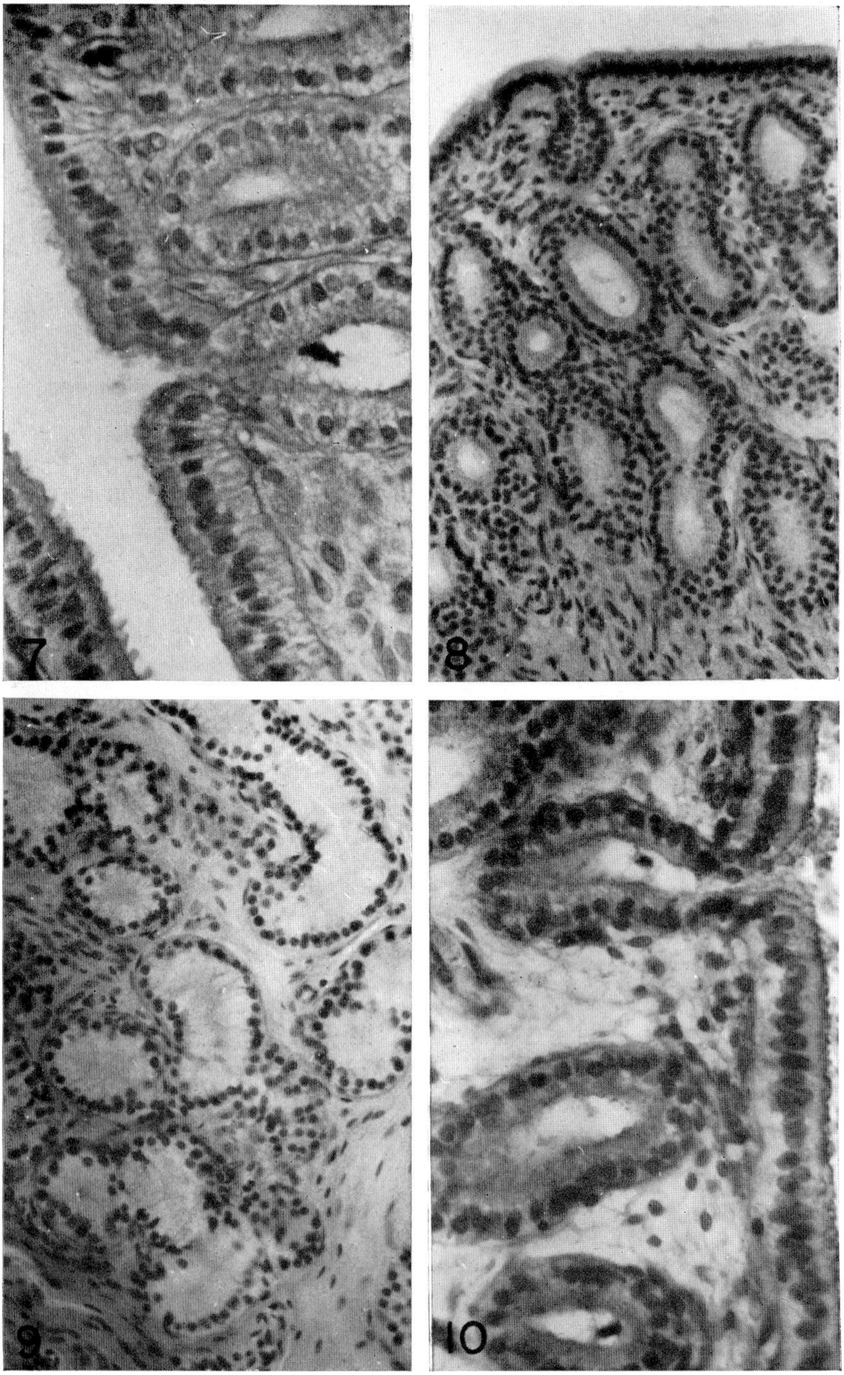

7, Uterus of bear with delay blastocysts killed on August 30, showing character of surface epithelium. PAS and hematoxylin. ×600.

8, Uterus of bear with delay blastocysts killed in November, showing detail of surface epithelium and gland neck segments. Masson. ×300.

9, Same uterus as in *8* but showing detail of gland crypts. Masson. ×300.

10, Uterus of bear with delay blastocysts killed in November, showing nature of PAS reaction in gland neck segments. PAS and hematoxylin. ×600.

PLATE V

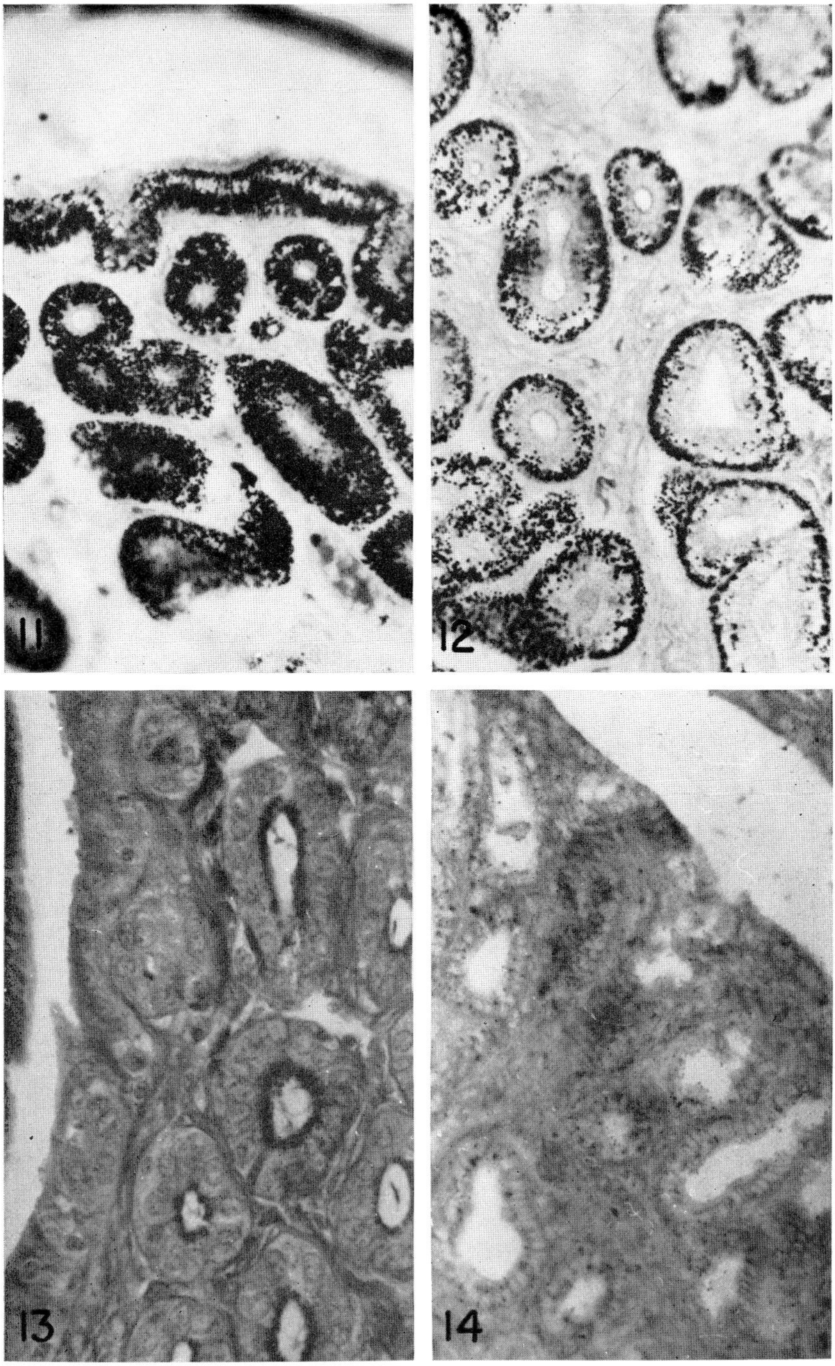

11, Uterus of bear with delay blastocysts killed on August 30, showing sudanophilic lipids in surface epithelium and gland neck segments. Sudan black B. ×300.

12, Same uterus as in *11* but showing sudanophilic lipids in glandular crypts. Sudan black B. ×300.

13, Uterus of "preovulatory" bear killed in late May, showing PAS reaction in epithelial components and gland lumina. Apical cytoplasm of gland cells is crowded with minute diastase-resistant granules. PAS and hematoxylin. ×600.

14, Same uterus as in *13*. Note absence of sudanophilic lipid in epithelial components in contrast to delay uterus as seen in *11* and *12*. Sudan black B. ×300.

PLATE VI

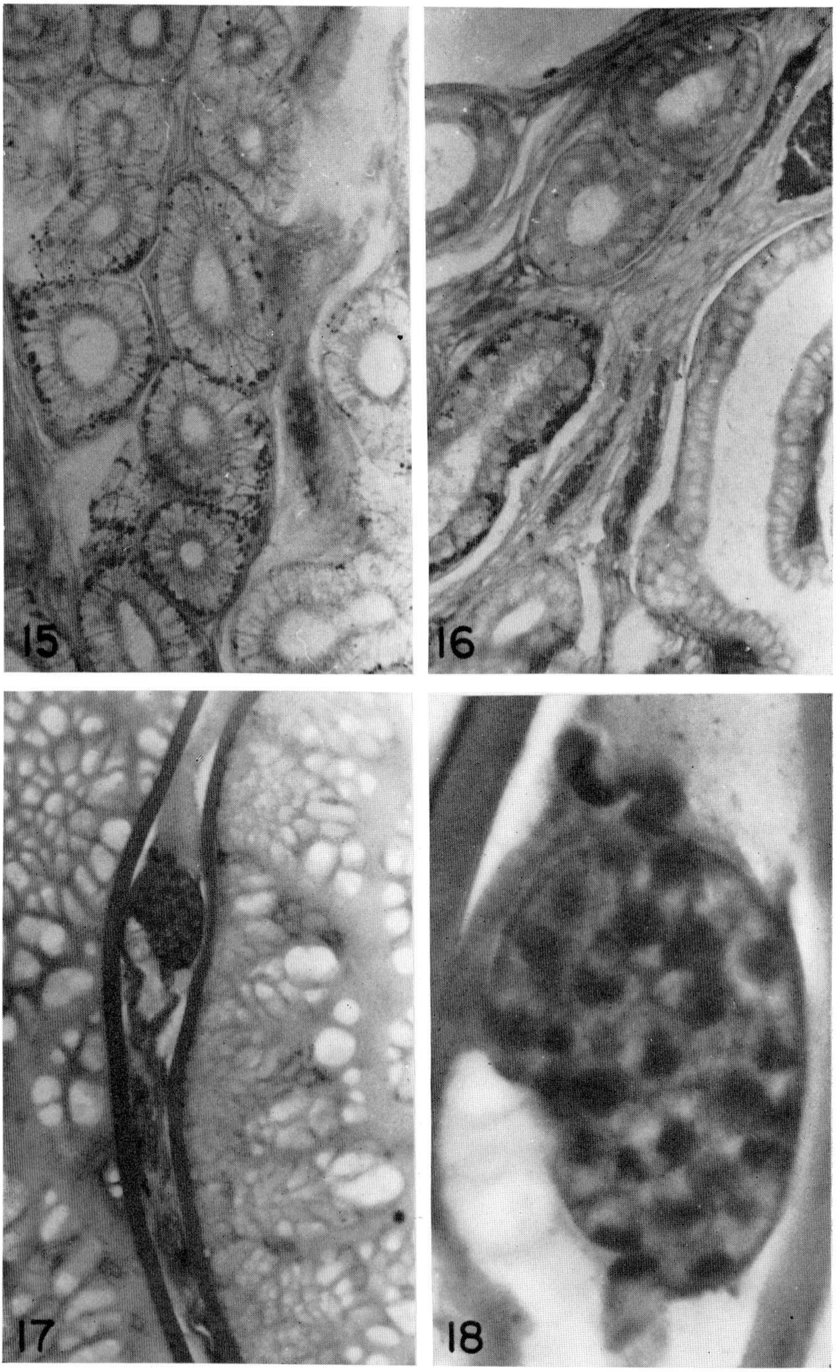

15, Uterus of "pregnant" December bear mesial to implantation cavity. Lipid droplets still abundant in necks and upper crypts of glands but now absent in gland fundi and surface epithelium. Sudan black B. ×300.

16, Implantation chamber of December bear beneath forming placenta showing lipid droplets in some gland fundi and absence of lipid in others. Sudan black B. ×300.

17, *18*, Central sections through inner cell mass of unimplanted blastocyst obtained from a bear killed in late August. Description in text. H. & E. ×300 and 600, respectively.

PLATE VII

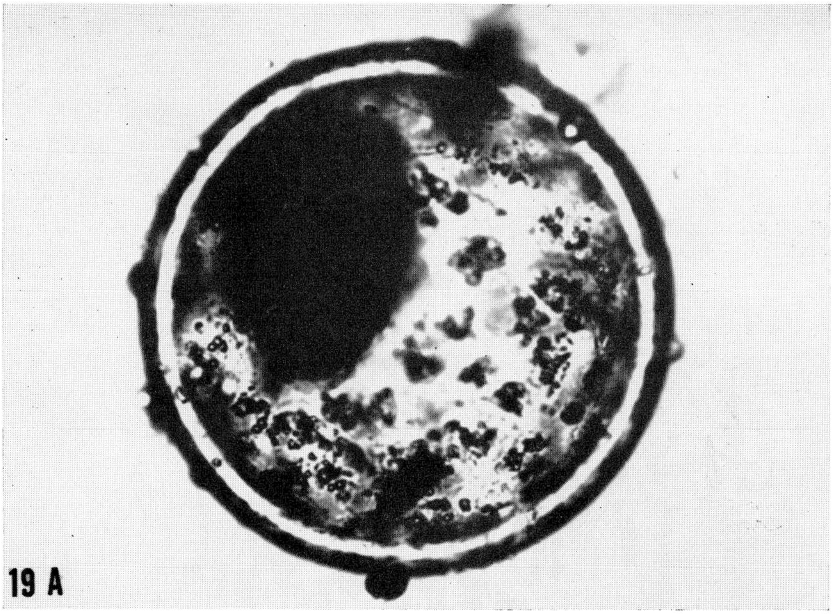

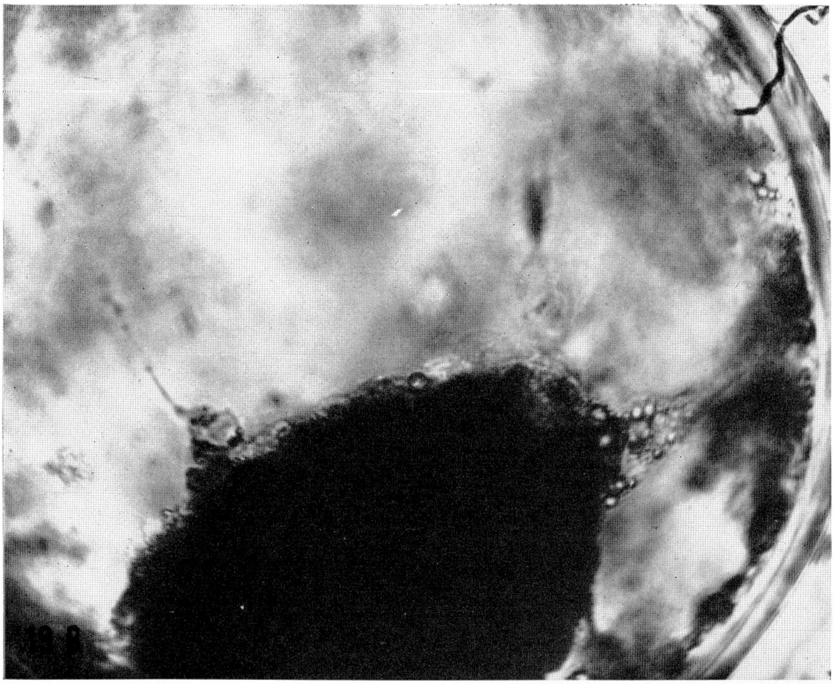

19A, *19B*, Intact blastocyst recovered from bear killed on June 22, shown at two different magnifications. The inner cell mass is the large dark body. In the high-power view (*B*) cellular retinacula joining cell mass and trophoblast are visible. Max. mag. ×200.

PLATE VIII

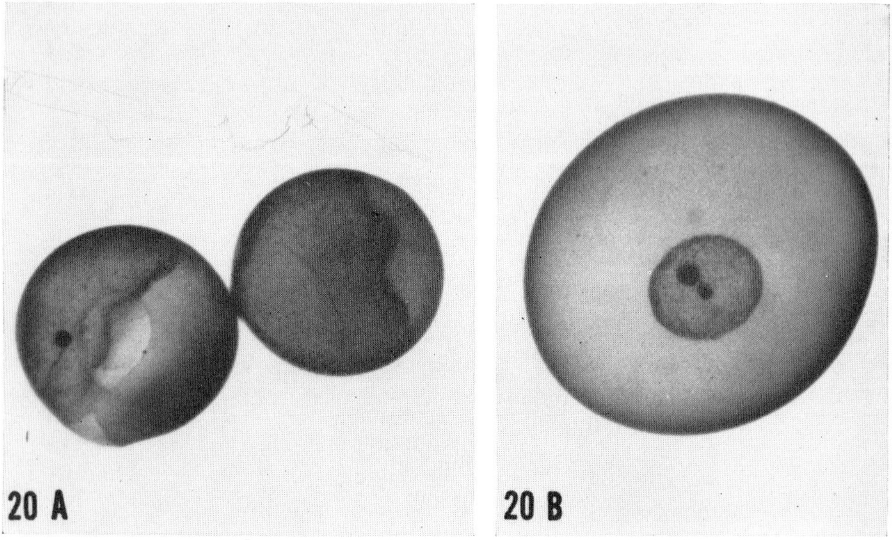

20A, *20B*, Unimplanted blastocysts recovered from bears killed in late August. In *A* there has been a minimum of shrinkage of the blastocyst within the zona. In *B* the blastocyst has shrunken appreciably. Note the unique double inner cell mass in *B*. (Description in text.) *A*, ×20. *B*, ×45.

It has been shown that in the bear the corpus luteum has a consistent structure throughout the delay period but that its structure, and presumably its function, are altered following implantation. The most obvious changes are a dramatic increase in total volume owing largely to hypertrophy of the lutein cells, an apparent great increase in vascularity, and a loss of the gross vacuolation that seems more or less characteristic of the corpora of delay. Marked vacuolation of the corpora lutea during the delay period has been reported in other carnivores, notably the wolverine (Wright and Rausch, 1955), the marten (Wright, 1942), and

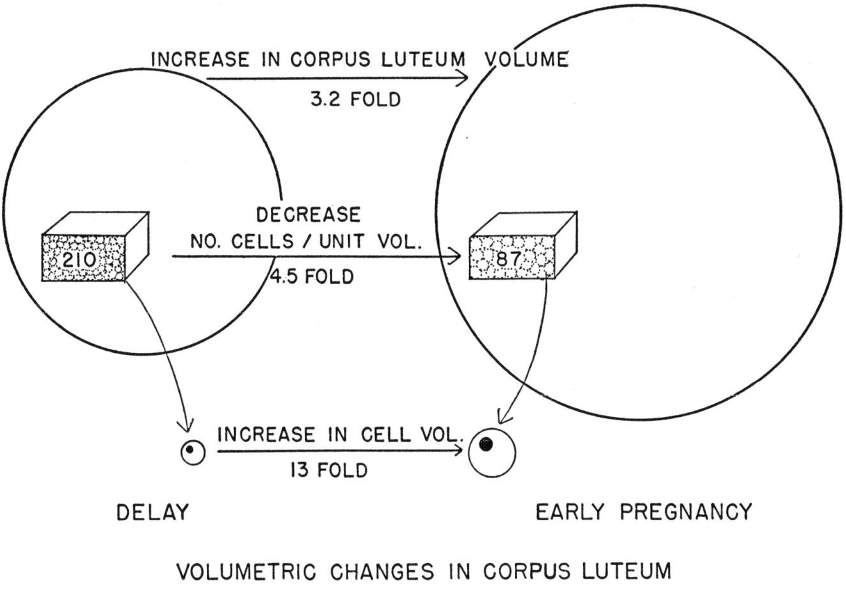

Fig. 1.—Volumetric changes in corpus luteum and individual lutein cells between delay and early pregnancy periods illustrating basis for postulated cell death (cf. text).

the fisher (Eadie and Hamilton, 1958). On the other hand, Rausch (1961), who examined the corpora of two Alaskan black bears in which the uterus presumably contained unimplanted blastocysts, makes the perplexing statement that the corpora do not "closely resemble the inactive corpora observed in the ovaries of the wolverine . . . nor those described from the ovaries of badgers, *Meles meles* . . ." (by Neal and Harrison, 1958); he did not indicate how they differed, however.

From figures cited earlier it is apparent that the increase in the volume of the corpus luteum between the delay and postimplantation periods is less than would be expected from the volume increase of the individual cells that compose it (Fig. 1). While the mean increase in volume of the corpus luteum was three-and-one-fifth fold, that of the individual cells was nearly thirteen fold. On the other hand, a numerical count of cells per unit volume in the corpus luteum of pregnancy showed a four-and-one-half-fold decrease over that in the corpus luteum of delay. The difference in volume increase for individual cells (×13) and the volume increase for a constant number of cells (×4.5) is caused by the supplementary tissues, principally vascular, which increase in volume but at an appreciably lower rate than the cells. The four-and-one-half-fold increase is thus the average of volume increases in cells and supplementary tissues and is the figure that should be compared with volumetric change in the corpus luteum as a whole for purposes of estimating changes in cell population. The fact that the mean volumetric increase of the corpus luteum is lower (about 3.2) suggests that the corpus luteum of pregnancy contains fewer cells than that of the delay period by about 30 per cent. The possibility of considerable cell death in the corpora during the delay period demands more critical investigation.

The present study, being necessarily descriptive, throws no light on the possible functional attributes of the corpora lutea of the delay and postimplantation periods.

Finally, my observations on summer bears suggest the possible occurrence of a phenomenon that, while not immediately related to the central theme of this paper, is nevertheless of considerable interest in regard to other aspects of reproductive physiology in bears, namely, that ovulation may not occur in the absence of a coital stimulus. My evidence that ovulation may be "induced" is not conclusive, but it is highly suggestive. Essentially, it is based on the finding of large graafian follicles in various stages of atresia in twelve bears, one a presumed yearling, the others adults, during the months of June and July. Such follicles were encountered only in early summer, never therafter. Since corpora lutea were not observed in the ovaries of any of these bears with atretic large follicles, it is evident that they had not ovulated. Whether any of these bears had borne young the preceding winter was unknown, but it seems unlikely, for Rausch (1961) found no follicles larger than 2 mm. in the ovaries of two adult black bears killed in early summer that had borne young some months previously. Furthermore, the presence of large follicles is inconsistent with the alternate-year breeding cycle of black bears accompanied by cubs.

The question, then, is Why had these animals not ovulated if this phenomenon occurs spontaneously in bears? It is tempting to consider that the animals in question, either from lack of opportunity or for other reasons, failed to breed and in the absence of the copulatory stimulus did not ovulate. The problem is one that could easily be resolved in captive bears; one need only isolate females during the period when ovulation normally occurs and examine the ovaries thereafter for the presence of large follicles or corpora lutea. It would be essential to the experiment not only that sexually mature females be used but that they had not borne cubs the preceding winter or that they had been deprived of their cubs in early spring.

Summary

This study is based on the analysis of the reproductive organs of 53 wild female black bears of various estimated ages killed between late May and early September in New York State, 1 adult specimen killed in late November in Wisconsin, and 2 adults in early pregnancy killed in mid-December. Unimplanted blastocysts were recovered in June, August, and November. The material provides proof that in the black bear, as in certain other carnivores, embryonic development is characterized by a period of developmental arrest or retardation at the blastocyst stage and that implantation is postponed for a period of approximately five months. Unimplanted blastocysts recovered from the uterus are described, together with changes in the structure of the corpus luteum and in the structure and histochemistry of the endometrium during the delay and early postimplantation periods. Evidence is also presented that suggests that in the bear, as in certain other carnivores, ovulation may not be spontaneous but may require a coital stimulus.

Acknowledgments

The bulk of the specimens on which this report is based was collected by Hugh C. Black and is a contribution in Federal Aid in Wildlife Restoration Project W-89-R of the New York State Conservation Department under contract with the Department of Conservation of Cornell University. It is a pleasure to acknowledge the co-operation of Professor Oliver Hewitt, through whose courtesy these specimens were obtained. Thanks are also due Professor Harland W. Mossman, who generously turned over to me sections of a "delay uterus" from a bear killed in Wisconsin in late November, 1958. The help of David Heimbach in making a preliminary gross and microscopic survey of the ovaries of the New York State bears is gratefully acknowledged. Finally, credit is due Anthony Guerriere for his expert technical assistance during all phases of this study. This study was supported in part by research grants (G-7474 and G-24043) from the National Science Foundation.

References

Asdell, S. A. 1946. Patterns of Mammalian Reproduction. Ithaca, N.Y.: Comstock Press.

Baker, A. B. 1912. Further notes on the breeding of the American black bear in captivity. Smithsonian Misc. Coll., **45**:175–79.

Canivenc, R. 1960. L'ovo-implantation différée des animaux sauvages. Pp.

33–86 in Les fonctions de nidation utérine et leur troubles. Paris: Masson & Cie.

EADIE, W. R., and W. J. HAMILTON, JR. 1958. Reproduction in the fisher in New York. N.Y. Fish & Game J., **5**:77–83.

ENDERS, A. C., G. D. BUCHANAN, and R. V. TALMAGE. 1958. Histological and histochemical observations on the armadillo uterus during the delayed and post-implantation periods. Anat. Rec., **130**:639–58.

ENDERS, R. K. 1952. Reproduction in the mink (*Mustela vison*). Proc. Am. Phil. Soc., **96**:691–755.

FISCHER, E. 1900. Zur Entwicklungsgeschichte des Dachses. Mitt. Bad. Pool. Vereins, Karlsruhe.

HAMLETT, G. W. D. 1932. Observations on the embryology of the badger. Anat. Rec., **53**:283–303.

———. 1935. Delayed implantation and discontinuous development in mammals. Quart. Rev. Biol., **10**:432–47.

HANSSON, A. 1947. The physiology of reproduction in mink (*Mustela vison*, Schreb.) with special reference to delayed implantation. Acta Zool., **28**: 1–136.

MARSHALL, W. H., and R. K. ENDERS. 1942. The blastocyst of the marten (*Martes*). Anat. Rec., **84**:307–10.

NEAL, E. G., and R. J. HARRISON. 1958. Reproduction in the European badger (*Meles meles* L.). Trans. Zool. Soc. London, **29** (Part 2):67–131.

PEARSE, A. G. E. 1960. Histochemistry, Theoretical and Applied. 2d ed. London: Churchill.

RAUSCH, R. L. 1961. Notes on the black bear, *Ursus americanus* Pallas, in Alaska, with particular reference to dentition and growth. Ztschr. f. Säugetierkunde, **26**:65–128.

WRIGHT, P. L. 1942. Delayed implantation in the long-tailed weasel (*Mustela frenata*), the short-tailed weasel (*Mustela cicognani*), and the marten (*Martes americana*). Anat. Rec., **83**:341–53.

WRIGHT, P. L., and R. L. RAUSCH. 1955. Reproduction in the wolverine, *Gulo gulo*. J. Mammal., **36**:346–55.

DISCUSSION (*Chairman:* R. J. HARRISON)

HARRISON: The zona pellucida is very resistant during delay in European badgers. You can almost bounce the blastocysts within the tough zona.

WIMSATT: I agree.

CANIVENC: Do you have any evidence of two estrous periods, a main estrus and an accessory estrus, as Lindeman wrote? Have you made any observation that gestation varies with latitude?

WIMSATT: My material is insufficient to determine this point; since I had only one specimen after August, I have no information as to the possibility of a "false" estrus in the fall. The period of parturition seems to be about the same everywhere and independent of latitude.

CANIVENC: Do they implant in winter?

WIMSATT: They implant late in November or early in December.

CANIVENC: Are the days shortest?

WIMSATT: Yes, and they are getting shorter all the time.

HARRISON: Is it known how long lactation lasts?

WIMSATT: No. Young bears are born in late January or early February. A lactating female bear was collected on September 6. How long it continues thereafter is not definitely known.

SHELESNYAK: Did you say that the zona of delayed blastocyst of the bear is less rugged than that of other species?

WIMSATT: I tried to create just the opposite impression. It is more resistant than normal zonas of other mammals.

DEANESLY: The endometrium was said to be more estrogenic than progestational during delay. This is not the case in the stoat.

WIMSATT: You may remember that the delay uterus showed certain changes over the preovulatory uterus in that the epithelial cells and glandular components are more prominent during the delay period. They become even more so after implantation. Whether the differences noted between the preovulatory and delay uteri could reflect to some degree a luteal effect I am unprepared to say, but certainly the further changes following implantation are clearly luteal in nature.

SHARMAN: You said that in August the blastocyst is 1.75 mm. in diameter and discussed possible increase in size during the delay period. Did you see any evidence of mitosis in the August blastocyst?

WIMSATT: No. The smaller size and differentiating status of the June specimens indicate that mitoses would have been found in these specimens had they been sectioned, but mitoses were not observed in the sectioned August blastocysts. I had no blastocysts from late in the delay period, but gave reasons for my belief that in the November specimen, in which the blastocysts were destroyed by sectioning, enlargement had not occurred over the August blastocysts. I believe it probable that significant enlargement does not occur during the delay period, but I do not have the material to prove it. Unimplanted blastocysts recovered in the late fall must be obtained in order to resolve the question.

DICKMANN: You showed a good-sized zona. Is this all zona?

WIMSATT: As far as I know or can see, yes.

DICKMANN: How wide is the zona?

WIMSATT: Seven or eight microns.

HARRISON: It definitely gets thinner in badgers as delay progresses.

WIMSATT: In the specimens from June it was thinner than it was in the ones from August.

HARTMAN: This reminds me of what Böving calls the "gloiolemma," the mucoid layer being the "mucolemma," the zona pellucida the "oölemma" (in the forthcoming volume, *Mechanisms Concerned with Conception* [Pergamon Press, 1963]). The gloiolemma is the mucoid layer that the ovum picks up in the uterus, notably in the bitch, as described 130 years ago by Bischoff in his monograph on the embryology of the dog.

Certain of Dr. Wimsatt's slides remind me of Dr. Alden's very delicate test for estrogen in the uterus, namely, the disappearance of basal fat in the cells of the rat uterine epithelium. The absence of such fat seems to prove the presence of estrogen at the stage in question.

WIMSATT: In dissecting the zona off, I got the impression that it was layered. I did not find inner and outer membranes.

DICKMANN: This layering could exist. The zonae of most species that have been studied have more than one layer.

WIMSATT: You can see fine fibrillation and striation.

PHILIP L. WRIGHT

Variations in Reproductive Cycles in North American Mustelids

When Hamlett summarized the status of our knowledge of delayed implantation in 1935, the only American mustelid for which he presented conclusive evidence of arrested development of the embryos was the badger (*Taxidea taxus*). He did suggest that delayed implantation probably occurred in the marten (*Martes americana*) as well as three Eurasian species of *Martes* and in the long-tailed weasel (*Mustela frenata*, called *Mustela noveboracensis* in 1935). Hamlett's paper stimulated the study of reproduction in several species of mustelids as well as other mammalian groups. We now know in considerable detail the nature of the reproductive cycles of some American mustelids that were not then suspected of displaying delayed implantation.

In this paper the work that has been done on the reproductive cycles of seven American mustelids will be summarized. Two of these species also occur in Eurasia (*Mustela erminea* and *Gulo gulo*). The former has been studied more thoroughly by Europeans than by Americans. Pertinent information for each species is summarized in Table 1. The material will be discussed under the species headings. I have studied each of these animals except *Taxidea* in some detail, and where references are not cited, the information has come from my own data.

American Marten (*Martes americana*)

The marten was the first of the American mustelids known to have a prolonged gestation period. Marten have been maintained in captivity since 1913 by biologists of the United States Fish and Wildlife Service, first in Idaho and later at Saratoga Springs, New York. Ashbrook and Hanson (1927) described the summer breeding season for the first time and indicated that breeding occurs in July and August and

DR. PHILIP L. WRIGHT is professor and chairman of the Department of Zoölogy, Montana State University, Missoula.

TABLE 1

COMPARISON OF REPRODUCTIVE CYCLES IN AMERICAN MUSTELIDS

	American Marten, *Martes americana*	Fisher, *Martes pennanti*	Wolverine, *Gulo gulo*	River Otter, *Lutra canadensis*	American Badger, *Taxidea taxus*	Short-tailed Weasel, *Mustela erminea* (N.A. Material)	Long-tailed Weasel, *Mustela frenata*
Age of female at first heat...	2 years	1 year	1 year	2 years	4 months	2–2½ months	3 months
Gestation period..........	259–76 days	327–58 days	?	9½–12 months	7½–8 months(?)	10–11 months	9 months
Parturition period..........	March–April	March–April	March	December–April	March–April	April–May	April–May
Breeding season............	July–August	l. March–April	July(?)	January–April	August–September(?)	May, June, July	July
Wt. of paired ovaries of females with unimplanted blastocysts..............	39.2	133	143–244	76–215	?	Not recorded	21
Wt. of paired ovaries during active pregnancy........	Not recorded	184–240	291–430	365	?	Not recorded	48–79
Diam. of corpus luteum during unimplanted stage....	1.12	1.47	1.65–2.00	2.60	?	0.484	0.385–0.600
Diam. of corpus luteum during active pregnancy......	?	2.95	3.49	5.00	?	0.868	1.150
Usual number of young at birth.................	2–5	3–4	304	2–4	2–3	5–9	6–9
Usual wt. of adult female...	600 gm.	3 lb., 12 oz.	18–22 lb.	10–20 lb.	13–18 lb.	50–75 gm.	130–220 gm.
Approx. diam. of inactive blastocysts in microns....	500–900	1,000	2,000	1,000	950–75	400–700	600
Thickness in microns of zona pellucida in fixed material.	6.9	14.4	7.8	?	3.8	4.5	4.7
Interval between implantation and parturition......	25–28 days	?	?	?	?	?	23–24 days

that the young are born the following April. The gestation period was determined to be from 259 to 275 days. Markley and Bassett (1942) summarized the results of further observation on the marten at Saratoga Springs. They described many aspects of the biology of animals as they live in captivity. Although some females came into heat during their second summer, the youngest female at the time of the birth of her first litter was three years old.

Enders and Leekley (1941) described a pronounced vulval swelling during estrus and indicated that, generally, copulation took place during maximal swelling. Wright (1942*a*) described the unimplanted blastocysts from trapper-caught animals taken in Montana, and Marshall and Enders (1942) described blastocysts from western marten (*Martes caurina*) taken in Idaho.

Pearson and Enders (1944) in a significant experiment showed that, by appropriate photoperiod manipulation, bred females could be induced to implant their embryos earlier than normal and to produce litters in December rather than the usual time in April. Wright (1953) showed that there was only one species of marten in continental North America when he found intergradation between *M. americana* and *M. caurina* in western Montana and concluded that both types should be called *Martes americana*.

During the course of a long-term ecological study involving live trapping of wild marten in Glacier National Park, Jonkel and Weckwerth (1963) made a concerted effort to determine whether females are normally bred during their second summer. They were unable to find clear-cut evidence that this species breeds until its third year of life. It was necessary to study this problem in animals originally marked as juveniles because it has not been possible to recognize the yearling class with certainty in trapper-caught animals by cranial or skeletal characters. By performing a series of laparotomies on pregnant females, they demonstrated that the interval between implantation and parturition was less than 28 days. This is considerably shorter than that estimated by previous workers.

Wright (unpublished) counted the number of corpora lutea in 44 tracts of pregnant marten obtained from trappers in Montana. The average number was 3.02. Most of these ovaries were serially sectioned, but an effort was made to hand-slice the ovaries and count the corpora lutea under a dissecting scope. The ovaries of pregnant marten during the early winter weigh about 20 mg. each and are so small that it is difficult to make the counts accurately. One series of 24 pairs was checked by serial sectioning after they were hand-sliced, and no errors had been made in distinguishing adult from immature marten. Three errors in counting corpora lutea were found in 26 ovaries of pregnant animals. About one-third of the adult marten had all the corpora in one ovary, none in the other. Approximately half the winter population of female marten consists of non-pregnant individuals, and it is supposed that these are both juveniles and yearlings. The paired weights of 44 sets of pregnant ovaries averaged 39.2 mg., and 39 pairs of non-pregnant ovaries weighed an average of 28.1 mg.

The reproductive tract of a parous female that was repeatedly trapped during the breeding season by Vernon Hawley on the Glacier National Park study area was preserved promptly when the animal died. Hawley had observed that the animal showed a swollen vulva some two weeks earlier. Serial sections of the ovary (Pl. I, *1*) and oviduct show that the animal had ovulated some time earlier, and two tubal embryos were located. These embryos (Pl. I, *2*), with counts of 13 and 16 nuclei, were found in the lower third of the oviduct. The remains of the old corpora of pregnancy were also visible. The luteal cells in the new corpora were without vacuoles. No large follicles were found in the ovary, as would be seen in the mink at this stage. Large masses of interstitial cells made up the larger portion of the ovary. Another parous female that died in September during the live trapping on the same area was preserved by Richard Weckwerth. This animal, with blastocysts in the upper third of the uterus, showed the vacuolated corpora found earlier by Wright (1942*a*) in winter-caught marten. No stages with implanted embryos are available. Hawley and Newby (1957) describe other deaths during the summer of parous females on this study area and emphasize that these females are generally in poor condition after nursing a litter in the spring and breeding during midsummer.

Pelts of marten were much more valuable during the twenties and thirties than they are today, and there is less interest in marten-trapping generally. The marten was seriously depleted in the northeastern states and in eastern and central Canada by the early part of the century. This species has not made the striking recovery in the eastern portion of the continent that has been made by the fisher. Commercial marten-raising has never been financially profitable, in part because of small litter size and the prolonged delay in reaching sexual maturity, but also because the majority of marten bred in captivity do not produce litters.

FISHER (*Martes pennanti*)

The reproductive cycle of *Martes pennanti* is quite well known from the studies of Hall (1942), Enders and Pearson (1943), Hamilton and Cook (1955), Eadie and Hamilton (1958), and Wright and Coulter (1963). The evidence by Hall on the gestation period was from captive animals on fur farms in British Columbia. The findings of the other workers are largely from study of trapper-caught animals taken in New

York and Maine. In these states the animal has again become relatively common after a period of near extinction during the early part of the century (Hamilton and Cook, 1955; Coulter, 1960).

The fisher, most valuable of the terrestrial mustelids in terms of the quality of single pelts, is rigidly protected except during a winter trapping season, and summer specimens are not available. This animal has a gestation period just short of a full year. The parous female apparently comes into heat within a week or so after parturition. All adult females taken in the fall and early winter carry unimplanted blastocysts. Implanted embryos are found in February and March, and the young are born in March or April. Young females breed for the first time at one year of age. Coulter obtained a series of fishers from Maine in late March and early April that included two nulliparous females that had recently bred. Tubal embryos (Pl. I, *3*, *4*) were found in each. The corpora lutea were inactive in appearance. No lactating or recently bred parous females are available. The reproductive tracts of trapper-caught pregnant adult females that includes parous and nulliparous animals cannot be distinguished, but Eadie and Hamilton (1958) believe that these two classes can be distinguished from their skulls, the older animal having longer sagittal crests. The average number of corpora lutea found in New York fishers was 2.72, and in Maine specimens 3.28. Since the nulliparous female fisher appears to breed one year earlier than the marten, it appears that the former species has a significantly higher reproductive potential than the latter.

WOLVERINE (*Gulo gulo*)

A recent taxonomic study of nearctic and palearctic wolverines by Kurten and Rausch (1959) confirms the earlier view of Rausch (1953) that there is only one circumpolar species of wolverine with the Eurasian form called *Gulo gulo gulo* and the North American form called *Gulo gulo luscus*. No additional material seems to have been published since Wright and Rausch (1955) described the general nature of the reproductive cycle from material collected from trappers in Alaska. Adult females taken in October, November, and January showed unimplanted blastocysts. Implanted embryos were found in late January and February, and lactating females were collected in April.

One of the points not determined from this study was the time of the breeding season. No specimens were available from late April until October, but the ovaries of the two lactating April specimens showed little sign of estrus. It seemed reasonably certain that the breeding season was delayed until after the lactation period. Mohr (1938–39) described breeding in a pair of captive wolverines in the Copenhagen Zoo between July 17 and 22, 1915, followed by birth of a litter on February

17, 1916. This case represented a gestation period of 215 days and is complementary to the findings of Wright and Rausch. Biologists working during the summer months in areas where wolverines occur should be alert to the possibility of obtaining precise information on the breeding time. Ovaries of adult females taken during any of the warmer months of the year could be studied to yield valuable information on this point.

River Otter (*Lutra canadensis*)

The nature of the reproductive cycle in *Lutra canadensis* has been largely unknown, but the species was once reported to have a gestation period of about 2 months. Liers (1951), who had for many years raised otters in Minnesota as a hobby and for business purposes, reported a winter breeding season in his tame otters and gestation periods ranging from $9\frac{1}{2}$ to $12\frac{1}{2}$ months. Hamilton and Eadie (1963) have recently studied the reproductive tracts of 74 trapper-caught female otters taken from November to April in New York. They have very kindly permitted me to quote from their recently written unpublished manuscript. Unimplanted blastocysts were found in animals taken in November and December, and implanted embryos in February, March, and April. Their material shows a breeding season in March and April in which two-year-old females breed for the first time. After a gestation period of about 12 months the young are born. Recently parous females come in heat and are bred during the period of lactation; thus adult female otters, as with adult female fishers, are almost continuously pregnant. The otter differs from the fisher, however, in that the female fisher apparently mates for the first time at the age of one year and produces its first litter when two years old. In the otter, sexual maturity is generally delayed for one more year, and the female does not produce her first litter until she is three years old.

Liers (1951, 1958) describes a January and February breeding season in his tame otters and the birth of the young from January into February. In contrast, Hamilton and Eadie (1963) find that New York otters in the wild litter in March and April. It is possible that there is a difference in the timing of the events in the reproductive cycle in otters of the two regions, but I think it is more likely that Liers's captive otters experienced some acceleration of the events of the annual cycle as a result of the condition of captivity and an unnatural diet. I have seen a tendency for captive females of *Mustela frenata* to produce their litters earlier in the spring than they presumably would have if they had remained in the wild. This is discussed later in this paper.

AMERICAN BADGER (*Taxidea taxus*)

It is surprising that no one has followed up the fine study of reproduction in the American badger published almost thirty-one years ago by Hamlett (1932). He described unimplanted blastocysts from seven specimens taken in December and January in Kansas. Four animals taken in February and March had implanted embryos. Six of the twenty-two specimens, all taken during the winter months, were not pregnant. He did not describe the ovaries of these animals, nor did he know precisely when the breeding season was, but he thought it might be in August or September.

Hall (1946) described the general condition of the reproductive tracts of seven females taken in Nevada between November 7, 1940, and February 3, 1941. Two in January and one in February showed implanted embryos; the others may have had unimplanted embryos. He believed that one of the January specimens was less than a year old. Hogue (1955), in a short popular article, says that badgers breed in September, particularly the latter portion, and that juvenile animals may breed when four months old. He thinks the gestation period is between $7\frac{1}{2}$ and 8 months.

The badger is much more common in the western states now than it was thirty or forty years ago, when it was trapped intensively for its fur. Because of the great decline in the value of its pelt, there is little trapping of badgers now. We need a thorough study of this species based on extensive collections of wild-caught animals taken throughout the year.

SHORT-TAILED WEASEL (*Mustela erminea*)

Mustela erminea, a cirumpolar species, called the stoat in England, the ermine on the continent, and the short-tailed weasel in North America, has been studied by several European and two American workers. In England, adult males weigh about 300 gm. and adult females about 200 gm., while in the United States, although the various subspecies are quite variable in size, most males weigh less than 150 gm. and females under 90 gm. Watzka (1940) described the blastocysts and showed for the first time that a long delay in implantation was present. This was confirmed in England by Deanesly (1943) and in the U.S.S.R. by Lavrov (1944), both from studies of large numbers of females taken in the wild. Evidence for a long gestation period had been provided from captive animals by Mallner (1931), Mathis and Psenner (1938), Grigoriev (1938), and Müller (1951). This species as studied in Europe is apparently unique in that young females come into heat while still not fully grown and may be impregnated by the adult males while less than two months old. This extremely precocious sexual maturity has been described by Deanesly (1943) and Müller (1954). The recently parous females mate during or shortly after lactation, and the gestation period may be as long as 10 months or perhaps longer.

The description by Watzka (1940) of a spring breeding season in *M. erminea* followed by a direct development of embryos with a gestation period of eight weeks has not been confirmed by the other European workers. Both Deanesly (1943) and Lavrov (1944) indicate that virtually all the female weasels, young and adult, are impregnated during the late spring or early summer breeding season.

In 1933 Hamilton presented evidence that there was a delay in implantation in a North American example of *M. erminea* (then called *M. cicognanii*), and in 1942 Wright described the blastocysts in several wild-caught females taken in fall and winter (Pl. I, 5). Information on the reproductive tracts of female *M. erminea*, taken mostly in Montana from late winter until midsummer, is summarized in Table 2. This information is entirely in agreement with findings of Deanesly and Lavrov. Additional data from females taken in the wild from late summer through fall and early winter are not shown in Table 2. I have seen no non-pregnant fall or winter specimens except the one animal described in 1942, and in this case a complete serial section of both ovaries was not obtained. Most females of this species have from two to five corpora in each ovary, but one female had no corpora in one ovary and six in the other. Hamilton (1958) demonstrated that unimplanted blastocysts can be recovered from fresh reproductive tracts of *M. erminea* by flushing the uterine horns with a syringe.

A female of *M. erminea* captured in August, 1948, and isolated in my laboratory from that time on, produced a litter of five on March 24, 1949, after a gestation period of at least 205 days. I have been unsuccessful in obtaining matings of captive animals of this species. There is no evidence for an early spring breeding season followed by a short gestation period in *M. erminea* in North America.

The smallest North American weasel (*Mustela rixosa*) apparently does not have the long periods of gestation characteristic of the two larger species. Litters may be born at various times of the year, even during the winter months (Hall, 1951). In England the female reproductive cycle of the closely related European weasel, *Mustela nivalis*, has been adequately studied by Deanesly (1944). She finds no evidence of delayed implantation in this species. Litters are usually born in April or May, with some as late as August. Some females may produce two litters in the same year, and some early-born females may bear young during the summer of their first year.

Whether or not *M. rixosa* and *M. nivalis* are properly regarded as belonging to the same species seems not to have been definitely determined. It is of interest that *M. rixosa*, which ranges to the northern limit of the North American continent, well within the Arctic Circle, has been able to adapt itself to the arctic without the benefit, if one wishes to consider it a benefit, of delayed implantation. Prell (1927, 1930)

TABLE 2

CONDITION OF WILD-CAUGHT SPRING AND EARLY SUMMER FEMALES OF *Mustela erminea*. SPECIMENS TAKEN IN WESTERN MONTANA EXCEPT AS NOTED

Date	Condition of Pelage	Condition of Oviduct and Uterus	Condition of Ovaries	Remarks
February 20, 1941	White	Unimplanted blastocysts	Small corpora lutea	
February 24, 1941	White	Unimplanted blastocysts	Small corpora lutea	
March 20, 1946	Two-thirds brown	Embryos, 3+3	Large corpora lutea	
April 30, 1950	Brown	Full-term fetuses, 3+3	Large corpora, 4+2	
May 15, 1930	Brown	Tubal morulas, 3+3	Recent corpora, 4+4	Lactating female, carrying food to young when shot by H. W. Mossman in Wisconsin
May 24, 1950	Brown	Oviduct much enlarged	Large mature follicles	Lactating female, approaching estrus
June 29, 1952	Brown	Small blastocysts	Recently formed small corpora	Juvenile, caught June 17, kept alive for 12 days
July 10, 1960	Brown	Blastocysts	Inactive corpora	Juvenile
July 20, 1945	Brown	Blastocysts	Inactive corpora	Juvenile
July 22, 1945	Brown	Blastocysts	Inactive corpora	Juvenile
July 22, 1945	Brown	Blastocysts	Inactive corpora	Juvenile
July 23, 1945	Brown	Tubal morulas	Recent corpora	Juvenile
July 28, 1949	Brown	Blastocysts	Inactive corpora	Parous
July 28, 1949	Brown	Blastocysts	Inactive corpora	Juvenile
July 30, 1960	Brown	Blastocysts	Inactive corpora	Juvenile

believed that delayed implantation was primarily a trait of mammals originating in the arctic and that the summer was too short for such species to rear their young unless the young were born immediately after the winter season.

LONG-TAILED WEASEL (*Mustela frenata*)

Apparently Warren (1932) was the first to suspect a summer breeding season in *Mustela frenata*, on the basis of the reproductive condition of three summer specimens taken in Colorado. In New York, Hamilton

(1933) obtained additional information when a captive female gave birth to a litter on May 1 after having been isolated since February 20. Hamlett (1935) found tubal embryos in two females taken in Indiana in July. Wright (1942*a*) showed that corpora lutea and unimplanted blastocysts could be found in fall and winter females. From captive animals maintained in the laboratory it was determined (Wright, 1942*b*, 1948*a*) that breeding occurs in July and that the young are born the following spring. Estrus is marked by a swollen vulva, and ovulation is induced by copulation. Unmated females may remain in heat for several weeks if not bred. At the end of the breeding season the ovaries of unmated females are without corpora. The average duration of pregnancy in 20 cases of animals bred in captivity was 279 days. Representative stages in the female reproductive cycle from wild animals taken throughout the year are available.

Fertilization stages were found during the third day postcoitum (Wright, 1948*b*). Cleavage proceeds at a rather slow rate, since morula stages were found still in the oviduct on day 11 and early blastocyst stages were found on day 15. After the expansion of the blastocysts that follows, no significant changes occur until shortly before implantation. By a series of exploratory laparotomies it was determined that implantation occurs about 23 or 24 days prior to the birth of the young. In the wild, litters are usually born from mid-April until mid-May. Parous females do not come in heat during lactation, as may occur in *M. erminea*, but heat is usually delayed until after July 1. At this time young females are essentially full grown, and breeding by adult males of both parous and young females is accomplished. All wild females appear to be impregnated during this summer breeding season.

In weasels from the northern states a molt to white winter pelage occurs in the fall and another molt to brown occurs in the spring before the birth of the young. The onset of the spring molt takes place about 25 days prior to implantation and the spring molt is usually completed a few days prior to parturition. This relationship provides a very convenient means of determining when implantation is about to occur because the molt to brown can be observed without disturbing the animal. In males the period of the molt from white to brown is accompanied by gradual development of the testes to breeding condition from the winter inactive state. It was suspected that in both sexes the spring molt was brought about by increased levels of gonadotrophic hormone (Wright, 1942*b*). Further evidence to support this theory was provided when a series of recently molted white weasels injected with gonadotrophic hormone in early winter grew brown hair during the course of the injections. Controls injected with water showed no molt at this time (Wright, 1950).

PLATE I

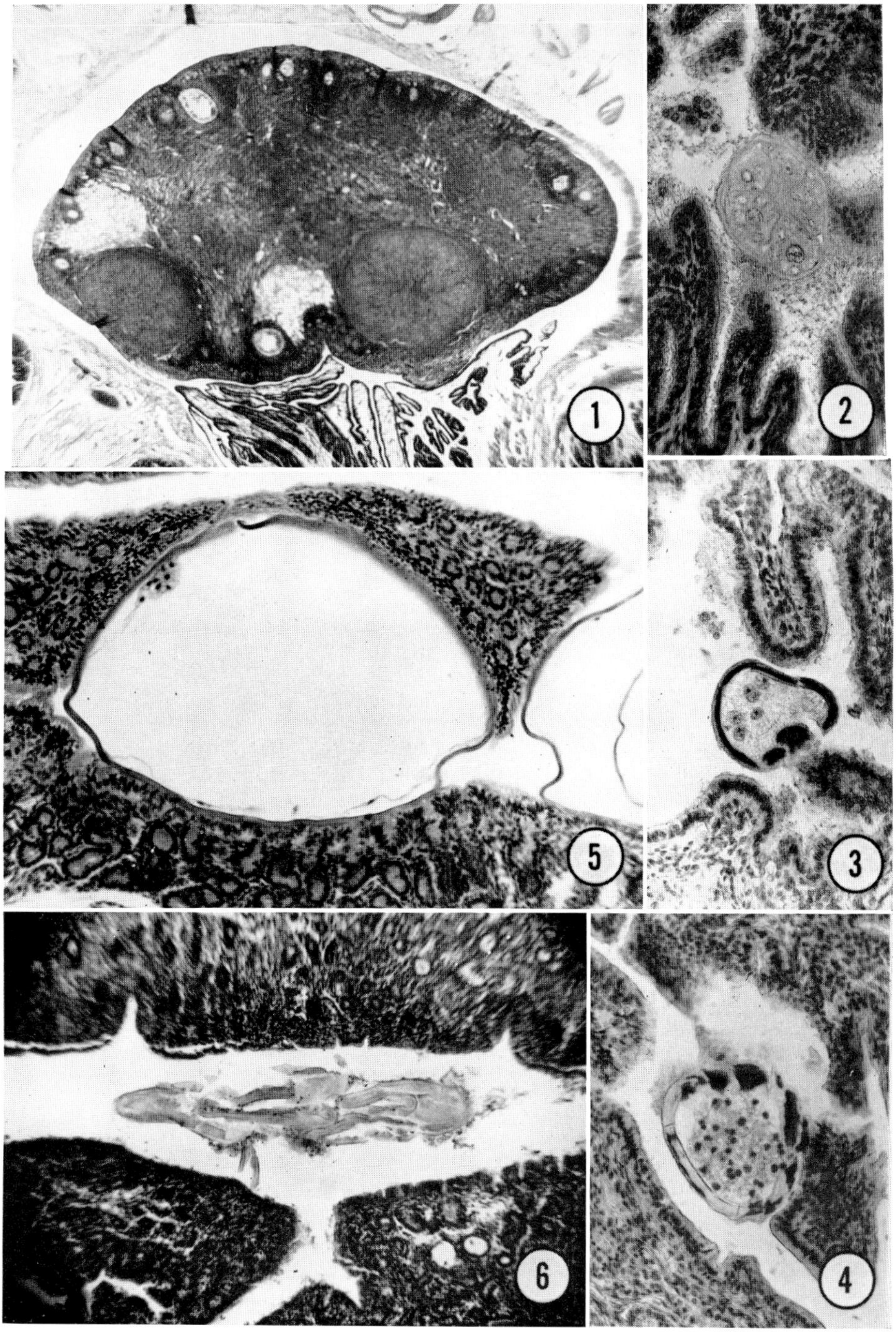

1, Ovary of parous female *Martes americana* with tubal embryos of 13 and 18 cells. Obtained July 22, 1954. Two recently formed corpora are clearly visible, as are two degenerating old corpora with highly vacuolated cells.

2, Tubal embryo from lower third of oviduct from the same animal as shown in *1*.

3, Tubal morula with about 20 cells from *Martes pennanti* from a nulliparous animal; taken April 4, 1957.

4, Tubal morula with about 230 cells from *Martes pennanti* from a nulliparous animal; taken March 28, 1957.

5, Unimplanted blastocyst from parous *Mustela erminea*. Obtained July 28, 1949. There are about 25 nuclei in the inner cell mass and about 100 nuclei in the trophoblast.

6, Dead blastocyst from *Mustela frenata* 14 days after ovariectomy.

PLATE II

All the following are from captive specimens of *Mustela frenata.*

7, Ovary at estrus. Note the mature Graafian follicles and the tremendous development of oviduct. Obtained on August 17.

8, High-power view of the same ovary as shown in *7*, to show thin thecal gland of scattered mature cells, embryonic and mature interstitial gland cells (*upper right*).

9, Newly formed corpus luteum 8 days after mating, to show maximum development of corpus luteum prior to delayed implantation stage. Mature interstitial gland cells also visible.

10, Uterine mucosa of animal with unimplanted blastocysts stained by the Bauer-Feulgen method. The luminal epithelium is abundantly supplied with glycogen. Specimen obtained in September.

PLATE III

All the following are from captive specimens of *Mustela frenata.*

11, Ovary obtained in September during inactive stage of pregnancy. Notice the reduced corpora lutea and oviduct and the massive interstitial gland cells.

12, High-power view of same ovary as shown in *9*. Notice the reduced luteal cells and the mature interstitial cells.

13, Ovary obtained in April prior to implantation. This animal produced a litter of 4 young 27 days after this ovary was removed; thus implantation occurred about 3 days after this stage was obtained. Note the well-developed, active corpora lutea and the medium-sized Graafian follicles.

14, High-power view of the same ovary as shown in *13*, to show a functional corpus luteum and reduced interstitial cells.

PLATE II

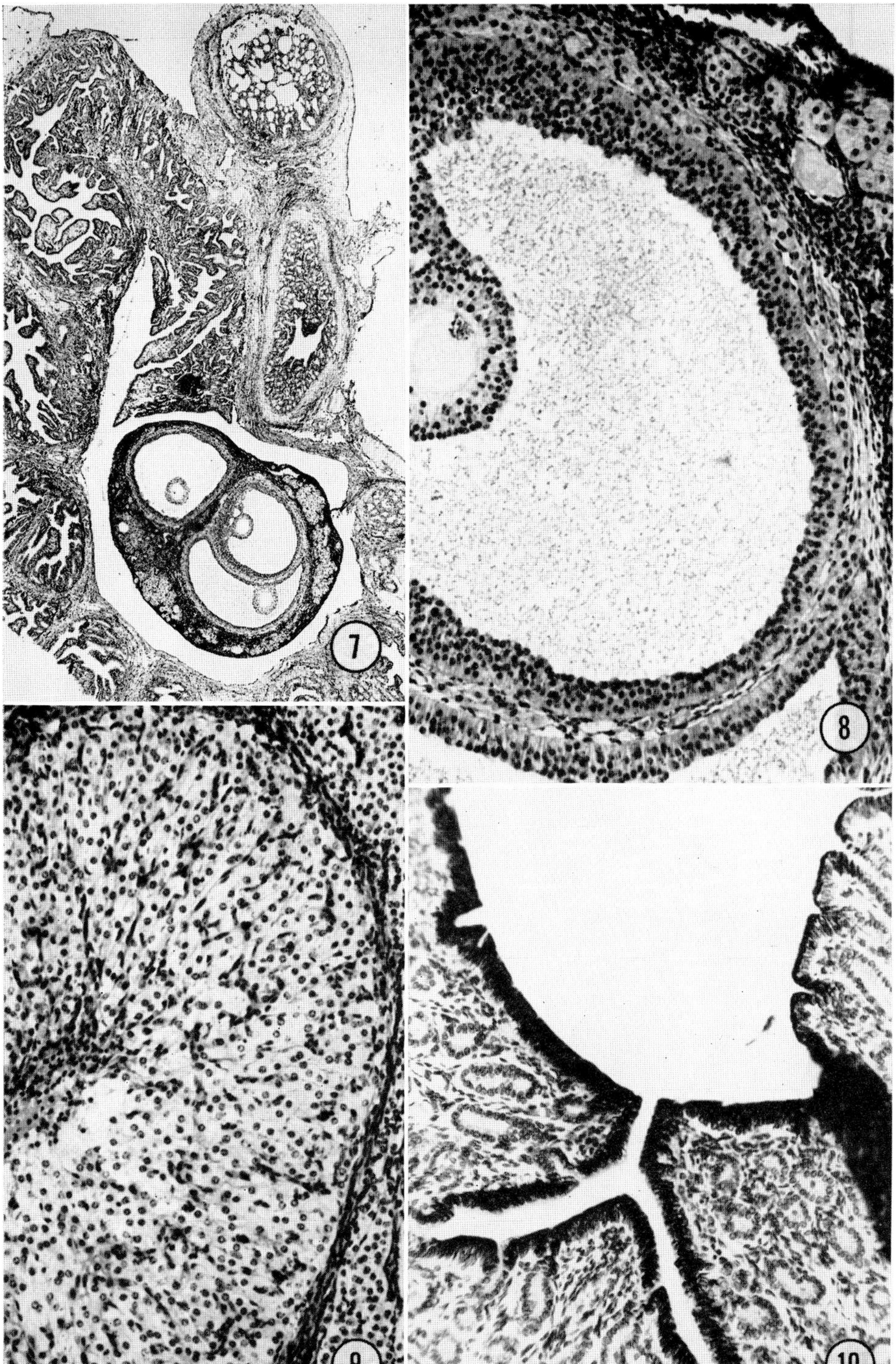

PLATE III

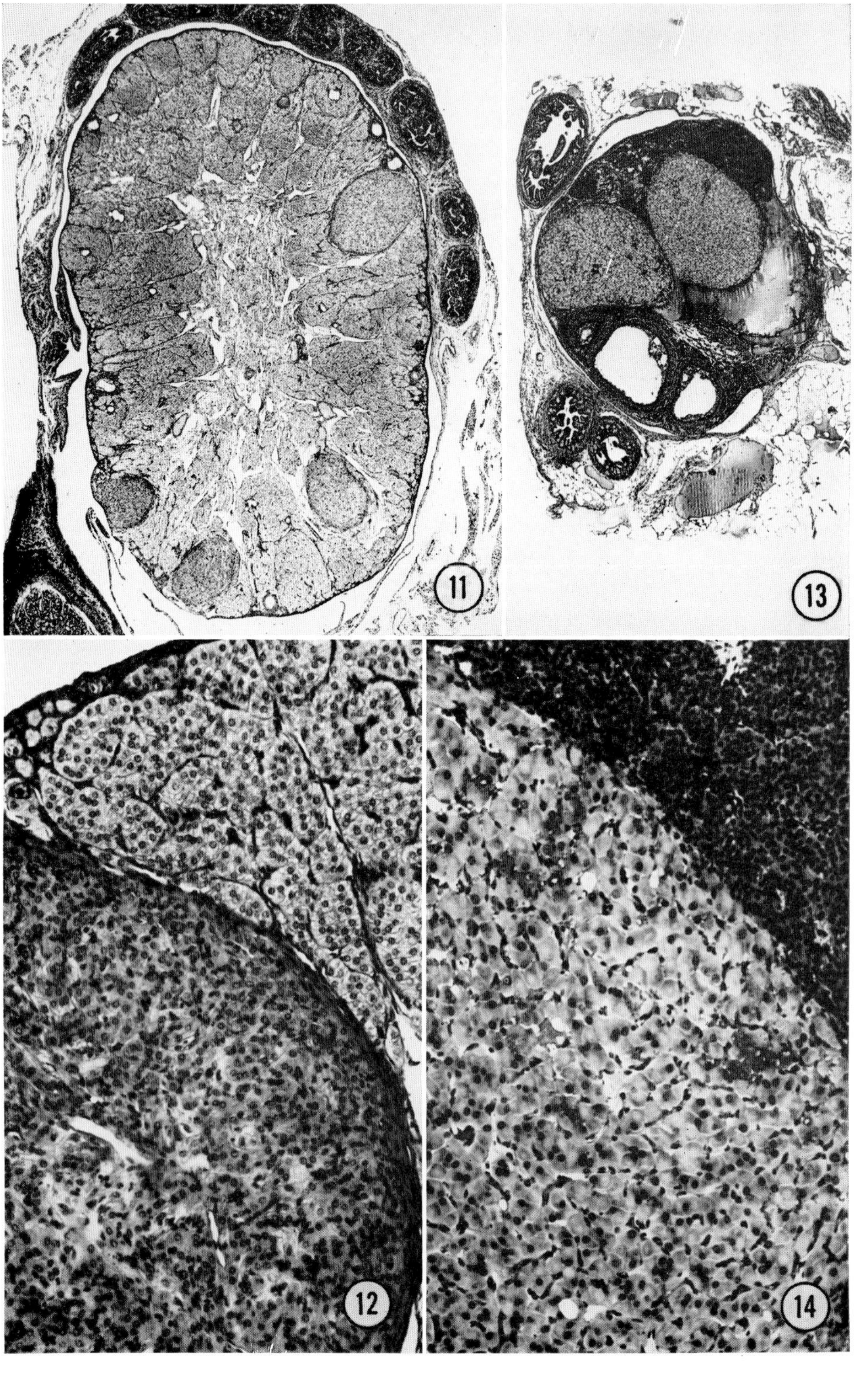

The relationship of the fall and spring molts to normal reproduction in females is further borne out by the fact that if a captive-bred female weasel does not undergo the normal molts she will generally not produce a litter the following spring. Normally, in adult males the testes fully regress during late summer to the size of those of immature animals. If adult males do not undergo the fall molt to white at the usual time, it is generally found that their testes are not fully regressed. Although we do not know very much about the factors causing the molt to white, it seems clear that the white winter weasel of both sexes is one in which the reproductive tract is at its lowest level of activity.

Cyclic changes in the ovary of this species are reasonably well known from many stages obtained at critical times from both captive and wild animals. These stages have been intensively studied by Dr. H. W. Mossman and me, but this information has not been published. Cyclic changes in the ovaries of *M. erminea* that are generally similar are described in some detail by Deanesly (1935).

The ovary at estrus (Pl. II, *7*, *8*) has large graafian follicles, and the corpora lutea that form after ovulation develop fairly mature luteal cells, but the corpora do not become as large as the ripe follicles. About the time the embryos enter the uterus, the luteal cells become elongate or stellate in shape and assume an inactive appearance that continues for several months (Pl. II, *9*). Unlike the mink, in which additional ripe follicles may develop after ovulation (Enders, 1952; Shackelford, 1952), no mature graafian follicles appear at this time in the weasel. However, extensive areas of interstitial tissue develop, and the ovary becomes a solid mass of very active glandular-appearing interstitial cells. The luteal cells during late summer are smaller than the interstitial gland cells (Pl. III, *11*, *12*). The interstitial cells remain active until spring, when, about the time of implantation, they decrease in size and many become pycnotic and degenerate (Pl. III, *14*).

The corpora lutea remain small throughout the summer and regress even more during the fall and winter. Just prior to implantation they increase in size markedly as a result of hypertrophy of the luteal cells (Pl. III, *13*, *14*) and remain active until late in the period of active pregnancy. The ovaries of this species, as with most of the others considered in this paper, approximately double in size prior to implantation. The increase in size is largely due to the increase in the corpora lutea, although there may be some follicular development at this time also. During late pregnancy the corpora begin to regress somewhat; after parturition they continue to degenerate quickly, and within a month no sign of them can be found.

Hormonal Injections

Both the weasels, *M. frenata* and *M. erminea*, have a useful quality from the standpoint of experimental work, in that all the wild-caught females taken from July through the winter can be regarded as pregnant. Experiments in injecting ovarian hormones have been conducted in captive females of *M. frenata* in an effort to determine more precisely the hormonal picture involved in the maintenance and implantation of the blastocysts. In general, these procedures were conducted on a small number of animals as pilot experiments, with the hope that leads would be forthcoming that could be applied to larger series of animals.

EFFECT OF OVARIECTOMY

A female in white winter pelage obtained from a trapper on February 23, 1950, was bilaterally ovariectomized on February 28. Serial sections of the ovaries showed 4 inactive corpora lutea in each. One uterine horn was removed on March 6 and serially sectioned. Blastocysts were found that had lost a good deal of their staining capacity. One March 14 the animal was killed and autopsied, and the remaining uterine horn was serially sectioned. The blastocysts appeared to be dead (Pl. I, *6*), since no nuclei could be detected, and they were recognized only from the collapsed and disintegrating zona pellucida. The regression of the uterus after ovariectomy seen in this and in other ovariectomized animals, together with the dead appearance of the blastocysts, suggests that the ovaries are essential for the maintenance of the unimplanted blastocysts. This, of course, is contrary to the findings of Canivenc and Laffargue (1958) for *Meles*.

EFFECT OF PROGESTERONE

Administration of progesterone both by daily injection and by periodic implantations of the cystalline hormone has been carried out in both intact and recently ovariectomized females during the period of inactive pregnancy. When injected in doses of 2 mg. per day in females ovariectomized at the start of the injection, progesterone markedly stimulates the uterus, but no clear-cut evidence was obtained to suggest that implantation can be induced in this way. After 8 days of progesterone treatment, blastocysts that appeared to be living were found in the uterus of a female ovariectomized at the start of injections.

In one intact female, implantation occurred after about 8 days of injection of progesterone during the month of February, but, when additional females treated in the same way failed to show implantation, it was concluded that implantation in the first animal had occurred as a result of natural factors.

Another female ovariectomized on the day that the embryos appeared to be implanting was injected with progesterone together with estrogen. One near-term fetus was still alive when the animal was autopsied 19 days later. Five resorption sites were found at this time.

Histochemistry of Uterus

The late William B. Atkinson studied the histochemistry of several stages of normal and hormonally treated castrate weasel uteri that I sent him. The following experimental stages were studied in castrate females: untreated; estrogen treated for 9 and for 13 days; progesterone treated for 10 and for 15 days; estrogen for 11 days, followed by androgen for 10 days; and estrogen followed by progesterone for 8 days. These stages were compared with those from normal estrus, fall and winter inactive pregnancy, and pre- and postimplantation.

The only normal uterus that was similar to the injected series was the normal estrous stage, which resembled precisely the estrogen-treated ones with respect to the distribution of mucin, glycogen, alkaline phosphatase, and lipase. The early fall delayed-implantation stage showed an abundance of glycogen in the tall columnar cells of the luminal epithelium (Pl. II, *10*). No glycogen was demonstrated at that site in any of the injected animals. The normal stages at the time of implantation are under considerable stimulation over the delayed implantation stage, but none of the injected animals were similar to the implantation stages. We did not study the histochemistry of uteri injected with various proportions of estrogen and progesterone simultaneously, and this technique is still available to gain further insight into the hormonal picture involved in the maintenance of the blastocyst and the uterus during the period of arrested development and the obviously altered hormonal picture involved at the time of implantation.

Maintenance of Uterus and Blastocysts during Period of Arrested Development

The remarkably developed interstitial glandular tissue characteristic of the ovaries of *M. frenata* and *M. erminea* during the summer, fall, and winter and the reduced size and inactive appearance of the corpora lutea at this time strongly suggest that the uterus and blastocysts are being maintained by hormones produced by the former tissue rather than by the corpora lutea. The fact that the uterine histology and histochemistry at this time are so different from that induced by injections of progesterone further suggests that the hormone being secreted by this interstitial glandular masses is not progesterone. Extensive series of summer ovaries of the other species considered in this paper are not available, but it is apparent that most, if not all, have well-developed areas of interstitial cells during the period of delayed implantation.

Advantages of *Mustela frenata* for Laboratory Work

All these species are ferocious and largely intractable when compared with the usual laboratory animals. *Mustela frenata* is perhaps the most useful of the seven species for experimental work. It is relatively common, can be bought from trappers, and is unprotected in most states. After a few days in captivity, it becomes adjusted to life in a cage and is quite hardy. Individuals have lived for as long as eight years in my laboratory. It takes ether anesthesia well and is a good subject for surgery. Operated individuals do not disturb the incision, and infections after surgery are uncommon. It will breed readily in captivity, and the majority of bred animals become pregnant and produce young the following spring. Only small cages for housing are required. I never attempted to handle the live animals without anesthesia. The only serious difficulty I encountered was that many of the young succumbed prior to weaning.

Evolution of Delayed Implantation in Mustelids

Hamlett (1935) discussed various theories concerning the evolutionary development of this type of reproduction in some mammals. The suggestion of Fries (1880) with regard to *Meles* and *Capreolus* is the only one of these theories that he considered to have merit.

Fries proposed that delayed implantation had arisen as an adaptation favoring the survival of young, since early-spring birth provides them with a maximal period of growth before winter and thus increases their chances of survival through the winter. If the usual reproductive sequence were followed, a breeding season in the winter would be required for early spring parturition. Fries considered that climatic conditions and a shortage of food would make this an unfavorable time, whereas in late summer the animals should be in prime physical condition for breeding, so that would be the most favorable time for the rut. Hamlett pointed out that this and other theories depend on the supposed effects of winter cold on survival of the young as an evolutionary factor in bringing about this type of cycle and thus do not explain its occurrence in tropical species, such as the armadillo. Because of this and also the fact that related species living in the same climatic conditions do not have discontinuous development, Hamlett suggested that perhaps this is a "useless character" without survival value to the species.

Delayed implantation in the mustelids is not necessarily related to the same phenomenon in rodents, artiodactyls, edentates, and other distantly related species. I do not see that the occurrence of the condition in tropical species or the absence of it in related species rules out the possibility that it is an adaptive character rather than a "useless" one.

It seems important to distinguish between the *proximate* and *ultimate* factors involved, as Baker (1938) and Farner (1955) have in discussing the evolution of breeding seasons in birds. The *ultimate* factors in this case are those which have been responsible for a strong positive selection of individuals that developed a reproductive pattern favorable to survival and a negative selection of individuals that failed to develop patterns most favorable to survival. Favorable climatic conditions and the abundance of food during spring and summer might be considered *ultimate* factors in the evolution of this reproductive pattern, characterized by both breeding and rearing of the young during this season. Lack (1954) considers delayed implantation an adaptation to avoid rutting in an inclement season. He states that mammalian breeding seasons are "sometimes correlated directly with the food supply."

Apparently not previously mentioned is the possibility that the female heat period during lactation, as occurs in three of these species, might result in a temporary family relationship at the time the young are being weaned. The young of these mustelids may be weaned at about five or six weeks of age and reach full growth at three months, a considerably shorter period than is the case for many carnivores. They require a relatively large volume of food, and if the male actively co-operated in bringing food to the young this would be distinctly advantageous to their survival. Generally we think of these animals as largely solitary and unsocial at times other than the breeding season. However, a number of authors (Seton, 1929; Hamilton, 1933; and Grigoriev, 1938) have mentioned males of *M. erminea* in attendance at the nest and carrying food to the young. Since females of this species have been found to be pregnant when only two months old, it may be that they are also bred by the same adult male before breakup of this family relationship. In none of these mustelids do the juvenile males reach sexual maturity during their first summer.

Whatever may have been the factors responsible for the evolutionary development of this type of reproductive cycle in northern mustelids, it seems reasonable to consider it an adaptive character having survival value to these species.

The *proximate* factors are the environmental stimuli to the reproductive system that regulate the particular seasonal pattern of reproductive activity. The experiment of Pearson and Enders (1944) in inducing implantation of the embryos of *M. americana* several months earlier than usual by increase in photoperiod during the fall months was of interest for two reasons. In the first place, they demonstrated that the embryos did not require all the usual long period of rest before they were capable of being implanted, and, second, they suggested a mechanism by which the timing of implantation might be accomplished in this species. *Mustela frenata* may also respond to changes in photoperiod (Wright, 1948*a*), and in one case a litter was born after a gestation period of only 103 days. This animal, however, did undergo a partial molt to white and another molt to brown during the relatively short gestation period. The same animal had gestation periods of 229 and 336 days in successive years.

In most of the species discussed here implantation normally occurs after the winter solstice. Implantation generally occurs several weeks after the day length has begun to increase in both species of *Mustela* and both species of *Martes* and in *Taxidea*. In the captive otters studied by Liers (1951) implantation took place in several animals when the days were still shortening, but the wild-caught otters studied by Hamilton and Eadie (1963) had not undergone implantation until February. In the wolverines obtained in northern Alaska by Rausch, implantation took place in January under conditions of very little light. Increased photoperiod may well be an important proximate factor involved in the timing of parturition in these mustelids generally.

In my experience with *M. frenata* several litters were born to captive females in January, February, or March, whereas in the wild all evidence points to the usual period of birth in the Montana region from mid-April to mid-May. Most of the females that produced litters earlier than usual were captured in the wild during the fall or winter and were generally brought indoors after having been caught but were not subjected to increased photoperiod. I originally attributed the early birth to the exposure to warm temperatures during the winter months. There was also some evidence that the unusually rich diet fed the captive weasels may have accelerated spring molting and the early birth of litters. It was not possible to study these factors under controlled conditions. Other factors involved in keeping these animals under confinement may affect their normal cycles. Although increased photoperiod is probably the more important of the *proximate* factors in these species generally, we should not rule out other factors, such as increasing temperature during the spring, until further studies have been made.

Acknowledgments

This work was financed by grants from the National Research Council Committee for Research in Problems of Sex, the Society of the Sigma Xi, the Montana State University Research Committee, and the Montana Cooperative Wildlife Research Unit. Many colleagues and former students have co-operated by furnishing valuable specimens. Dr. H. W. Mossman took many of the colored slides used to illustrate the talk and also took several of the black-and-white illustrations. I am especially indebted to my wife, Margaret H. Wright, who did most of the microtechnique. She further helped materially in the preparation of this manuscript.

References

Ashbrook, F. G., and K. B. Hanson. 1927. Breeding martens in captivity. J. Hered., **18**:498–503.

———. 1930. The normal breeding season and gestation period of martens. U.S. Dept. Agric. Circ. 107.

Baker J. R. 1938. The evolution of breeding seasons. In G. R. de Beer (ed.), Evolution. London: Oxford University Press.

Canivenc, R., and M. Laffargue. 1958. Action de différents équilibres hormonaux sur la phase de vie libre de l'œuf fécondé chez le blaireau européen (*Meles meles* L.). C.R. Soc. de Biol., **152**:58–61.

Coulter, M. W. 1960. The status and distribution of fisher in Maine. J. Mammal., **41**:1–9.

Deanesly, R. 1935. The reproductive processes of certain mammals. Part IX. Growth and reproduction in the stoat (*Mustela erminea*). Phil. Trans. Roy. Soc. London, **225**(528):459–92.

———. 1943. Delayed implantation in the stoat (*Mustela mustela*). Nature, **151**:365–66.

———. 1944. The reproductive cycle of the female weasel (*Mustela nivalis*). Proc. Zool. Soc. London, **114**:339–49.

Eadie, W. R., and W. J. Hamilton, Jr. 1958. Reproduction in the fisher in New York. N.Y. Fish and Game J., **5**:77–83.

Enders, R. K. 1952. Reproduction in the mink (*Mustela vison*). Proc. Am. Phil. Soc., **96**:691–755.

Enders, R. K., and J. R. Leekley. 1941. Cyclic changes in the vulva of the marten (*Martes americana*). Anat. Rec., **79**:1–5.

Enders, R. K., and O. P. Pearson. 1943. The blastocyst of the fisher. Anat. Rec., **85**:285–87.

Farner, D. S. 1955. The annual stimulus for migration: experimental and physiological effects. Recent Studies in Avian Biology. Urbana: University of Illinois Press.

Fries, S. 1880. Über die Fortpflanzung von *Meles taxus*. Zool. Anz., **3**:486–92.

Grigoriev, N. D. 1938. On the reproduction of the stoat. Zool. Zhur., **17**: 811–14.

Hall, E. R. 1942. Gestation period in the fisher with recommendations for the animal's protection in California. Calif. Fish & Game, **28**:143–47.

———. 1946. Mammals of Nevada. Berkeley: University of California Press.

———. 1951. American Weasels. Lawrence: University of Kansas Pub., **4**: 1–466.

Hamilton, W. J., Jr. 1933. The weasels of New York. Am. Midland Naturalist, **14**:289–344.

———. 1958. Early sexual maturity in the female short-tailed weasel. Science, **127**:1057.

Hamilton, W. J., Jr., and A. H. Cook. 1955. The biology and management of the fisher in New York. N.Y. Fish & Game J., **2**:13–35.

Hamilton, W. J., Jr., and W. R. Eadie. 1963. Reproduction in the otter, *Lutra canadensis*. J. Mammal. (In press.)

Hamlett, G. W. D. 1932. Observations on the embryology of the badger. Anat. Rec., **53**:283–301.

———. 1935. Delayed implantation and discontinuous development in the mammals. Quart. Rev. Biol., **10**:432–47.

Hawley, V. D., and F. E. Newby. 1957. Marten home ranges and population fluctuations. J. Mammal., **38**:174–84.

Hogue, J. 1955. Badger. Colo. Conserv., **4**:28–29.

Jonkel, C. J. and R. P. Weckwerth. 1963. Sexual maturity and implantation of blastocysts in the wild pine marten. J. Wild. Mgmt., **27**:93–98.

Kurten, B., and R. Rausch. 1959. Biometric comparisons between North American and European mammals. I. A comparison between Alaskan and Fennoscandian wolverine (*Gulo gulo* Linnaeus). Acta Arctica, **11**:5–20.

Lack, D. 1954. The Natural Regulation of Animal Numbers. London: Oxford University Press.

Lavrov, N. P. 1944. Biology of ermine reproduction (*Mustela erminea* L.). People's Commissariat for Procurement, U.S.S.R. Trans. Cen. Lab. of Biol. of Game Animals, **6**:124–49.

Liers, E. E. 1951. Notes on the river otter (*Lutra canadensis*). J. Mammal., **32**:1–9.

———. 1958. Early breeding in the river otter. *Ibid.*, **39**:438–39.

Mallner, F. 1931. Neues über Roll- und Tragzeit der echten Marder. Folia Zool. hydrob., **2**:145–63.

Markley, M. H., and C. F. Bassett, 1942. Habits of captive marten. Am. Midland Naturalist, **28**:604–16.

Marshall, W. H., and R. K. Enders. 1942. The blastocyst of the marten (*Martes*). Anat. Rec., **84**:307–10.

Mathis, J., and H. Psenner. 1938. Beobachtung über die Tragzeit des Hermelins (*Putorius ermineus* L.). Anat. Anz., **85**:292–99.

Mohr, E. 1938–39. Vom Järv (*Gulo gulo* L.). Zool. Gart. Lpz., **10**:14–21.

Müller, H. 1951. Zur Biologie von Hermelin (*Mustela erminea* L.) und Mauswiessel (*M. nivalis* L.). Rev. Suisse Zool., **58**:421–27.

———. 1954. Zur Fort pflanzunfsbiologie des Hermelins (*Mustela erminea*). *Ibid.*, **61**:451–53.

Pearson, O. P., and R. K. Enders. 1944. Duration of pregnancy in certain mustelids. J. Exp. Zool., **95**:21–35.

Prell, H. 1927. Über doppelte Brunstzeit und verlängerte Tragzeit bei den einheimischen Arten der Mardergattung *Martes* pinel. Zool. Anz., **74**:122–28.

———. 1930. Die verlängerte Tragzeit der einheimischen *Martes*-arten: Ein Erklärungsversuch. *Ibid.*, **88**:17–31.

Rausch, R. 1953. On the status of some Arctic mammals. Arctic, **6**:91–148.

Seton, E. T. 1929. Lives of Game Animals. New York: Doubleday, Doran & Co.

SHACKELFORD, R. M. 1952. Superfetation in the ranch mink. Am. Naturalist, **86**:311–19.

WARREN, E. K. 1932. When do weasels mate? J. Mammal., **13**:71–72.

WATZKA, M. 1940. Mikroskopisch-anatomische Untersuchungen über die Ranzzeit und Tragdauer des Hermelins (*Putorius ermineus*). Ztschr. Mikro.-anat. Forschung., **48**:359–74.

WRIGHT, P. L. 1942*a*. Delayed implantation in the long-tailed weasel (*Mustela frenata*), the short-tailed weasel (*Mustela cicognani*), and the marten (*Martes americana*). Anat. Rec., **83**:341–53.

———. 1942*b*. A correlation between the spring molt and spring changes in the sexual cycle in the weasel. J. Exp. Zool., **91**:341–53.

———. 1948*a*. Breeding habits of captive long-tailed weasels (*Mustela frenata*). Am. Midland Naturalist, **39**:338–44.

———. 1948*b*. Preimplantation stages in the long-tailed weasel (*Mustela frenata*). Anat. Rec., **100**:593–607.

———. 1950. Effects of gonadotrophic hormone on the pelage of white winter long-tailed weasels. *Ibid.*, **106**:130.

———. 1953. Intergradation between *Martes americana* and *Martes caurina* in western Montana. J. Mammal., **34**:74–86.

WRIGHT, P. L., and M. W. COULTER. n.d. Reproduction in Maine fishers. Unpublished manuscript.

WRIGHT, P. L., and R. RAUSCH. 1955. Reproduction in the wolverine, *Gulo gulo*. J. Mammal., **36**:346–55.

DISCUSSION (*Chairman:* R. K. ENDERS)

DEANESLY: The mole (*Talpa europaea*) has much the same cyclic changes in ovarian interstitial cells as those Dr. Wright described, although it does not have delayed implantation, so there is no necessary connection between the two conditions.

ALDEN: In the last picture showing the glycogen, the appearance of it and the stromal nuclei suggest to me that progesterone was not present. I wonder whether the embryo in this animal was about to implant?

WRIGHT: The stage that you saw was obtained in October. Implantation would not occur until February or March. It was a long time from implantation.

ALDEN: Would it have been implanted if you had injected progesterone?

WRIGHT: No, it would not. Injections of progesterone alone do not induce implantation during the delay period.

ALDEN: Is there any effect on the uterus with the injection of progesterone?

WRIGHT: In general, progesterone affects, most surprisingly, the deeper portions of the glands. A similar histological picture is seen in the uterus after injection of progesterone into a castrated animal.

WIMSATT: Am I correct in saying that these are all induced ovulators?

WRIGHT: Yes, as far as we know. We really know only about *Mustela frenata*. In this species if you isolate females in the summer there are no corpora in the ovaries in the fall or winter.

WIMSATT: Do you have any information on the survival of follicles at the time of breeding or ovulation? Do you find evidence of atresia?

WRIGHT: There may be atresia in large follicles. We do not have very much evidence on this.

WIMSATT: I am interested because of my work on bats. I did not see the structural changes one would see in bats.

WRIGHT: This particular stage was obtained fairly soon after the animal came into heat. There was not very much opportunity for atresia to have occurred in this animal.

BUCHANAN: At what time of year was the weasel, in which a dead blastocyst was found, ovariectomized?

WRIGHT: February.

BUCHANAN: Was that at a time when implantation could have been imminent?

WRIGHT: We could tell by the lack of molting that implantation was not imminent in that animal.

BUCHANAN: You did not do this in the fall?

WRIGHT: No, I did not think this was of particular importance at that time. The degeneration of the uterine mucosa was so striking after ovariectomy that it seemed extremely unlikely that the blastocyst could remain alive for any length of time.

NUTTING: Does molting occur in the absence of the ovaries?

WRIGHT: It may occur in castrated animals. The castrated weasel may turn white in the fall and may also turn brown in the spring.

ORSINI: I was interested in the cited precocious sexual maturity of the females. Do you have any measure of the male sexual maturity?

WRIGHT: Males do not reach sexual maturity until the second year in any of the seven species discussed here.

ORSINI: Does the male come back and breed with his young?

WRIGHT: Adult males breed both adult and young females.

MAYER: Does the corpus change after the time of implantation or some time before?

WRIGHT: We have no adequate information on this for most of these species. In *Mustela frenata* the corpora increase in size just before implantation. We had a stage obtained by operation 27 days before the animal produced young from the remaining horn. The embryos were not implanted at this stage, but they must have done so three or four days later. The corpora were at maximum size in this animal.

CLEWE: I was interested in the unusually long time the zygote spent in the oviduct in the long-tailed weasel. Are there any data to indicate whether or not this is general in mustelids?

WRIGHT: As far as I know, the problem has not been studied in any other mustelid that exhibits delayed implantation. Robinson studied cleavage and tubal transport in the ferret. Both cleavage and tubal transport were considerably delayed in *Mustela frenata*.

NOYES: I am confused about the genetic situation. Is the male that brings the food the father? Does he mate his daughters?

WRIGHT: He could be, but the chances are very unlikely. These animals are solitary at other times of the year. The male is probably feeding another male's young.

BUCHANAN: I would like to ask a question on taxonomy. *Mustela rixosa* is similar to what other species?

WRIGHT: *Mustela nivalis.*

BUCHANAN: What about *Mustela putorius*, the polecat? Do we know whether this has delay or not?

DEANESLY: Not as far as I know.

HARTMAN: To quiet Bob Noyes's mind on the effect of father-daughter matings, may I remind him that at the Wistar Institute in Philadelphia the geneticist Helen Dean King, after a hundred brother-sister matings, produced by selection the famous "Wistar" rat.

RICHARD J. HARRISON

A Comparison of Factors Involved in Delayed Implantation in Badgers and Seals in Great Britain

It is now known that the badger (*Meles meles*) and the common and gray seals (*Phoca vitulina* and *Halichoerus grypus*) in Britain or off British coasts exhibit delayed implantation. It also seems highly likely that the reproductive pattern varies in its timing in different localities and in its manifestations in animals of different ages. A description of what has been found to date about reproduction in these three species and some discussion of possible factors affecting the reproductive pattern, delay in implantation, and the initiation of attachment seem relevant to this symposium.

Material and Methods

Common seals (over 300) were obtained from the area of the Wash, East Anglia (see Fig. 1 for various regions mentioned in the text) at different times of the year from 1949 to 1962. The seals were either shot, clubbed, or captured alive. They aggregate as the tide falls on sandbanks in herds of up to 400 animals. Despite their nervousness toward man, they can be stalked on land and their behavior observed through field glasses. The great majority were obtained between the months of March and September; navigational difficulties, fog, and storms make long trips into the Wash somewhat hazardous in winter months. The seals do not come ashore in snow or gales and appear to seek warmer or sheltered waters in inclement weather (Harrison and Venables, 1963). Each animal was measured and weighed when possible, and notes were taken of its state of maturity. The reproductive and endocrine organs were then removed and fixed in the field except when the seals were taken back alive or as complete carcasses to the labora-

DR. RICHARD J. HARRISON is professor of anatomy in the University of London, at the London Hospital Medical College, England.

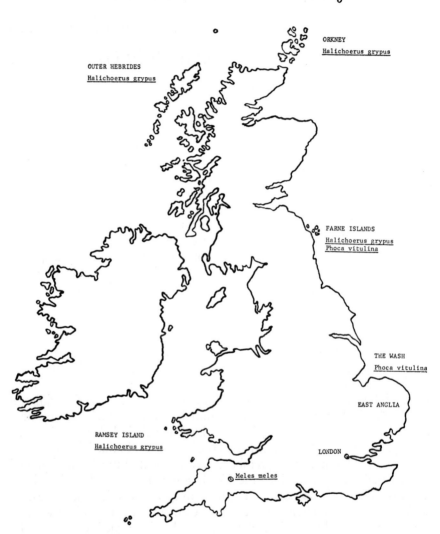

FIG. 1.—Map to indicate the principal places in the British Isles where seals and badgers have been obtained by us and other authors (see also Hewer in references for gray seal studies).

tory. The histological appearances of the ovaries, testes, and accessory reproductive organs of many of the particularly interesting animals in the series have been described by Amoroso, Harrison, Matthews, and Rowlands (1951), by Harrison, Matthews, and Roberts (1952), and by Harrison (1960). Details of the growth and structure of the thyroid glands from the majority of these animals have been given by Harrison, Rowlands, Whitting, and Young (1962).

Reproduction in gray seals has been studied by us at Ramsey Island, Pembrokeshire, in 1951 and in a scanty number of seals that have invaded the Wash during the last ten years. These last were usually shot in the water by fishermen in mistake for common seals. More information has been obtained by Davies (1949) and Hewer (1957*a*, 1957*b*, 1960), whose findings and conclusions will be given later.

The great majority of the badgers (80 females and 17 males) examined were from southwest England, Somerset and Devon. Some had been knocked over by cars; others had been killed by badger-diggers, keepers, or pest-control officers. The circumstances under which the animals were obtained often made histological examination difficult. Whenever possible, the reproductive organs were removed and fixed. It soon became apparent that the number of corpora lutea often exceeded that of the uterine blastocysts or implantation sites. All ovaries were therefore sectioned serially (Neal and Harrison, 1958; Harrison and Neal, 1959). Numerous observations on badgers in the wild have been carried out by E. G. Neal and his collaborators (Neal, 1958). In addition, with the skilled assistance of J. H. P. Sankey some twelve badgers have been kept alive in captivity in specially constructed runs and dens for many years at Juniper Hall, Dorking, Surrey (Sankey, 1955), and also at the London Hospital Medical College. During the last four years a mating pair was kept in an underground concrete-lined cellar containing earth and straw (Pl. I). A sloping entrance was constructed in an attempt to provide artificially an environment similar to that in the wild. Females known to have mated in captivity were given progesterone alone (50–150 mg.) and also an orally active progestogen, Nor-ethisterone (20 mg. daily for 3 weeks), together with 1 mg. daily of an orally active estrogen during the period of delay. Methyl testosterone (2.5 mg. daily) was also administered to another mating pair during the same period. One female recovered from the wild in May was isolated in captivity, ovariectomized bilaterally in September, and sacrificed in November.

The Common or Harbor Seal (*Phoca vitulina*)

The pupping season of common seals in the Wash, East Anglia, extends from about June 6 to June 25, with little annual variation. For the years investigated (1949–61) the majority (85 per cent) of pups were born between June 19 and 23. Local fishermen believe that all pups are born by Midsummer Day. The earliest a pup has been seen was on May 10, but it was dead and isolated on a bank. The earliest a live pup has been observed is May 28. Several pups have been recovered dead, still within their chorionic sacs, suggesting that fright may cause precipitate and premature labor. Figure 2 shows diagrammatically the reproductive events in any year.

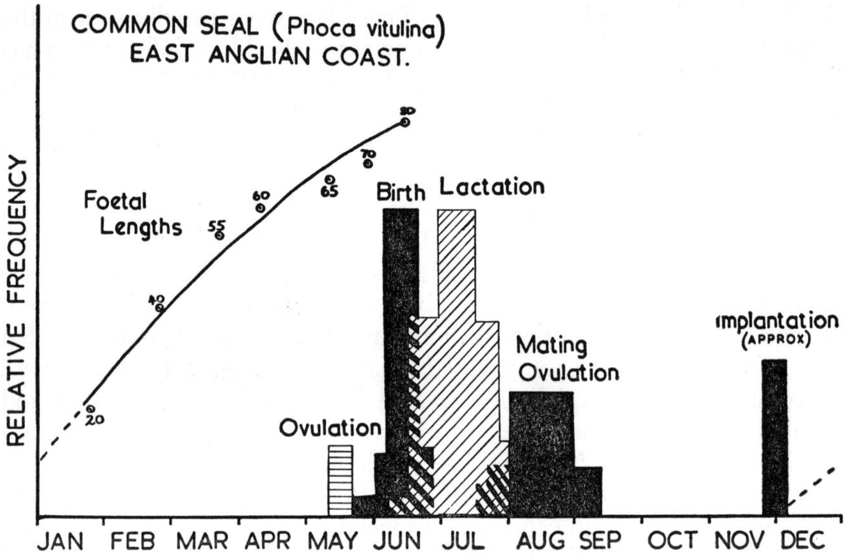

FIG. 2.—Diagram to indicate the time of year the principal events occur in the reproductive cycle of common seals in the Wash, East Anglia. For evidence of spring mating (not shown) in Shetland common seals see text.

Lactating females have been shot during the four weeks between June 20 and July 18. Involutionary changes were present in the mammary glands of adult female seals shot on July 25. In captivity females have suckled their pups between three and four weeks: the pups were between three days and a week old at the time of capture. It therefore seems likely that the length of lactation is from four to six weeks.

Copulation has been seen by us in shallow water at the edges of banks in late July and early August. Local fishermen confirm that this is the usual time of mating, and, in twelve years of personal observation and questioning those who go out daily into the Wash, we have not seen or heard of mating at any other time of the year (but see Venables and Venables, 1959). Several adult females killed late in July and in August have had large single follicles 2–2.5 cm. in diameter in one ovary. A

PLATE I

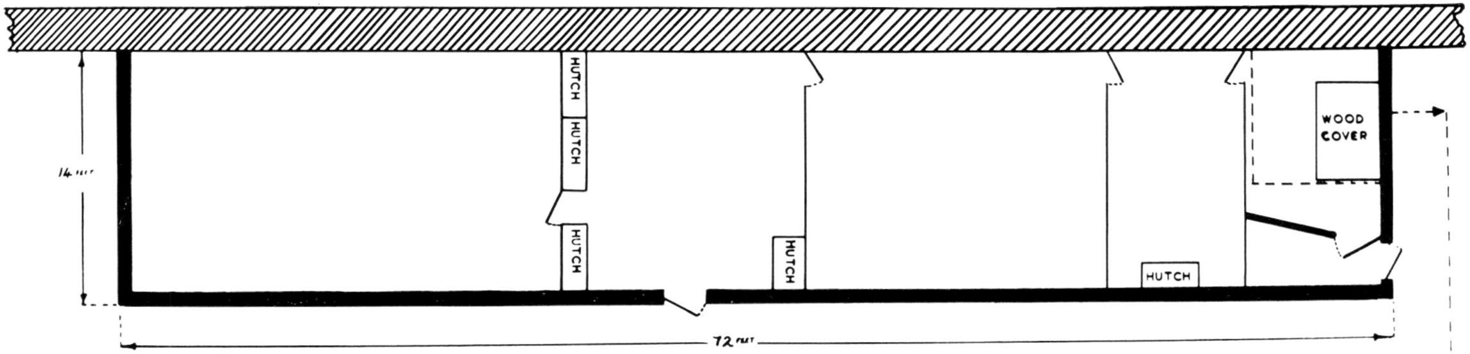

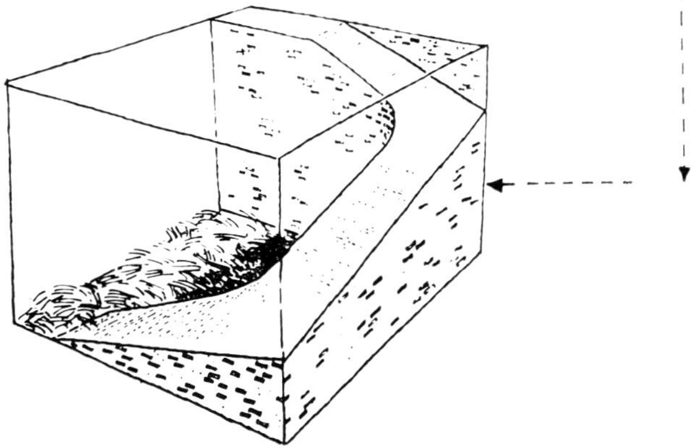

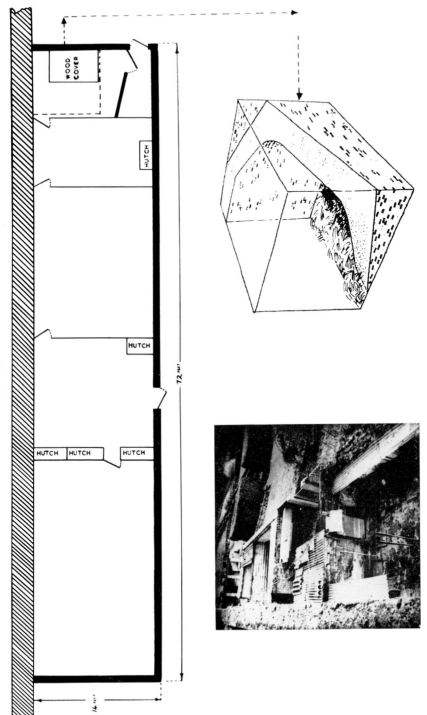

Diagram of pens in which badgers have been kept successfully for many years at Juniper Hall, Dorking, Surrey, by J. H. P. Sankey, warden of the Field Centre. Photograph of the pens, constructed in an old greenhouse. Diagram (*right*) of the specially constructed underground chamber, filled at first with earth but replaced with hay by the badgers.

recently ruptured follicle was present in the ovary of a cow killed in captivity on July 27, two weeks after lactation had ceased. A young corpus luteum, probably about two weeks old, was found in the ovary of a cow killed on August 30. Another cow was known to have pupped on June 23; it was kept in captivity, suckling its own (our hope) and occasionally two other pups for four weeks. It was killed on August 30, and a large, healthy, and apparently mature follicle 2.5 cm. in diameter was present in the right ovary. It appears that both in the wild and in captivity ovulation occurs about two to three weeks, possibly longer, after lactation has ceased and during the latter part of July through August. In no animal has more than one corpus luteum been found, and twinning has not been observed. In two cows kept in captivity ovulation occurred spontaneously in the absence of an adult male.

Ovulation can, however, occur in May. Recently ruptured follicles, still with a central cavity, were found in two females killed in early May and a cow killed on May 15 had a young corpus luteum in one ovary and several 1-cm. follicles in the other. These females were killed at sea and were apart from any large herd; they were young adults with no evidence of having previously been pregnant.

It is not known exactly when implantation occurs in East Anglian common seals. A number of fetuses ranging in size from 15 cm. to 65–80 cm. at term have been recovered between February and June (Fig. 3). Their size at particular dates suggests that implantation could occur in November or early December. It is perhaps significant that no adult female seals killed by us or by local fishermen who have made observations for us for over ten years has been found to be pregnant in September, October, or November. This suggests that the length of delayed implantation is of the order of two to three months.

Other information on the reproductive behavior of the subspecies of *P. vitulina* (Scheffer, 1958) agrees, on the whole, with that observed in the Wash. Venables and Venables (1957) find that the pupping season of common seals in Shetland is from June 14 to July 5. The mating season lasts from early September to mid-October and mating takes place in the water after molting has been completed. The Venables also discuss the possibility of spring matings, which they think not unlikely in view of the high degree of sexual excitement exhibited by adult seals. In a subsequent paper (1959) they report definite, but not frequent, vernal coition in May in seals that they considered to be subadult pairs. Havinga (1933) states that in Dutch waters common seals pup from June 14 to July 14, and, although he did not witness mating, it is reported to occur during August and September. Fisher (1954) observed mating in *P. vitulina concolor* on Nova Scotia and New Brunswick immediately after a pupping season in May and early June. Implantation is considered to occur in late September, with a period of delayed implantation of two to three months. The pupping season in *P. vitulina richardii* of Alaska and British Columbia begins in May and lasts until late June (Scheffer and Slipp, 1944; Imler and Sarber, 1947; Fisher, 1952). Mating has been reported in August and September, and early implantation sites have been observed during late October. Sleptzov (1943) reports that *P. vitulina largha* in the Okhotsk Sea mates after molting in June and July.

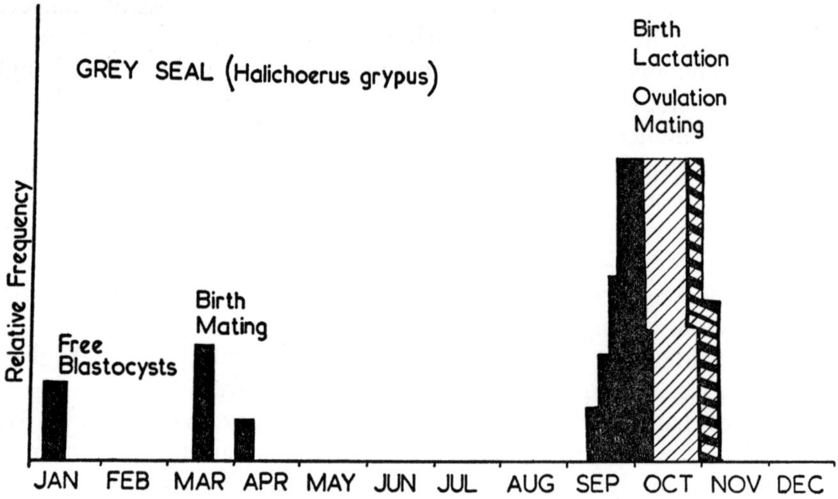

FIG. 3.—Diagram to indicate the time of year the principal events occur in the reproductive cycle of British gray seals, compiled from personal observations and those of K. M. Backhouse and H. R. Hewer (see references to each in the text).

THE GRAY SEAL (*Halichoerus grypus*)

Observations on the reproductive pattern in the gray seal are still very scanty. Hewer and Backhouse (1960) observed mating in a colony of gray seals on the southern inner Hebrides on September 24. The cow taking part had given birth on September 11. Mating occurred frequently at the end of this month. The first birth was seen on September 1, and most pups were born in the subsequent three weeks (Fig. 3). Pupping occurs later on Shillay, starting on September 10–15 and continuing until early October (Hewer, 1957*a*). Mating was first seen on October 8. Davies (1949) considers that copulation occurs when the pups are twelve days old; Darling (1947) gives the interval between birth and copulation as eleven to fourteen days. Hewer considers these intervals to be too short and puts the *average* interval at sixteen days. He states that this is not inconsistent with his findings at Ramsey Island, Pembrokeshire (Hewer, 1957*b*).

On January 3 Backhouse and Hewer (1956) killed a gray seal cow on the Pembrokeshire coast that had a corpus luteum with a central cavity in the left ovary. A blastocyst 2.3 mm. by 1.8 mm. was present, lying free in the left uterine horn. Three bulls killed at the same time showed no evidence of spermatozoa in the testes or epididymides. An adult bull killed by us on March 6 had inactive testes and lacked spermatozoa. Backhouse and Hewer conclude that fertilization must have taken place earlier than January, probably at the time of mating during September and October. They assume that delayed implantation occurs in this species and point out that Turner (1870) found a corpus luteum but no conceptus early in March. An adult cow, shot on May 13 in the Wash, was pregnant, but the conceptus was macerated and the fetal membranes were degenerating. It was difficult to assess the age of the conceptus, but it could hardly have been more than three months old. These scanty observations suggest that implantation occurs after early January and that the length of delayed implantation is of the order of at least three months. It is interesting that Backhouse and Hewer (1957) have found newborn pups in the spring; they estimate the total of spring pups in any one year in the region to be about twenty to thirty. Birth was reckoned to have taken place about the middle of March, which, assuming fertilization to have occurred in the autumn, would give a "true" gestation period of six to seven months. It is suggested that these spring pups were from "virgin" cows that possibly came into estrus early in the absence of parturition and lactation. Backhouse (1960) has reported mating in April; possibly the cow was one of those that had pupped in March. An adult cow killed in the Wash on April 11 was not pregnant but had a large corpus luteum in the left ovary.

It seems highly likely that delayed implantation is the rule in pinnipeds, except perhaps *Odobenus*. It has been reported in *Callorhinus Arctocephalus*, *Mirounga*, *Pagophilus*, *Leptonychotes*, and *Cystophora*, as well as in the species discussed above (see Harrison, Matthews, and Roberts, 1952), for references.

The European Badger (*Meles meles*)

The appearances of the reproductive organs of the series of badgers obtained from southwest England are reported on in the publications quoted on p. 101. Since 1958 some fourteen more animals have been obtained, and several have been observed in captivity and subsequently sacrificed. Investigation of these animals has revealed findings that confirm for the most part those already described. The following general observations may be made, but there would seem to be even greater variation in the pattern of events than was thought at the time of our first reports (see also Canivenc, 1957).

Birth of cubs in southwest England occurs most frequently during the first three weeks of February (Fig. 4). A few births have been recorded during the latter half of January in milder regions. March births are not infrequent but are very exceptional after mid-April. The exact date of birth is difficult to ascertain because parturition always occurs in an underground chamber. Observations on births in captivity, the sizes of very young cubs and the times of their first appearance above ground, the lengths of fetuses and circumstantial evidence from examination of sets,

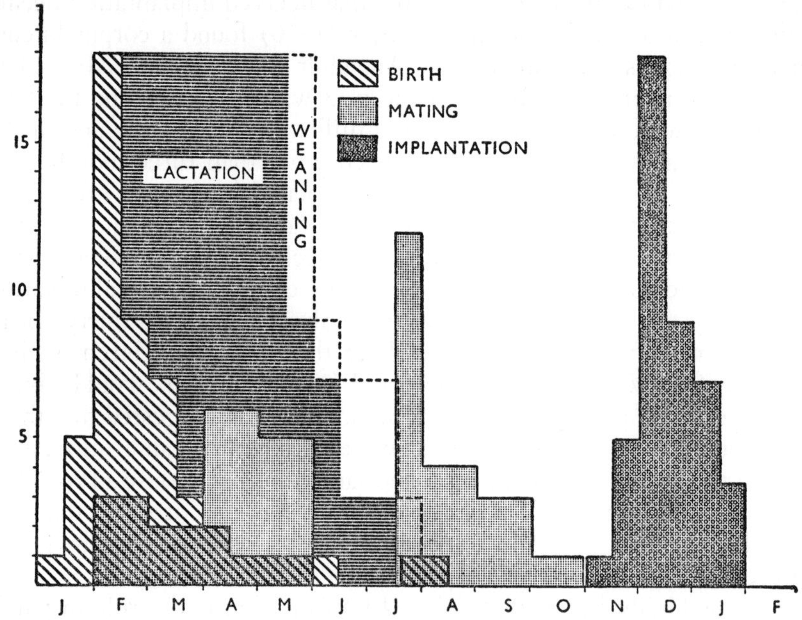

Fig. 4.—Diagram of events in the reproductive cycle of female badgers in southwest England. From E. G. Neal and R. J. Harrison, *Trans. Zool. Soc. London*, 29 (1958), 89. Reproduced by permission of the Zoological Society of London.

have all confirmed the statements made above. The number of cubs in a litter is most frequently either two (50 per cent) or three (20 per cent). There is one authentic record of a litter of five. The cubs appear above-ground eight weeks after birth. Female cubs reach sexual maturity at the age of twelve to sixteen months, though a few do not mature until later in the second year. Little histology has been done on the testes of male cubs owing to lack of material. Observations on male cubs in the wild and in captivity suggest that they do not mature sexually until they are over two years old.

After reaching maturity, all female badgers display a sequence of events that varies between two extreme patterns. A considerable deficiency in our knowledge is that we have little idea of what happens to any one female in successive years, and observations on animals in captivity are vitiated by the prolonged delay in implantation that seems characteristic of such restraint and by the difficulty of guaranteeing that a pair in captivity will mate. Females may ovulate as early as February, then exhibit a series of cycles of follicular activity, vaginal cornification, and ovulation in either June, September, or October or even successively in all three months. Implantation occurs most frequently in December, but also in November and January.

Some females killed in October have unattached blastocysts in the uterine horns, apparently unfertilized eggs with corona radiata cells in the uterine tubes, and corpora lutea of different ages in the ovaries and exceeding in number that of both eggs and blastocysts combined. Some of these corpora have appearances similar to recently ruptured follicles earlier in the spring and can be only a few days old. Several females killed just before the expected time of implantation have had four times as many corpora in the ovaries as blastocysts in the uterine horns. At this time the average number of corpora is 6.2, but the number of blastocysts per animal averages three. By contrast, a female may ovulate for the first time in September or October, with implantation again in the period from November to January. Females have been killed in September and October with large healthy follicles but with no corpora or blastocysts; the vaginal epithelium was thick and cornified. Other females showed recently ruptured follicles and blastocysts in the uterus but no old, established corpora.

Once the corpora have lost their fluid-filled central cavity, which they do after two to three weeks, their age is difficult to judge. Corpora of pregnancy are large, well vascularized, with large cells. The marked activity of the uterine glands throughout pregnancy suggests that these corpora may well be active. They retrogress rapidly after parturition and can be detected only with difficulty after a few weeks. A post-parturient ovulation can follow within some two or three weeks of parturition, but it is not known whether every cow ovulates so early. In at least two females in our series it did not appear to have occurred within an estimated eight weeks of parturition. During delay the corpora can shrink to as small as 1 mm. in diameter, though 2 mm. is the usual size at this time. They are remarkably ill developed; the luteal cells are small and their cytoplasm finely vacuolated. These corpora are poorly vascularized, and what capillaries there are contain little blood. Some cells appear so shrunken, with "fibrous" cytoplasm and pycnotic or fragmenting nuclei, as to be considered degenerate. It appears that the gland was hardly established sufficiently to maintain its total cell population. After implantation there is little doubt that the corpora are subject to a strong rejuvenating stimulus. They enlarge rapidly to 4 mm. in diameter and many in early pregnancy contain leucocytes, apparently removing cellular debris from degenerating luteal cells.

During delay the uterine mucosa shows remarkably consistent appearances; the uterine glands are straight and exhibit little secretory activity. The lining epithelium of the uterine horns is of the tall columnar, palisade type, varying in height from 25 to 45 μ and with cytoplasm that stains palely. The vaginal epithelium, however, exhibits considerable differences during delay. Females with a thick, stratified squamous epithelium have been killed in early spring, in June, August, and September. Healthy mature follicles were present in the ovaries of these animals. In females in which ovulation had occurred, either in early spring or later, the vaginal epithelium was either sloughing or was of a low transitional type. It would seem that these successive estrous manifestations during delay affect the vaginal epithelium more dramatically than the uterine mucosa.

Comparison of the appearances of the reproductive organs with mating behavior is also interesting. It is thought that, as in other mustelids, only long-duration matings result in fertilization. These occur mostly in the period from February to May but have also been observed in September. Short-duration pairing occurs from February to May and also from mid-July to October. The majority of females in our series contained blastocysts by June, and spring, in fact, seems to be the fertile mating period. The number of boars killed is not enough to allow a confident statement of precisely when the testes are active. It does, however, appear that boars are fertile from late January until at least July and probably longer (Fig. 5). There is a decline in activity after late September, and full activity is not restored until January.

In all, 73 blastocysts were recovered from 25 animals; they were often clustered at one end of the horn. Spacing definitely occurs almost immediately before implantation. The over-all zonal diameter showed an increase from 0.7–0.8 mm. in March–May to 2–3 mm. in October and just before implantation. There appeared to be a definite and consistent increase in the number of cells in the blastocysts as delay advanced (in June blastocysts possessed 900 $\pm$ 100 cells, whereas in December the number had increased to between 2,000 and 2,250).

Several attempts were made to procure implantation earlier in delay. Administration of progesterone alone or of progesterone with estrogen (see p. 101 for doses) failed to precipitate implantation; methyl testosterone neither affected the behavior of sows or boars nor procured implantation. Pairs known to have mated were provided with a special underground chamber (Fig. 1), but again implantation did not occur. Ovariectomy early in delay did not cause implantation but did result in considerable enlargement of blastocysts to 3.5 mm. at a time when those of delay recovered in the wild averaged 2.3 mm. It is not known, unfortunately, what would have happened if the animal had been allowed to remain alive until the expected time of implantation. Lack of live animals prohibited further experiments.

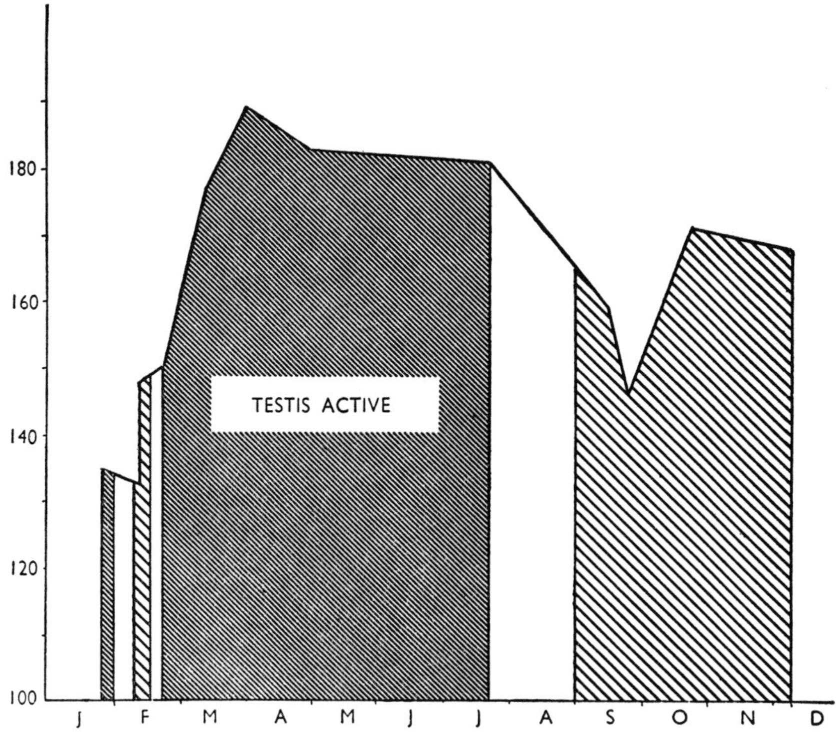

Fig. 5.—Table to show the average diameters of the seminiferous tubules from testes of animals killed January to December. Dark hatching indicates full testicular activity with marked storage of epididymal spermatozoa; lighter hatching indicates reduced testicular activity with few spermatozoa in the epididymides. Compare with Fig. 5 and with statements on matings of long and short duration in the text. From E. G. Neal and R. J. Harrison, *Trans. Zool. Soc. London*, 29 (1958), 89. Reproduced by permission of the Zoological Society of London.

Discussion

It seems, even if the evidence is not all that could be wished for, that there are several features about the delay in implantation in the species investigated that can be considered comparable or at least comparatively similar in pattern. Implantation in the European badger usually occurs in December before the shortest day in the year; in the common seal it probably occurs in late November or early December, that is, at about the same time. It seems to occur a little later in the gray seal, though the evidence for this must be considered meager. The badger exhibits the widest range of variation in its reproductive pattern. Ovulation may occur as early as February, and blastocysts have been recovered from March to December. In many animals the number of corpora lutea is greater than the number of blastocysts, and it is maintained that this is due to additional ovulations that occur during delay. It is not known for certain, though it seems unlikely, whether ova liberated at these additional ovulations are fertilized. Perhaps these ovulations during delay could be considered comparable to those of pseudopregnancy in other mammals. There is also evidence in our series that pseudopregnancy does in fact occur, although it is just possible that there may have been blastocysts that did not survive the "bleak" conditions of delay and were absorbed. Several animals killed early in the year possessed young corpora but no tubal eggs or intrauterine blastocysts.

It does not, however, seem necessary that there be an additional number of corpora in order to precipitate implantation. If all animals *had* to have corpora to provoke implantation, then one would expect the ratio of corpora to blastocysts in December to be at least twice the number from February to June. This is not so; the ratios are 6:2 and 4:2. Apart from the early ratio's being possibly affected by true pseudopregnancy, perhaps initiated by short-duration matings, two other factors may influence affairs.

The time of birth of a badger in any year affects the time of onset of maturity in the subsequent year. An animal born in February can exhibit a pattern later in its second year quite different from that seen in a cub born in April. It cannot be ascertained how much this affects matters in adulthood; even observations on badgers in captivity have failed to reveal further information. There is definite evidence that a small number of gray seals are born in March, six months before, or after, the normal breeding season. The subsequent pattern of events in these pups is not known. In any event, it now seems fairly certain that seals (Laws, 1956) take up to four or more years longer to reach maturity than do badgers, and thus early or late birth of a seal may not affect its subsequent reproductive history. It should be emphasized that we have never seen more than one corpus luteum in the ovary of any seal.

The time of year at which parturition occurs may affect events in the badger sow or the seal cow. There is a suggestion that younger females may not exhibit such lengthy periods of delay, but it is often difficult to assess accurately the age of badgers and seals killed in the wild. At least much of the aberrant "out of season" mating behavior appears to be indulged in by the younger females, though it must not be assumed that the males are necessarily fertile at this time.

An important point that may well have considerable bearing on the pattern is that there is growing evidence that not all females (either badgers or seals) become pregnant every year, though they may ovulate. The proportion that do not cannot be assessed other than to state that in our series it amounts to only one or two females shot each year, particularly in recent years. There could be many explanations why these females have not become pregnant, not least of which may be the depredations of man.

All the factors mentioned above would be enhanced by a variation in length of lactation and by the actual time of the year it occurs. All three forms ovulate fairly soon after parturition, but there is little evidence that a few female badgers do not do so at once. Gray seals ovulate soonest after parturition (within 12–16 days) and badgers within about three weeks; both forms are lactating during these periods. Common seals appear to ovulate only after lactation has ceased. Some badgers seem to delay the postparturient ovulation until several weeks later. One of these, at least, had four cubs. Is it possible that the number of cubs suckled influences the time of the postparturient ovulation and even of the whole pattern of events in the subsequent year?

It has been shown that light is of some significance in obtaining implantation in certain mustelids (Pearson and Enders, 1944). Exposure to increasing day length by use of artificial light shortens the gestation periods in the American marten and also in mink. It seems unlikely that light can have much effect on implantation in badgers. Most blastocysts have become attached before the shortest day, and badgers are strictly nocturnal during winter months in southwest England. Much the same can be said about common seals, which, although not nocturnal, spend much of the day in winter months at sea diving in murky waters, and when on land spend much of the time asleep. Increasing length of day might be a factor in gray seals with their suspected later implantation.

Notini (1948) has considered the effects of climate and temperature on implantation in badgers, but his experiments were inconclusive. Implantation does, however, occur a month later in Swedish badgers than in British, not quite so late in German ones (Fischer, 1932), and perhaps a little earlier in those from southern France (Canivenc and Laffargue, 1956). Births in northern Britain occur later than in the milder southwest (Neal, 1948). The American badger appears to implant later in the year at high altitudes (Grinnell, Dixon, and Linsdale, 1937). What information there is suggests that pupping and mating occur earlier in common seals the farther north they breed, and, although the evidence is not conclusive, it seems that implantation is also earlier, in September and October (see p. 102).

The record length of delay in implantation in badgers seems to be 15 months (J. Freeland, Hull Zoo, quoted in *The Field 1860–67*). Many of the abnormally long periods of delay reported have been in animals isolated in captivity as adults. Neal is firmly of the opinion that adult badgers captured as adults never become adapted to captivity. They do not settle down but mope and behave abnormally. An adult female was still of a ferocious and aggressive disposition after five months' careful tending. In the wild, activity diminishes during December; badgers spend less time aboveground and sleep for long periods in a chamber filled with hay or other heat-insulating material. The temperature in the nesting chamber at different times of the year has been investigated by Neal, who reported a rise in temperature of as much as 14° F during the period immediately before implantation would be expected to occur. This rise in the temperature prevailing in the nesting chamber could be associated with the simultaneous diminished activity caused by colder seasonal conditions. Both these factors could play an important part in precipitating implantation. On the assumption that they did, we provided a mating pair with an artificially constructed underground nesting chamber containing earth in which the animals could make a burrow. Hay was provided outside. The badgers settled down quickly to their new surroundings and ate well. They soon removed most of the earth and replaced it with hay; no pregnancy ensued. All these pairs were brought up by hand from the time they were cubs. They became extremely friendly toward man and were almost domesticated. They were well conditioned to having meals at regular times and to being petted. Perhaps this interfered with the diminished-activity state that we suggest may be an important factor in precipitating implantation.

Acknowledgments

Grateful thanks are expressed to all those who helped to collect animals, particularly to the Eastern Sea Fisheries Joint Committee, to the crews of their vessels and the skipper, J. M. Bray, and also to the late J. Thomas, badger-digger of Clayhidon; all did their utmost to obtain animals at critical times of the year, often under unpleasant conditions. The expenses were generously defrayed by the Royal Society, the Zoological Society of London, and the Yarrow Research Fund of the London Hospital Medical College. Grateful acknowledgments are also expressed to E. G. Neal, J. H. P. Sankey, and R. F. Birchenough.

References

Amoroso, E. C., R. J. Harrison, L. H. Matthews, and I. W. Rowlands. 1951. Reproductive organs of near-term and newborn seals. Nature, **168**: 771–72.

BACKHOUSE, K. M. 1960. The grey seal (*Halichoerus grypus*) outside the breeding season: A preliminary report. Mammalia, **24**:307–12.

BACKHOUSE, K. M., and H. R. HEWER. 1956. Delayed implantation in the gray seal *Halichoerus grypus* (Fab.). Nature, **178**:550.

———. 1957. A note on spring pupping in the grey seal (*Halichoerus grypus* Fab.). Proc. Zool. Soc. London, **128**:593–94.

CANIVENC, R. 1957. Étude de la nidation différée du blaireau européen (*Meles meles*). Ann. Endocrin. Paris, **18**:716–36.

CANIVENC, R., and M. LAFFARGUE. 1956. Présence de blastocystes libres intrautérins au cours de la lactation chez le blaireau européen (*Meles meles*). C.R. Soc. Biol., **150**:1193–95.

DARLING, F. F. 1947. Natural History of the Highlands and Islands. Chap. 11. London: Collins.

DAVIES, J. L. 1949. Observations on the gray seal (*Halichoerus grypus*) at Ramsey Island, Pembrokeshire. Proc. Zool. Soc. London, **119**:673–92.

FISCHER, E. 1931. Early stages in the embryology of the badger. Verh. Anat. Ges. Jena, **40**:22–34.

FISHER, H. D. 1952. The status of the harbour seal in British Columbia with particular reference to the Skeena River. Bull. Fish. Res. Board, Canada, No. 93.

———. 1954. Delayed implantation in the harbour seal, *Phoca vitulina* L. Nature, **173**:879–80.

GRINNELL, J., J. S. DIXON, and J. M. LINSDALE, 1937. Fur-bearing Mammals of California. Berkeley.

HARRISON, R. J. 1960. Reproduction and reproductive organs in common seals (*Phoca vitulina*) in the Wash, East Anglia. Mammalia, **24**:372–85.

HARRISON, R. J., L. H. MATTHEWS, and J. M. ROBERTS. 1952. Reproduction in some Pinnipedia. Trans. Zool. Soc. London, **27**:437–540.

HARRISON, R. J., and E. G. NEAL. 1959. Delayed implantation in the badger (*Meles meles* L.). Mem. Soc. for Endocrin., **6**:19–25.

HARRISON, R. J., I. W. ROWLANDS, W. H. WHITTING, and B. A. YOUNG. 1962. Growth and structure of the thyroid gland in the common seal (*Phoca vitulina*). J. Anat. Lond., **96**:3–15.

HARRISON, R. J., and L. S. V. VENABLES. 1963. Common Seals. Sunday Times Pub.

HAVINGA, B. 1933. Der Seehund (*Phoca vitulina* L.) in den Hollandischen Gewassem. Tijdschr. ned. dierk. Ver. (Leiden), **3**:79–111.

HEWER, H. R. 1957*a*. A Hebridean breeding colony of grey seals, *Halichoerus grypus* (Fab.) with comparative notes on the grey seals of Ramsey Island, Pembrokeshire. Proc. Zool. Soc. London, **128**:23–66.

———. 1957*b*. Notes on the marking of Atlantic seals in Pembrokeshire. *Ibid.*, **125**:87–95.

———. 1960. Behaviour of the grey seal (*Halichoerus grypus* Fab.) in the breeding season. Mammalia, **24**:400–421.

HEWER, H. R., and K. M. BACKHOUSE. 1960. A preliminary account of a colony of grey seals *Halichoerus grypus* (Fab.) in the southern inner Hebrides. Proc. Zool. Soc. London, **134**:156–95.

IMLER, R. H., and H. R. SARBER. 1947. Harbour seals and sea lions in Alaska. Spec. Sci. Rep. U.S. Dept. Interior Fish Wildlife Serv.

LAWS, R. M. 1956. Growth and sexual maturity in aquatic mammals. Nature, **178**:193–94.

NEAL, ERNEST. 1958. The Badger. Pelican Books A140. A reprint of The Badger, 1948. London: Collins.

NEAL, F. G., and R. J. HARRISON. 1958. Reproduction in the European badger (*Meles meles* L.). Trans. Zool. Soc. London, **29**:67–130.

NOTINI, G. 1948. Biologiska Undersoknigar over Gravlingen. Uppsala.

PEARSON, O. P., and R. K. ENDERS. 1944. Duration of pregnancy in certain mustelids. J. Exp. Zool., **95**:21–35.

SANKEY, J. 1955. Observations on the European badger *Meles meles meles* (L.). South Eastern Nat. & Antiq., pp. 20–34.

SCHEFFER, T. H., and J. W. SLIPP. 1944. The harbour seal in Washington State. Am. Midland Naturalist, **32**:373–416.

SCHEFFER, V. B. 1958. Seals, Sea Lions and Walruses. California: Stanford University Press.

SLEPTZOV, M. M. 1943. On the biology of reproduction of Pinnipedia of the Far East. Zool. Zhur. Moscow, **22**:109–28.

VENABLES, U. M., and L. S. V. VENABLES. 1957. Mating behavior of the seal *Phoca vitulina* in Shetland. Proc. Zool. Soc. London, **128**:387–96.

———.1959. Vernal coition of the seal *Phoca vitulina* in Shetland. *Ibid.*, **132**: 665–69.

Discussion was deferred until after Dr. Canivenc's paper.

R. CANIVENC AND M. BONNIN-LAFFARGUE

Inventory of Problems Raised by the Delayed Ova Implantation in the European Badger (Meles meles *L.*)

In all species of mammals one can discern with some accuracy a relationship between the fixed and the free stages of the egg. Species that have deferred implantation of ova are characterized by the alteration of this relationship. The prolonging of the free stage is responsible for this situation.

In 1953 we studied superfetation in the rat. We showed that localized administration of progesterone can hasten implantation of ova. In this way two generations of embryos of very different ages are obtained. It was our intention to study the conditions of birth, using this method. However, the prolonging of the free phase of life responsible for the delay in implantation of ova seemed to us to be of too little importance to continue the work in the rat.

In 1954 we became interested in the reproductive physiology of the badger, which possesses, as Fisher (1931) has shown, a nidation delayed by several months. We had great difficulties in obtaining the animals needed for this work, but, after having studied six hundred animals between 1955 and 1962, we can report here some personal impressions about the implantation of ova in this animal.

In order to present faithfully the difficulties of this work and our thoughts at the time of these studies, we shall give the different parts of our research in sequence. All our researches should be the synthesis of solutions to the problems that developed progressively. A large portion of this work has been presented in a European symposium.

DR. RENÉ CANIVENC is professor of histology and embryology in the Faculty of Medicine, Bordeaux, France.

Problems and Their Solutions

1. *When are blastocysts in the uterus?* First by paraffin sections, then by study with a magnifying glass after opening the uterine horn lengthwise, we were able to find fertilized eggs at any time after February. Thus, our results differed from those of Fries (1880), Fisher (1931), and Neal (1948), who placed coitus between July and August. However, Neal, in collaboration with Harrison (Neal and Harrison, 1956), shortly after hearing from us, discovered free blastocysts in April.

From our research we can conclude that there is a fertile postpartum coitus. This coitus results in a new ovular generation. When the tables of Fisher and Neal and our own tables are consulted, it is apparent that there can be only one period during which embryonic development takes place. In France, in the county of Gironde, implantation of ova occurs in the last days of December. Birth takes place in the first fortnight of February.

At the conclusion of this first problem, a second one presented itself—can the eggs, fertilized at the postpartum coitus, remain unimplanted for ten months in the uterus in the blastocyst stage and still result in a normal gestation, or are they eliminated and replaced later by a new generation that has a better future?

2. *Can the ova from the postpartum coitus start their development again and become implanted at the normal date?* The experiment showed that we could give an affirmative reply to this question. This was how we proceeded: females captured in March were operated on; we proceeded to mark all the corpora lutea in each ovary by putting a non-absorbable silk thread through every one of them. We cut the uterine horn between two ligatures at the tubouterine junction. We then released the animals into their burrows with their males and their young.

In the following January, we captured these animals again and examined them. They had obviously gravid uteri. Under the microscope only the corpora lutea marked in the spring were found (Pl. II, *1*). There were no other luteal formations. From this, one can draw two conclusions: (*a*) The ova fertilized postpartum are capable of starting their development again ten months later. (*b*) The progestational corpora lutea of postpartum can become gestational and insure normal gestation.

3. *Are the latent blastocysts hormonally independent, and what are the relationships between the survival of blastocysts and the hormonal condition?* In our district, parturition is followed by ovulation. Eighty-four per cent of the postparturient females ovulate, and fertilized eggs at every stage of development (morulae of 2, 4, 16, etc., blastomeres) are found.

Generally, the ova are in a blastocyst state, unimplanted in the uterine cavity without a clear distribution. Apart from some very small variations in size during the stage of free life, they seem to remain quiescent until autumn. A short time before implantation, the ova suddenly increase in size; their diameter may reach 5 mm. We have classified blastocysts in two categories: latent blastocysts and preimplanted blastocysts. Luteal changes occur in the ovaries simultaneously with the increase in blastocyst size.

We should note that it is possible to discover blastocysts of different sizes in the preimplanted stage. After the ligature of the uterine horns, blastocysts that have all come from the same springtime ovulation can be of unequal size at the moment of implantation. It is possible that successive generations (as in the case of the mink) bring about the appearance of blastocysts of different sizes, but blastocysts of different sizes are found in the same badger after only one ovulation.

From the information given above, it is apparent that the length of the free life may reach ten months. However, animals kept in captivity for a year and a half in the Natural History Museum in Paris still had unimplanted intrauterine blastocysts, and corpora lutea in excellent latent condition were still present in the ovaries.

Bilateral castration (Canivenc and Bonnin-Laffargue, 1956) has no effect on the morphology of blastocysts; they remain the same size and do not implant. The hormonal relationships at different periods of the year, indicated by standards discussed later, do not modify it in any way. The vaginal structures are very sensitive to estradiol benzoate during the latent period, but progesterone has no effect in this site.

It appears, therefore, that there is an independence, which may be relative, between the unimplanted blastocysts and their immediate environment.

4. *Do corpora lutea undergo any morphological changes during pregnancy?* We have seen that a corpus luteum can, in the badger, pass through stages of very different functional value. The morphological studies that we have carried out have shown that the timing of these phases follows the schedule in Table 1.

The measurement of corpora lutea and the cytometry are convincing. Table 2 reveals the facts better than a long commentary would. Special cytological studies show that the function of the luteal cells varies considerably. From all this one can conclude that the corpora lutea pass through a very long latent phase but that the recommencement of their activity comes about well *before* the implantation of the blastocysts (Pl. I). It is certain that maternal phenomena guide the recommencement of ovular development.

To complete these morphological results, biochemical determinations

TABLE 1

DEVELOPMENT OF THE CORPORA LUTEA

Progestation			Gestation
Beginning of progestational stage	Latent progestational stage	Active progestational stage	Gestational stage
Formation of corpus luteum	Latent life of corpus luteum	Preimplantation	Gestation

TABLE 2

DIMENSIONS OF THE DIFFERENT CORPORA LUTEA DURING THE REPRODUCTIVE CYCLE

No. of Animal	Size of Corpora Lutea (mm.)	Size of Cells (μ)	Period of Pregnancy	Stages of Corpora Lutea
Bl 79	0.54	13.80	January	Metaplasia
Bl 340	0.88	12	February	
Bl 333	2.10	14.64	February	
Bl 195	2	15	February	
Bl 204	1.85	12.18	March	Latent progestational stage
Bl 353	1.90	12	March	
Bl 203	1.80	10.86	March	
Bl 211	1.87	11.76	April	
Bl 2	1.80	11.40	May	
Bl 382	1.72	10.50	May	
Bl 384	1.87	8.60	May	
Bl 220	1.95	10.44	June	
Bl 223	1.80	9.78	June	
Bl 388	1.27	11.30	June	
Bl 234	1.70	11.40	July	
Bl 235	1.95	9.60	September	
Bl 66	1.76	15.60	October	Preimplantation
Bl 301	1.87	14	October	
Bl 302	1.90	15.36	October	
Bl 304	1.65	14	October	
Bl 414	1.90	17.16	November	
Bl 416	1.81	17.22	November	
Bl 420	2.49	19.56	November	
Bl 48	2.03	24.60	December	
Bl 10	2.67	24.41	December	Implantation
Bl 422	2.30	24	December	
Bl 312	2.92	26	December	

PLATE I

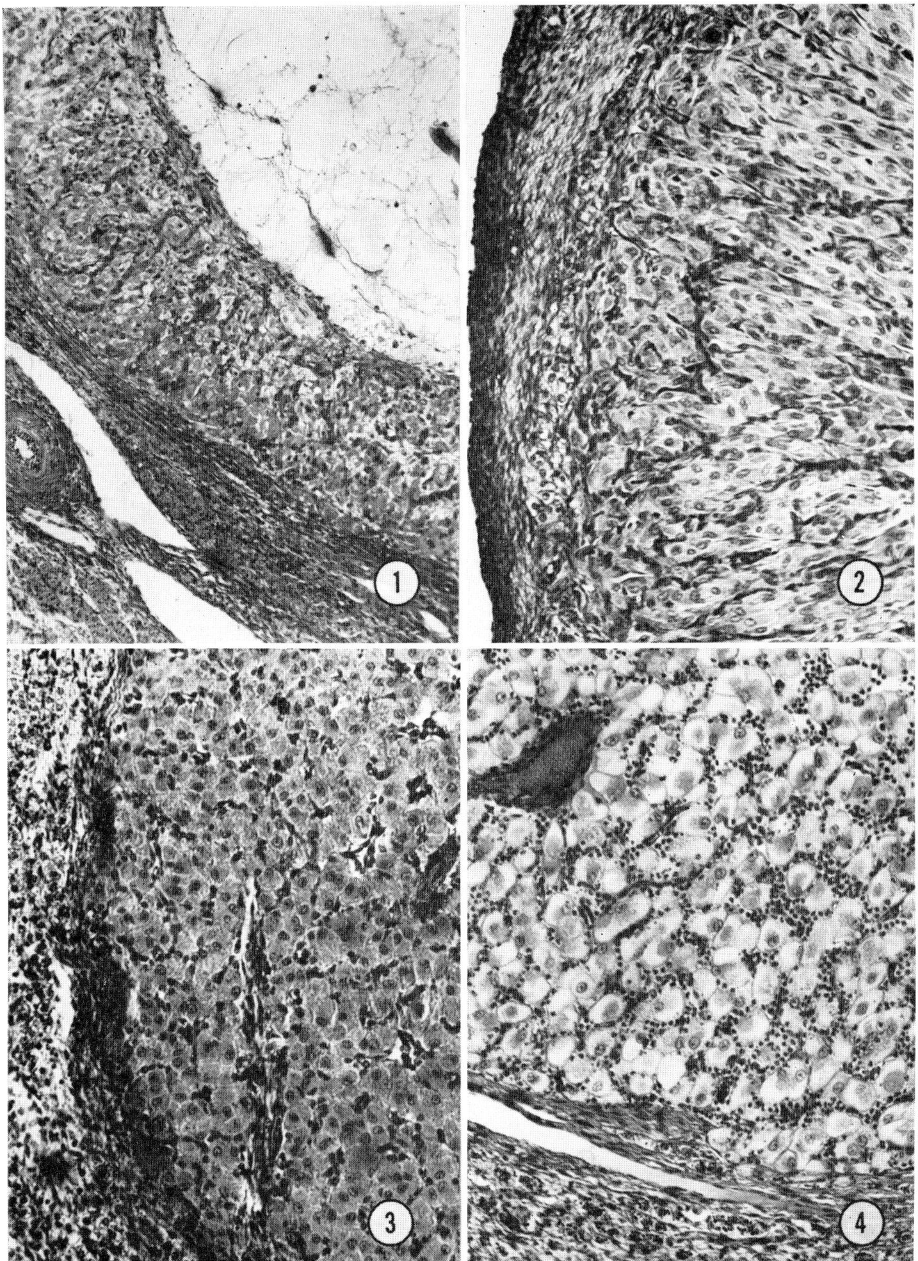

The four types of corpora lutea of the European badger: *1*, Progestational metaplasia; *2*, Latent corpus luteum, progestation; *3*, Active corpus luteum, preimplantation; *4*, Corpus luteum, gestation.

PLATE II

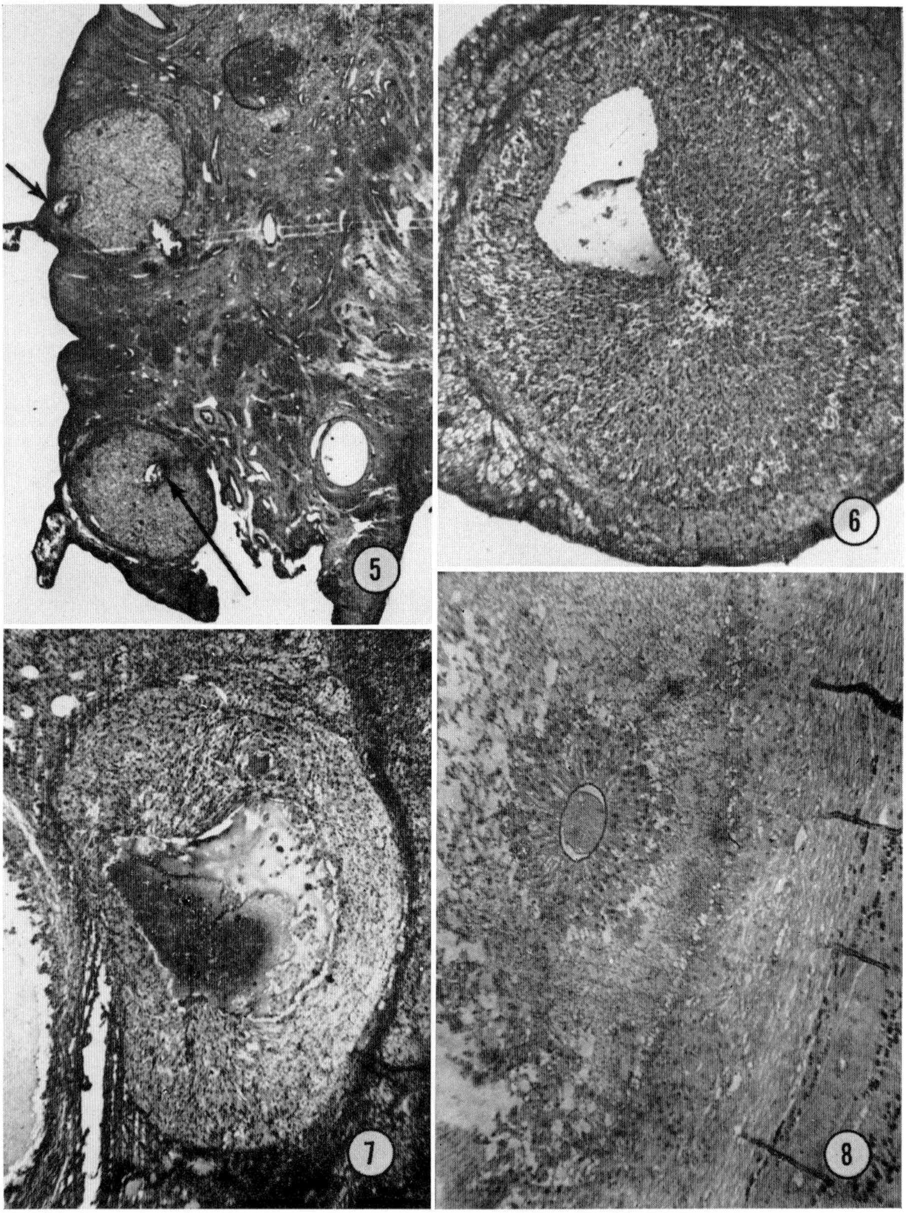

5, Corpora lutea marked in the spring (*arrows*). Female killed the following winter, 10 months later.

6, Ovary of an animal having received large doses of gonadotrophins during the latent phase of the corpus luteum. New corpora lutea appear, but they are of the latent type.

7, Ovarian graft in the spleen of a female killed in January, showing a new corpus luteum.

8, Ovarian graft in the spleen of a female killed in May, showing a new atretic follicle.

have been carried out. If the method of Jayle and Crepy (1952) for the determination of urinary pregnandiol is valid when applied to the European badger (checks in progress seem to show that it is), the variations of this metabolite of progesterone can be determined biochemically in relation to the variations in the morphology of corpora lutea (Ruffié, Bonnin-Laffargue, and Canivenc, 1961).

5. *Does the latent period apply to luteal activity alone or does it apply to all ovarian formations?* Here we encountered the very controversial problem of the interstitial ovarian gland. The existence of follicular atresia is one of the most remarkable phenomena that we have encountered. It persists during gravidity and during the latent stage of the corpora lutea, showing that the ovarian inactivity applies only to luteal formations. We shall later have to explain this in relationship to hypothalamo-hypophyseal factors.

Therefore, follicles grow during the entire latent stage, and the real problem is to know whether this growth regularly terminates in ovulation, occasionally terminates in ovulation, or never terminates in ovulation.

6. *Is there a pituitary latency?* It is normal in the case of an ovarian failure to look for pituitary causes. We did this with the badger by comparing its pituitary cytology at different periods of reproduction. We used the polychromatic technique that Herlant (1960) perfected recently. It gives very good results, and we compared the pictures coming from animals during the active luteal phase (gestation) and at different periods of the progestational stage.

During the active gestational luteal stage the pituitary cells are very numerous, large, with finely granulated cytoplasm of lilac violet color, and always in direct relationship to the vessels.

During the period of latent life these cells are smaller, they have smaller nuclei, and their cytoplasm is strongly colored lilac violet. It is obviously a debatable point whether this is pure coincidence or whether it in fact shows a pituitary insufficiency. It should theoretically be possible to substitute experimentally for the deficiency. This is what we have done. The administration of considerable doses of the two pituitary gonadotrophic hormones, whether alone or mixed in different proportions, produced great ovarian changes. When the administration of these substances results in ovulation and the appearance of new corpora lutea in the ovary, the new corpora are always of the non-functional type, identical to those of the latent stage (Canivenc, Bonnin-Laffargue, and Relexans, 1962) (Pl. II, *2*).

This would seem to show that the luteotrophic factor is at fault or that it is produced in insufficient amounts by the pituitary or, yet again, that it is not released into the system. It now seems logical to bear in mind a seventh problem—the part played by the hypothalamus in the determination of luteal behavior.

7. *Is there an external factor that might stimulate the luteal factor through a hypothalamic pathway?* Placing under the skin of a female a short-wave transistor, we registered and compared the behavior norms of the free animal and in this way drew up a program of its acts, covering almost a year. The badger is a night animal, living an underground life. The analysis of more than five hundred meters of recording, concerning the period from March to December, shows that the activity is strictly correlated to the nocturnal period of the day. It is at its greatest around December, that is to say, at a time contemporaneous with the stage of the implantation of ova. We think that this is not a mere coincidence. We believe that in the badger the prolonging of the nocturnal phase conditions the luteal activity in the same way as prolongation of the length of the day stimulates ovarian activity in the mink or the marten (cf. Enders and Pearson, 1943; Pearson and Enders, 1944; Hansson, 1947).

We have also considered, so far without very much success, the part played by the external temperature. As have Notini (1948) and Neal and Harrison (1958), we have noted behavioral changes in the badger at the approach of winter. The animal brings into its burrow at that time great quantities of fresh grass. We think that the fermentation of this grass brings about a considerable increase in the temperature of the burrow. The problem remaining to be solved is whether this increase in the interior temperature in turn brings about a hypothalamic change or whether this behavior is only the result of a former resumption of luteal activity. Personally, we are in favor of the latter hypothesis.

We have also explored hypothalamic activity by the ovarian intrasplenic graft technique. In animals receiving an intrasplenic ovarian graft at the end of winter, one notices the presence of one or two large follicles in the graft. Besides these, one finds new corpora lutea, but these do not have the morphology of an active corpus luteum. They are identical to the latent progestative corpora lutea (Pl. II, *3*). In animals receiving an intrasplenic ovarian graft during the period of rest, one finds only large follicles (4–5 mm.), without metaplasia of the granulosa. We have not seen luteal formations (Pl. II, 4).

Because of difficulties in obtaining animals, we have not done the same experiments during the active luteal phase (October–December). However, experiments already show that a true active corpus luteum cannot appear outside the normal period (October, November, December).

Integration of Results

Let us note, first of all, that the majority of species with deferred implantation of ova have an annual cycle. Let us also note that the postpartum estrus that we have described for the badger is a very consistent phenomenon. Eighty-four per cent of females are fertilized after March. This phenomenon has been identified in other species with deferred implantation of ova. In wild animals it is certain that the appearance of any estrous condition is always taken advantage of by the species, and a pregnancy begins.

In species that have deferred implantation of ova the problem becomes more difficult when several estrous stages are apparent. In the roe deer (Stieve, 1950), in the bear (Lindemann, 1954), in the marten (Prell, 1927), in the mink (Hansson, 1947; Enders, 1956), and in the badger (Neal and Harrison, 1958) there are several estrous stages. It seems vital to us to know whether one can identify (1) a main estrus, (2) a secondary or accessory estrus, as Stieve (1950), Prell (1927), and Lindemann (1954) stress, or (3) whether the two estrous stages have the same functional value. This is fundamental. Estrus and the consequent appearance of corpora lutea determine the occurrence of a normally active pregnancy. In our opinion, the appearance of a second luteal generation seems to be due to an absence of blocking of FSH activity by the existing corpora lutea or to the absence of a luteotrophic factor.

Morphological and physiological examinations of the luteal activity of the badger show that the progestational corpora lutea are insufficiently active, or are inactive, during the period of latency. Numerous authors have already noticed this. Hamlett (1935), with the armadillo, noticed it when interpreting the aspect of uterine mucosa; Talmage and his collaborators (1954) affirmed it and suspected a relative insufficiency. Deanesly (1954) made the same remarks about the stoat. Hansson (1947) and Enders (1956) later found this same inactive aspect of the corpora lutea with the mink and, similarly, Wright and Rausch (1955) with the wolverine. On the other hand, Stieve (1950) affirms that in the roe deer the progestational corpora are more active than are the gestational ones. We shall certainly have to talk about all this again in the discussion of this paper so as to draw together the common lines, if there are any.

If the corpora lutea are insufficient, the cause would, in our opinion, lie with a lack of the LH or LTH factor or its inability to be released into the system. In fact, Greenwald (1962) has recently shown that in the lactating mouse this latter mechanism seems the most likely. Certain writers, of whom Talmage (1954) is one, thought that the quantity of progesterone was insufficient or that another factor must come into play and be added to progesterone to set off the implantation of ova. Hammond (1951) has the same opinion about the mink. The experiments of the group at Rice University on the armadillo give reason to believe that there is an extra-ovarian factor, but what is it? On the other hand, not all animals have implantation of ova after ovariectomy. One fact remains sure: the implantation of ova is preceded by an increase in the activity of the corpora lutea, both in the mink (Enders, 1956; Hansson, 1947) and in the badger (Canivenc and Bonnin-Laffargue, 1956).

However, to our knowledge, all attempts to hasten the implantation of ova by the addition of progesterone alone, or together with estrogen, have been unsuccessful in all species tried (cf. Hansson, 1947; Cochrane and Shackelford, 1962; Canivenc and Bonnin-Laffargue, 1956; Harrison and Neal, 1956). All those using for the same purpose the addition of pituitary hormones (heterogeneous, it is true) have been equally unsuccessful (with the armadillo, Hamlett, 1935; with the mink, Hansson, 1947, and Enders, 1956; with the European badger, Canivenc and Bonnin-Laffargue, 1956). It would take too long to relate to you all the failures we have experienced with the addition of extra-ovarian hormones (thyroid, adrenal, hypophyseal) or vitamins.

This is our present interpretation: we believe that the progestational hormone can be active only if it is transformed by another factor, perhaps enzymatic. This factor may be liberated by LTH, and the latter is probably under the influence of the hypothalamic centers. In our opinion, there can be no question of a quantitative effect of progesterone. Instead, the kind of progestin may be important.

In each species having deferred implantation of ova, the period during which progesterone becomes active is clearly defined in time. It is unchanged, which explains why there are species whose ova are implanted regularly in the spring (the period of the lengthening of the days—the marten, mink, stoat, and roe deer), and, on the other hand, there are species whose ova are implanted when the day is at its shortest (the badger and the bear).

In November we have encountered ovaries having recent generations of corpora lutea, but we have not encountered ovaries having two generations of corpora lutea. This shows that a second active luteal period is present in the autumn. This would explain our observations, those of Harrison and Neal, and those which Dr. Short recently told us about (recent corpora lutea in autumn). So as to obtain greater accuracy in our common studies, we should have to know the gestational history of every wild animal at the moment of its capture. To eliminate mistakes, one would have to know exactly when the first gestation took place, in the spring or in the autumn. This seems to me to be of prime importance. Let us not forget, however, that the placental scars remain for a very long time in the uterus of multiparous females and that one can therefore differentiate between primiparous and nulliparous animals.

We cannot conclude with certainty in favor of an ovarian cause in the implantation of ova in the European badger because we have always failed in our efforts to hasten implantation. Perhaps one should consider in the badger that a second coitus, if it is constant (which we do not yet know), might be regarded as the equivalent of the remating system

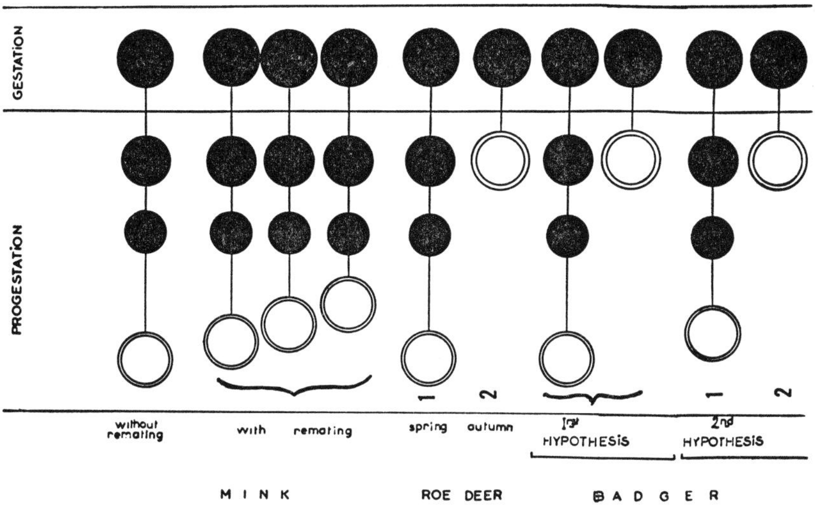

FIG. 1.—Position of the reproductive cycle of the European badger among the different systems found in the animals with deferred implantation. In the first hypothesis: some new corpora lutea appear in the animals that had ovulated previously. That is, ovulation during delay. This pattern is identical to that of the mink (Harrison and Neal, 1956). In the second hypothesis: ovulation appears in some animals (*1*) in February (postpartum estrus), in other animals (*2*) in autumn. In each case the corpora lutea can become gestational. This pattern is identical to that of the roe deer or marten (Canivenc and Bonnin-Laffargue, 1956).

used by breeders of mink. We have shown that the second mating is not indispensable, but its true meaning remains to be discovered. Stieve (1950) has, for instance, noticed in the roe deer that the second heat (autumn heat) corresponds to a true and not an apparent heat and that it happens only with older females having had their young late, with females fertilized for the first time, or with females that have not been fertilized. This observation is very similar to that of Watzka (1949). Taking this into consideration, one might perhaps provisionally relate the reproductive physiology of the badger to the schemes shown in Figure 1.

Concerning the biology of the badger, the problems remain, as a French literary author, Condorcet, said in 1900: "En histoire naturelle, des expériences détermineraient jusqu'à quel point dans les différentes espèces vivipares le temps de la gestation est variable ou constant, quelles sont les causes de ces variations, la possibilité et les moyens de faire agir ces causes à volonté, les effets qui en résulteraient pour l'individu dont la naissance est accelerée ou retardée."

References

CANIVENC, R. 1960. L'ovo-implantation differée des animaux sauvages. In G. MASSON (ed.), Les fonctions de nidation utérine et leurs troubles, pp. 33–68. Bruxelles. Masson.

CANIVENC, R., M. BONNIN-LAFFARGUE, and M.-C. RELEXANS. 1962. Sensibilité de l'ovaire du blaireau aux hormones gonadotropes. C.R. Acad. Sci. Paris, **254**:1677–78.

CANIVENC, R., and M. LAFFARGUE. 1956. Présence de blastocystes libres au cours de la lactation chez le blaireau européen *Meles meles* L. C.R. Soc. Biol., **150**:1193.

COCHRANE, R. L., and R. M. SHACKELFORD. 1962. Effects of exogenous oestrogen alone and in combination with progesterone on pregnancy in the intact mink. J. Endocrin., **25**:101–6.

DEANESLY, R. 1943. Delayed implantation in the stoat (*Mustela mustela*). Nature, **151**:365–67.

ENDERS, R. K. 1956. Delayed implantation in mammals. In Gestation: Transactions of the 2d Conference Josiah Macy, Jr., Foundation, pp. 113–31.

ENDERS, R. K., and O. P. PEARSON. 1943. Shortening gestation by inducing early implantation with increased light in the marten. Am. Fur Breeder, **15**:18.

FISHER, E. 1931. Die Entwicklungsgeschichte des Dachses und die Frage der Zwillingsbildung. Verh. Anat. Ges., **40**:22.

FRIES, S. 1880. Über die Fortpflanzung von Meles Taxus. Zool. Anz., **3**: 486–92.

GREENWALD, G. S. 1962. Luteinizing hormone content of the pituitary of the lactating mouse. Gen. & Comp. Endocrin., **2**:453.

HAMLETT, G. W. D. 1935. Delayed implantation and discontinuous development in mammals. Quart. Rev. Biol., **10**:432–47.

HANSSON, A. 1947. The physiology of reproduction in mink (*Mustela vison* Schreb) with special reference to delayed implantation. Acta Zool. **28**: 1–136.

HARRISON, R. J., and E. G. NEAL. 1956. Ovulation during delayed implantation and other reproductive phenomena in the badger (*Meles meles* L.). Nature, **177**:977–79.

HERLANT, M. 1960. Étude critique de 2 techniques nouvelles destinées à mettre en évidence les différentes catégories cellulaires présentes dans la grande pituitaires. Bull. Micr. Appl., **10**:37–44.

JAYLE, M. F., and O. CREPY. 1952. Technique de dosage du pregnandiol. Bull. Soc. Chim., **34**:435.

LINDEMANN, W. 1954. Zur Rassenflage und Fortpflanzungsbiologie des karpatischen Braubaren *Ursus arctos arctos* L. Saugetirk. Mitteil., **2**:1–8.

NEAL, E. 1948. The Badger. COLLINS (ed.), New Naturalist Monograph.

NEAL, E., and R. J. HARRISON. 1958. Reproduction in the European badger. Trans. Zool. Soc. London, **29**:67–131.

NOTINI, G. 1948. Biologiska Undersoknigar over gravlingen. Uppsala.

PEARSON, O. P., and R. K. ENDERS. 1944. Duration of pregnancy in certain mustelids. J. Exp. Zool., **95**:21–35.

PRELL, H. 1927. Über doppelte Brunstzeit und verlangerte Tragzeit bei den einheimischen Arten der Mardergattung *Martes pinel* L. Zool. Anz., **74**:122.

RUFFIÉ, A., M. BONNIN-LAFFARGUE, and R. CANIVENC. 1961. Le taux de prégnandiol urinaire au cours de la grossesse chez le blaireau européen (*Meles meles* L.). C.R. Soc. Biol., **155**:759.

STIEVE, H. 1950. Anatomisch-biologische Untersuchungen über die Fortpflanzungstatigkeit des europaischen Rehes (*Capreolus capreolus caprelus* L.). Ztschr. f. mikr. Anat. Forsch., **55**:427.

TALMAGE, R. V., G. D. BUCHANAN, F. W. KRAINTZ, E. A. LAZO-WASEM, and M. X. ZARROW. 1954. The presence of a functional corpus luteum during delayed implantation in the armadillo. J. Endocrin., **11**:44–49.

WATZKA, N. 1949. Über die Beziehung zwischen Corpus luteum und verlangerter Tragzeit. Z. Anat., **114**:366–74.

WRIGHT, P. L., and R. RAUSCH, 1955. Reproduction in the wolverine (*Gulo gulo*). J. Mammal., **36**:346.

DISCUSSION (*Chairman:* R. K. ENDERS)

WRIGHT: Did you see any evidence that the male badger is feeding young during the period of lactation? Does the male live with the female and bring food to the young at the time of weaning?

HARRISON: I should say Yes, but I should prefer that you consult Dr. Neal (see Neal, 1958, in References).

GLASSER: I am interested in the role of the secondary ovulation and of the relationship the secondary ovulation has to the hormonal conditions that are necessary for implantation in December. Do you believe that this is a form of restraint of luteal function? Perhaps the site of this restraint is interposed between hypothalamus and anterior pituitary, or pituitary and target organ, or, further, it may be an alteration of either kidney or liver function that results in metabolizing progesterone in such a fashion that it is less effective on a per molecule basis.

CANIVENC: We are progressing in that work now.

HARRISON: I am not convinced that it is the corpora that matter, but rather the follicles. I suspect that the follicles that develop during delay supply the uterus with just that amount of estrogen necessary to keep the lining epithelium active enough to supply the blastocysts, thus keeping the situation going. We should, of course, like more badgers in order to test this idea.

CANIVENC: Some estral phase appears during delayed implantation, but we have not found ovulation.

MAYER: Is there an endometrial factor responsible for the slow growth of blastocyst at the end of the lethargic stage, that is to say, in the preimplantation stage, and is there some interrelationship with an increase of the luteal tissue?

HARRISON: We thought at first that it might be the corpora lutea, but there is no correlation between the size of the blastocysts and the number of corpora at the end of delay. We think that the follicles and interstitial tissue are more important in this connection. The presence of many additional corpora means that there have been many follicles developing during delay and that they may be producing estrogens; there is also the possible action of interstitial tissue or adrenals during delay. Another point: Canivenc found postpartum ovulation in 84 per cent of the females. We found far less, hardly 35 per cent. This may be related to poor weather conditions in England in early spring and lack of food until later months. I should also emphasize that the corpora from the secondary ovulations soon resemble those from the first, and it is hard to differentiate them after a few weeks.

WILSON: You have successful ovulation but no fertilized eggs?

HARRISON: I do not think that these eggs are fertilized. In fact, in other specimens they are definitely degenerating.

WILSON: Are the males fertile?

HARRISON: They are fertile. They may be young males, probably in their second or third year, and may be individuals that were born late and so probably matured late. But other factors, which I have mentioned, may also operate.

WILSON: Can the rise and fall of estrogen make the female less receptive?

HARRISON: That is something we are working on.

DEANESLY: The corpus luteum of delay in the armadillo contains progesterone, so it may well be present at a low level in the badger. Do gonadotrophins produce small corpora lutea, and at what time of year?

CANIVENC: There is no difference between normal females and those with gonadotrophins.

Professor Harrison, how do you recognize the ovulation period in your badgers?

HARRISON: We can assess the time of ovulation from vaginal smears. In our series we serially sectioned all ovaries and also the uterine tubes, looking for ripe follicles, recently ruptured ones, and in the latter cases for eggs in the tubes. We found them consistently in those sows that had recently ovulated.

CANIVENC: Have you seen morulae?

HARRISON: Yes, ovulation occurred in the early spring, and can occur again in April, June, and October. We have several females that ovulated for the first time in October.

WIMSATT: Harrison spoke of the animal as entering semihibernation. This implied activity associated with the production of a 14° temperature rise in the burrow.

HARRISON: As the winter comes nearer and implantation time approaches, the badgers stay at home for longer periods—often remaining in the set for as long as three days. They may well be quite active underground. I am not sure how much Dr. Neal knows about this, but at least he thinks that it is the prolonged periods spent in the set that raise the temperature of the nesting chambers.

FISHER: In seals in Great Britain, you found blastocysts in January, and mating in March. Do you remember where these animals came from?

HARRISON: From the west coast (Wales) and the Hebrides. Backhouse and Hewer (1957) found very few spring births, about 20–30 in the regions they covered. Few spring matings have been observed, and this out-of-season activity is probably indulged in only by young cows that came into estrus early in the year.

FISHER: On the east coast of Canada, the gray seal breeds in winter, most pups being born in the last half of January, although pups have been found from late December to early March. At the other extreme of its range, in the Baltic, it is again a winter breeder. This species is most erratic in its breeding behavior. The ecological significance of delayed implantation is not nearly as clear for this species as it is for other northern phocids, particularly the harp seal. There is a tremendous mortality of young gray seals from drowning and exposure shortly after birth in the Gulf of St. Lawrence breeding area, unless there is an unusually severe winter with much ice, when they do well. It is better adapted to breeding on ice than on land, in my view.

I wonder whether Dr. Harrison would confirm that there is evidence of mating during lactation?

HARRISON: Yes. The average length of time from parturition to mating is 12–16 days.

FISHER: An interesting contrast in breeding behavior in gray seals between the population around the United Kingdom and the west Atlantic is that in the latter they are monogamous, from what observations we have, behaving much as the hooded seal does, whereas, in the United

Kingdom, there appears to be either incipient polygamy or promiscuity.

I should like to make the observation that the mechanism of delayed implantation not only is of ecological significance but is essential to the very survival of northern forms, such as the ringed seal and harp seal. Birth in the latter, for example, takes place at the only time of year (the end of February and mid-March for the northwest Atlantic shores) that a suitable "platform" is available in the form of dense pack ice. Mating is essential soon after birth because only then are the females concentrated and available. They are scattered over a tremendous region at sea for the rest of the year. Whether fortuitous or not, a surface bloom of zoöplankton occurs at the time the pups enter the water, forming immediately available food.

ROBERT K. ENDERS AND ALLEN C. ENDERS

Morphology of the Female Reproductive Tract during Delayed Implantation in the Mink

At least one aspect of the reproductive cycle of the mink was known to woodsmen and trappers long before mink were raised on fur farms. This was the very vigorous and prolonged copulation that is so characteristic of *Mustela vison*. Not much more was learned until about thirty years ago, when the rearing of mink for fur was well on its way to becoming a considerable industry. Breeding practice at that time was based on practical experience. Now breeding practice is based on a more or less complete knowledge of the reproductive processes, and more than six and one-half million kits were raised last year.

Mink breeders learned that the period of gestation varied from 42 to 79 days, and some fantastic explanations as to the cause of this variation were current. One such explanation was published, complete with illustrations, which claimed the longer gestations were due to the phenomenon that the ova had to reach the vagina, in which they were fertilized, then they journeyed back to the uterus for gestation! Short gestations were the result of the more usual process of fertilization and migration. Nor was it known that ovulation was not spontaneous but followed copulation by about 48 hours or that the blastocysts lay more or less quiescent in the uterine horns for a longer or shorter period. As these facts became known, the knowledge was incorporated into breeding practice. R. K. Enders (1939, 1952), Hansson (1947), Johansson (1951), and Shackelford (1948, 1950) were among the earlier workers in this field both in discovering the facts and in translating them into breeding practice.

DR. ROBERT K. ENDERS is the Isaac Clothier Professor and chairman of the Department of Zoölogy, Swarthmore College, Swarthmore, Pennsylvania.

Progressive mink breeders keep accurate records. From these records, statistically valid conclusions can be drawn. Breeders have been generous in permitting us to use their records; they have also donated animals for our use. Ralph Space has been particularly generous. Our work has been supported in part by the Department of Agriculture and by grants from the National Science Foundation.

Before discussion of various phases of the delay in implantation it is well to recall that reproduction in the mink differs from that of laboratory and domestic animals in many significant ways. For example, breeding early in the season may be followed by later breedings, and, in each subsequent breeding as well as in the first, follicles may develop to ovulation and the ova be fertilized. All or most of these ova develop into blastocysts that remain unimplanted until the increasing length of day stimulates the changes that bring about implantation (R. K. Enders, 1956). However, new follicles will not reach the stage of ovulation unless 6 days have elapsed since the previous mating. Not only will follicles fail to develop, but the size of the litter produced from the first breeding will be small. When a subsequent mating occurs more than 6 days after a mating, ovulation may follow. If the last copulation is fertile, it will contribute 80–90 per cent of the kits. Superfecundation and superfetation are normal in the mink. In superfecundation, when insemination is separated by a day, the first male sires approximately a third of the litter. In superfetation, as the interval between matings is increased, the proportion of kits from the first mating declines to 14 per cent in 7 days. If a sterile male is used, so that fertilization does not follow insemination, litter size is not affected.

The breeding season in mink in the northern states extends from late February to early April. Females that breed early or late are not as productive as those that breed in March. Copulations between March 10 and March 24 indicate that this is the height of the breeding season. There is some variation from year to year, but this appears to be independent of amount of sunshine and temperature. Artificial lighting may hasten the onset of breeding, but keeping mink in total darkness from January to May does not appear to alter breeding. This regimen resulted in one pregnancy of 92 days (Kirk, 1962).

Although breeding in total darkness was not later than breeding in controls, total darkness resulted in a longer delay in implantation in some of the experimental animals. Production under these conditions was poor; only 29 living kits were raised by 20 females. Some mink raisers report failure to breed in animals kept in the semidarkness of sheds, so this report is of great interest.

Genetic constitution plays some role in determining the date of estrus, although this is somewhat obscured by different breeding practices. "Yukon" mink are said to breed 2 weeks later than "Quebec" or "Eastern" mink, or, as some breeders state it, large mink "come in" slower than small mink.

There is a significant tendency for females to whelp on the same date each season but not to breed on the same date unless breeding practice exposes them only at that time. Single matings tend to produce larger litters than multiple matings, but there are more "misses" in single matings.

The mean length of gestation is approximately 51 days. Kits born before the forty-first day or after the seventy-ninth are not likely to survive for long. More than 20 per cent of the pregnancies fall outside the 45–55-day period delimited by the standard deviation. The embryos appear to implant about 28–30 days before parturition. This indicates that in a gestation of 92 days the blastocysts are at least 60 days old before they implant. Implantation in our stock seems to take place about April 10–12. In animals bred at or near the middle of the breeding season, implantation occurs about 20 days postcoitum or 18 days postovulation.

Both Hansson (1947) and R. K. Enders (1952) published histological descriptions of the reproductive tract of the mink. Recently, A. C. Enders (1961), in a comparative study, noted more variation in the endometrium of the mink during the delay period than in the other two animals studied. Since mink breed during the delay period, some variation in structure of the tract is to be anticipated. In the study reported here, attention has been focused on the correlation of structural changes in the ovary with its target organs, the uterus and vagina.

Over a period of several years, material was collected for histological examination from a large number of animals. Of a total of 39 of these animals included in this study, 17 were in the period of delayed implantation (blastocysts checked for in approximately half these animals), 11 were in a postimplantation stage of pregnancy, 6 were in postimplantation pseudopregnancy, 3 were anestrous, and 2 were unbred in the estrous period.

With the exception of three mink from the Texas wild population, the animals from which tissue was taken were ranch mink bred in Pennsylvania, then shipped to Houston just prior to necropsy. The histological and histochemical methods used were the same as those reported in A. C. Enders (1961). The tissue examined with the electron microscope was fixed in Caulfield's (1957) osmium tetroxide sucrose mixture and imbedded in Araldite following rapid ethyl alcohol dehydration.

Ovary

FOLLICULAR DEVELOPMENT

At all stages of delayed implantation, mature follicles can be found within the ovary. In a typical mature follicle the mural granulosa cells have a tightly organized columnar basal layer, the cells of which have a rounded distal end frequently containing lipid droplets. Two or three layers of spheroidal, less highly organized granulosa cells are also present. The discus proligerus and cumulus oöphorus are usually somewhat eccentrically placed, the follicles being slightly oval in general outline. As in the mural granulosa, the basal layer of cells of the cumulus oöphorus are highly columnar, with subsequent layers being less well organized. In any group of ovaries from delay animals the proportion of such mature follicles to atretic follicles varies, but some ovaries will have as few as a single mature follicle, whereas others will have several. Generally, follicles are most numerous at copulation and at the period of spacing prior to implantation. To the extent that animals mate several times during the delay period, there can be said to be a cycle of follicular development, but this does not have a fixed time relationship that can be determined for a single breeding population. That is, animals killed six days after mating, ten days after mating, and at other intervals after mating are not in a predictable stage of follicular development; different individuals show different stages of development on the same day post-coitum. It is probable that the differences may be influenced in part by the date.

Throughout the delay period, appreciable follicular atresia occurs, as mentioned previously. At this stage the cells of the theca interna hypertrophy and apparently form nodules of glandular interstitial tissue. After implantation, follicles undergoing atresia may form lutein plaques. In this instance the granulosa cells appear to contribute to the plaque formation rather than the cells of the theca. After implantation, numerous follicles are still present, but follicles of full preinseminal growth are rare.

CORPORA LUTEA

The mink, like the ferret, produces both secondary and tertiary follicular fluid at ovulation. After ovulation the granulosa cells become attenuated and are typically in strands forming a lacy network extending into the collapsed follicle. At this time the granulosa cells contain appreciable lipid, which exhibits both a positive Schultz test and evidence for carbonyl groups in fixed material. With vascular invasion and reorganization of the follicle into a corpus luteum, a number of changes occur. The granulosa cells round up, and their postovulatory pattern becomes obscured. The corpora formed in this fashion are quite cellular, with the lutein cells being 13–19 μ in diameter. Connective-tissue cells are numerous and there is relatively little intercellular space.

The corpora of delay, even following a single breeding, are not altogether uniform. Within a single ovary, two corpora may be different with regard both to cell size and shape and to lipid content (Pl. I, *6*). Furthermore, corpora may be different in different animals on the same day postcoitum (Pl. I, *2*, *4*, *5*). That is, corpora from two animals ten days after mating may be somewhat different in appearance. Generally speaking, the lutein cells of the corpora of delay contain relatively little lipid. In any single corpus luteum a few cells will have numerous lipid droplets, but the majority of cells do not. The more highly luteinized corpora of delay contain cells rather cuboidal in outline, occupying appreciably more space than the connective tissue and the sinusoids (Pl. I, *5*). These corpora have individual cells with lipid. In appearance, the more highly luteinized corpora of delay have lutein cells resembling those of the rat in early pregnancy. The lutein cells are indeed about the same size as rat lutein cells in early pregnancy but are only a fraction of the size of mature lutein cells of the mink. At the end of the period of delayed implantation, there is considerable change in the corpora lutea. Lutein cells from animals early in implantation are larger than the lutein cells of the delayed-implantation animals and may contain appreciable lipid.

The corpora lutea of the postimplantation period (Pl. I, *1* and *3*) are characterized by large lutein cells, highly dilated sinusoidal capillaries, and quite large fluid-filled spaces between the capillaries and the lutein cells. The lutein cells are not as uniformly acidophilic in this species as in some others. The edematous nature of the corpora is perhaps the most striking feature. In a few corpora, the accumulated fluid occupies close to one-third the volume of the corpus. Individual cells of the corpora contain numerous lipid droplets, but the majority are relatively free of lipid. The lipid droplets are both Schultz-positive and Ashbel-Seligman–positive. Some involution of the corpora lutea appears to take place prior to parturition, and after parturition the involution is rapid.

Some of the cytological characteristics of lutein cells have been enumerated recently (A. C. Enders, 1962). Characteristic of these cells are a folded margin, numerous mitochondria with villiform cristae, and a highly developed system of tubular and/or vesicular endoplasmic reticulum. Although ribosomes may be present in some abundance, most of the membranes of the endoplasmic reticulum do not have associated ribosomes. In contrast, the granulosa cells from preovulatory follicles contain numerous strands and cisternae of reticulum with associated ribosomes. The mitochondria are less irregular in outline and tend to have more lamelliform cristae. The margins of the granulosa cells have blunt projections rather than foldings. The contrast between these characteristics is of some importance in ascertaining the extent of luteinization of the corpora of delay.

As stated previously, lutein cells from delayed implantation are much smaller than those from the postdelay period. However, an examination of these cells with the electron microscope reveals the cytological characteristics of lutein cells (Pl. II, *8*). Lutein cells from the delay period show extensive marginal folding in relationship to the pericapillary space. The cytoplasm of these cells contains a variable number of ribosomes, but only in small areas are these ribosomes associated with membranes of the endoplasmic reticulum. The endoplasmic reticulum appears in cross-section to be highly vesicular, but the presence of numerous elongated profiles indicates that at least an appreciable portion is tubular. The mitochondria of the lutein cells of the corpora of delay show numerous villiform cristae, although some lamelliform cristae are also present.

The resemblance of these lutein cells of delay to the lutein cells of the pregnant rat is striking. In postimplantation animals the variation between individual lutein cells is marked. Both light and dark cells are present, and the amount of lipid in given cells varies. Although demonstrably inadequate preservation appears to enhance the differences between light and dark cells, a relative abundance of ribosomes in the latter indicates that there is a genuine difference between these cells. Both light and dark cells have the three typical features of lutein cells, but the dark cells have more highly folded margins, more irregular mitochondria with rather folded outlines, and a dense cytoplasm relatively rich in ribosomes. The light cells (Pl. II, *7*) closely resemble the lutein cells of delay and the lutein cells of other animals.

VAGINA

Our observations on the anestrous vagina confirm those of R. K. Enders (1952). The epithelium is stratified cuboidal, with occasional regions of low columnar cells. For the most part, it is only two or three cell layers thick. In periodic acid–Schiff preparations, a layer of strongly PAS-positive material is present on the luminal surface, and occasional cells show a distal accumulation of strongly PAS-positive material.

Animals in proestrus and unmated animals at the beginning of the breeding season have a stratified squamous vaginal epithelium. Neither mucus nor leucocytes are present within the epithelium, and there is a smooth transition from a polyhedral layer to the squamous layers. Animals killed within two hours after mating show a thick, cornified epithelium. In some regions there may be an amorphous non-cellular,

PLATE I

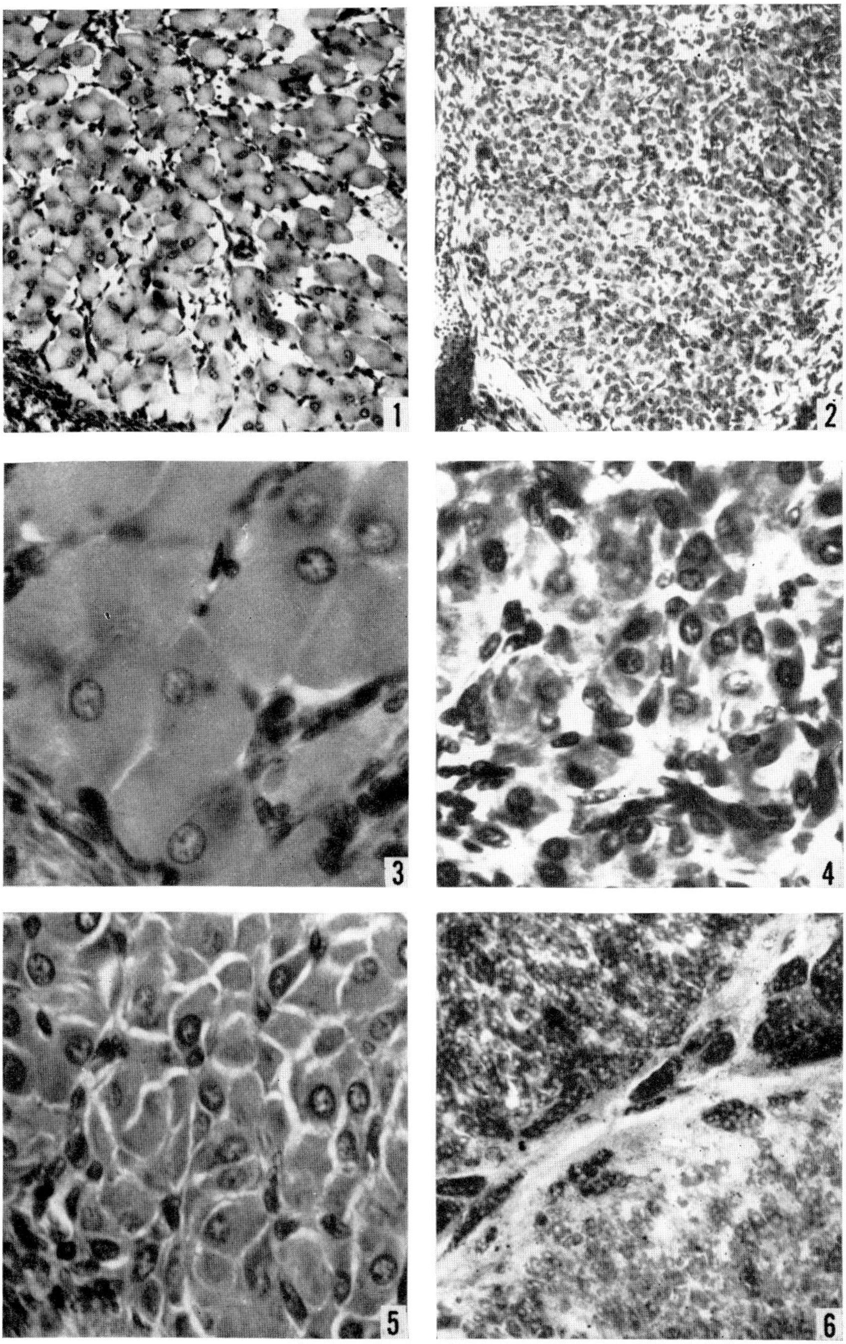

1, Corpus luteum of postimplantation. Note the intercellular space between the lutein cells. ×140.

2, Corpus luteum of delay. This is a relatively unluteinized corpus. ×140.

3, Corpus luteum of postimplantation. Note the large size of the lutein cells. ×440.

4, Corpus luteum of delay, showing small size of lutein cells. ×440.

5, Corpus luteum of delay, showing luteinization. ×440.

6, Two corpora of delay, showing different amounts of lipid. Sudan black B. ×135.

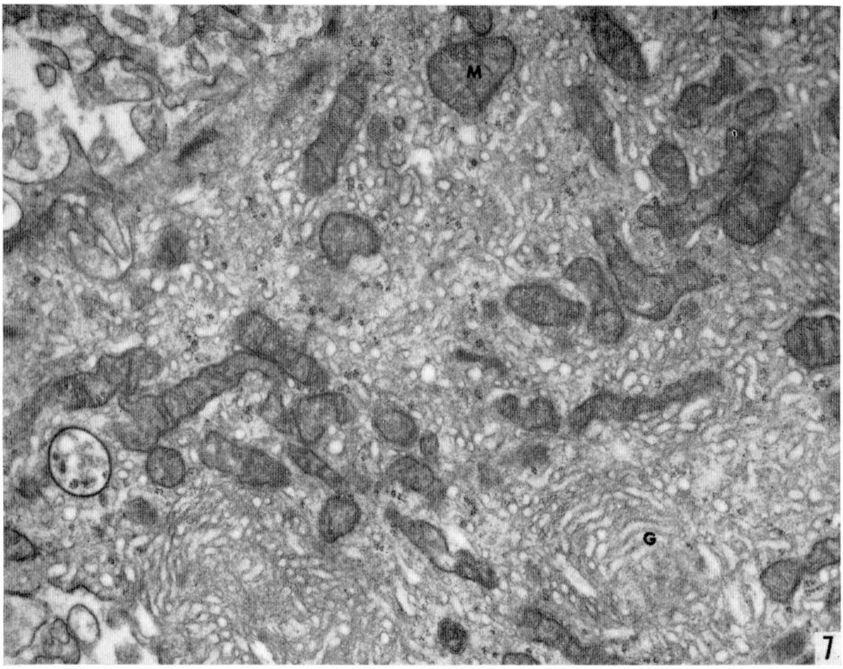

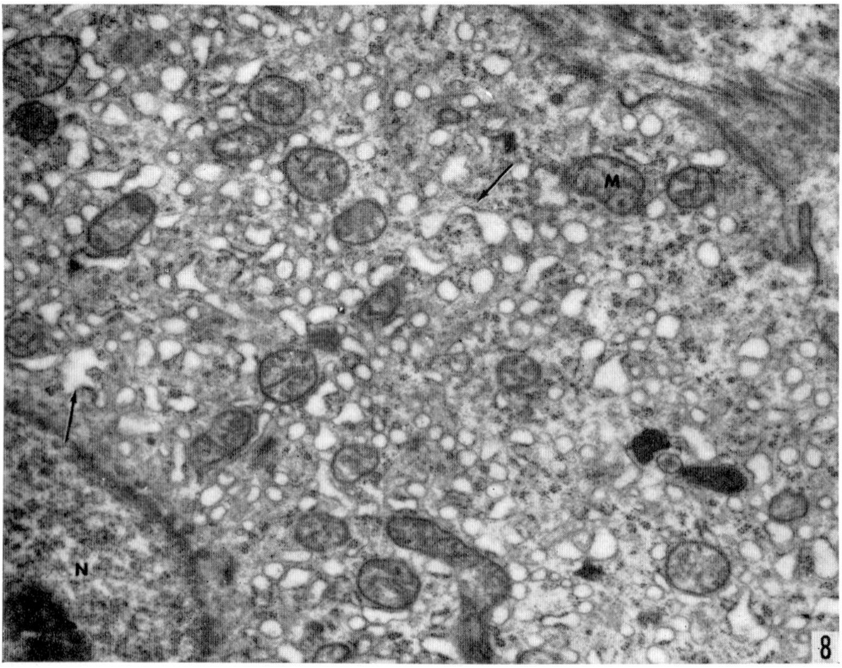

7, Lutein cell from postimplantation. Note abundance of agranular endoplasmic reticulum and the tubular cristae in the mitochondria (*M*). The margin of the lutein cell is at the upper and lower left. Golgi complex (*G*). ×15,000.

8, Lutein cell from delayed implantation. More ribosomes are present, but the characteristic forms of the endoplasmic reticulum and the cristae of the mitochondria (*M*) have already been established. The margin of the cell is at the upper right. Note that, although the endoplasmic reticulum appears to be vesicular, it is branching (*arrows*) and therefore tubular. Nucleus (*N*). ×15,000.

PLATE III

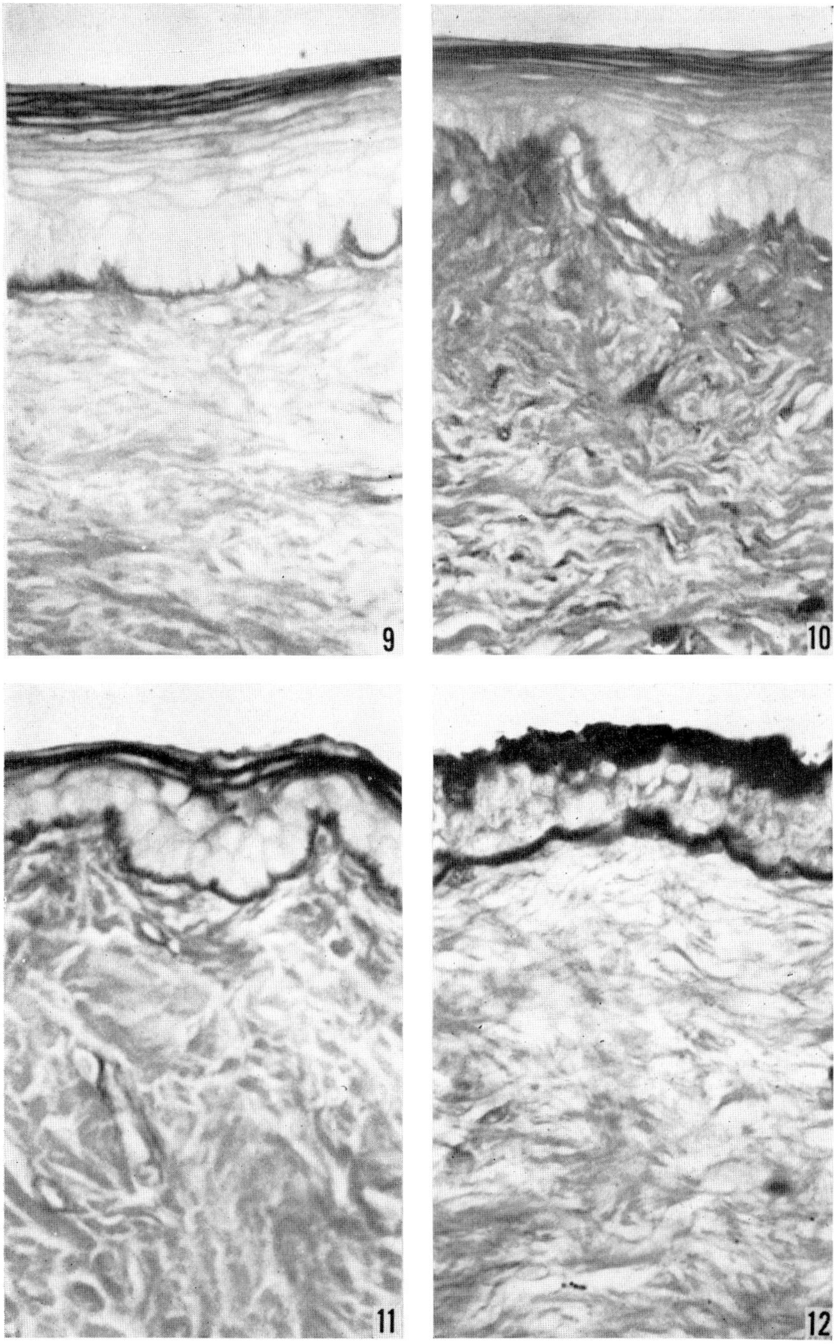

All photomicrographs in this plate are of sections stained by the periodic acid-Schiff technique. ×250.

9, Vagina of a mink at the time of ovulation. Note stratification.

10, Vagina of delay. Note stratification.

11, Vagina of late delay. Some PAS-positive material is present.

12, Vagina of postimplantation. Note heavy luminal layer of PAS-positive material.

PLATE IV

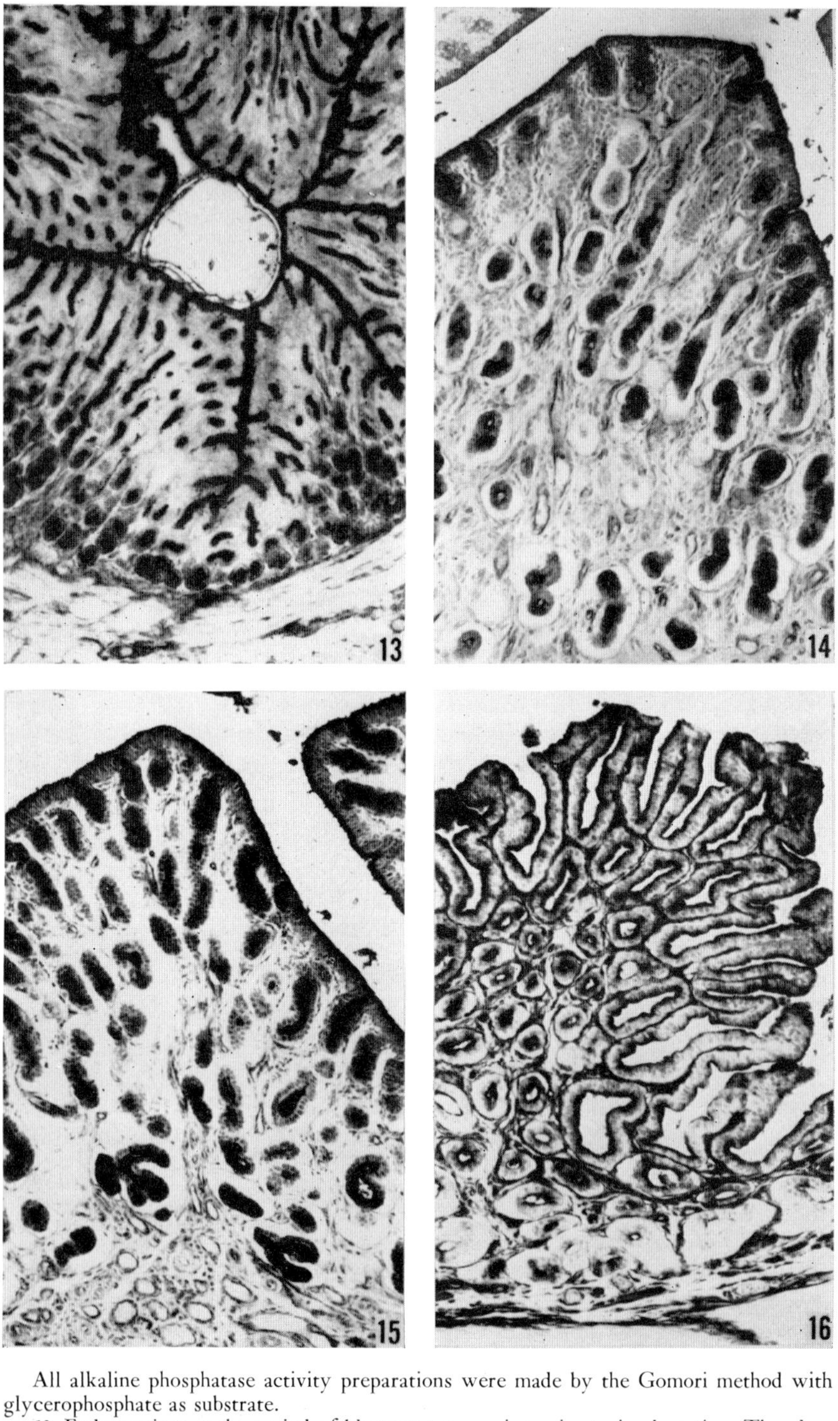

All alkaline phosphatase activity preparations were made by the Gomori method with glycerophosphate as substrate.

13, Endometrium at the period of blastocyst expansion prior to implantation. The clear central ring is the zona pellucida of the blastocyst. Frozen section. ×80.

14, Endometrium of delay. Note that there is relatively less activity in the intermediate region of the glands than in *13* or *15*. Cold alcohol fixation. ×130.

15, Endometrium of delay. Note the relatively greater activity in this endometrium compared to that in *14*. Cold alcohol fixation. ×130.

16, Endometrium from a pseudopregnant animal in the postimplantation period. Note dentate border of the endometrial fold. Cold alcohol fixation. ×130.

PLATE V

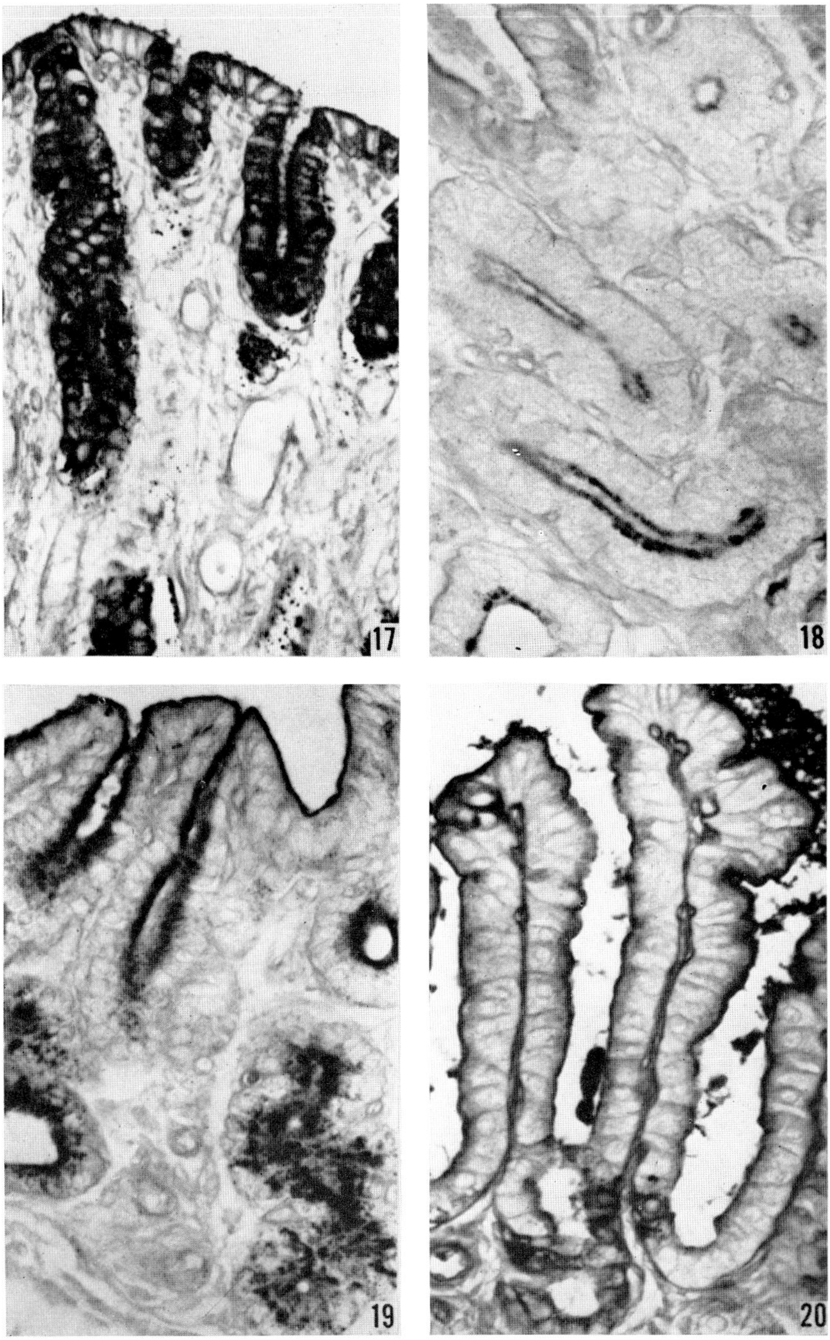

Periodic acid–Schiff-positive material in the endometrium. ×535.

17, Endometrium of an estrous animal. Note the great abundance of PAS-positive material in the glands. Most of this material is glycogen, since it can be eliminated by prior incubation in diastase.

18, Endometrium of delay. Only a fringe of diastase-resistant PAS-positive material is present.

19, Endometrium of delay. More diastase-resistant PAS-positive material is present. The granular material deeper in the gland cells is glycogen.

20, Endometrium from postimplantation animal. Only the dark material at the base of the luminal folds is glycogen.

weakly PAS-positive substance associated with the luminal surface of this epithelium. Leucocytes are only rarely encountered. One animal, two hours after its second mating, showed two or three patches of mucus adhering to the surface cornified layer, with a few leucocytes in this material. At the time of ovulation, two days after mating, the vaginal epithelium is also highly cornified (Pl. III, *9*). It is devoid of either leucocytes or mucus. There is a small amount of faintly PAS-positive material between the cells of the cornified layer.

In animals from 6 to 24 days postcoitus, the vaginal epithelium shows a wide variation, although always of the cornified type (Pl. III, *10, 11*). That is, some animals, such as one killed on day 6, had a heavily cornified vagina including a somewhat distinct surface layer of cornified cells about 4 cells thick. Another animal, killed 10 days postcoitus, had a cornified epithelium, but it was relatively thin, with numerous mitotic figures and a rather heavy PAS-positive substance between the cornified cells. In another animal, the cornified layer was thin, with appreciable sloughing from the surface. In only one animal from the delay period were cornified regions largely absent. In this animal, which had spaced blastocysts, there was a low, stratified epithelium with occasional sites of mucification. Intermediates between this last example and previously described examples were found in two instances. In one of these instances there were a few leucocytes in the epithelium, the stratification was only a few cells in thickness, and cornification of the surface layers was not universal. In the second instance there was a small amount of luminal mucus, although no mucous cells were found in the surface layers of the vagina per se. One animal that displayed the typical uterine motility of spacing and that was killed at the time of spacing exhibited a highly cornified vaginal epithelium. Another animal, in which the blastocysts were spaced and were distending the uterine lumen locally, also exhibited cornified squamous epithelium. In one instance, an implanting blastocyst was forcibly ejected from the uterus. The vagina of this animal was primarily stratified cuboidal, with squamous cells only in a few places. Leucocytes were common in the epithelium, but very little mucus was present. An animal with 5-somite embryos showed a greater amount of mucification, with numerous leucocytes.

In later stages of pregnancy and pseudopregnancy (Pl. III, *12*), the vaginal epithelium is stratified columnar, being 2–3 cells in thickness. The surface cells are elongated, with large amounts of strongly PAS-positive material in their distal portions. Although the vagina of pregnant mink is characterized by an abundance of PAS-positive material in the surface cells, not all the cells even at this stage are uniformly distended with PAS-positive material.

From the foregoing data, it appears that the vaginal epithelium is dependent on the follicular phase for stratification. It remains stratified during the greater part of the delay period, showing slight fluctuations in thickness that correspond to the variations in follicular development. At the end of the delay period and at early implantation, the progestational changes are marked, first, by the change to a stratified cuboidal rather than stratified squamous epithelium, then by progressive mucification.

Uterus

If variation in numbers of follicles and partial luteinization of the corpora lutea result in altered hormone titers, the variation seen in these aspects during the delay period should be reflected in the morphology of the uterus. Histological examination reveals some variation, which can be further extended by routine histochemical methods.

Tetrachrome procedures on Zenker's fixed material reveal the presence of a columnar, luminal epithelium, which in some animals is largely palisade, and in others tall columnar. The junction or mouth zone may be moderately dilated in some, less so in others. The intermediate zone is closed off, that is, the apical ends of the cells contact in some animals, while the lumen is patent in this region in other individuals. The extent of dilation of the basal portion of the gland also varies slightly, but, since some of these variations may be seen in different folds of endometrium in the same animal, it is not always clear that they result from more than local variation in structure.

A little more variation is seen in preparations demonstrating alkaline phosphatase activity (Pl. IV, *13*, *14*, *15*, *16*) and demonstrating polysaccharides (Pl. V, *17*, *18*, *19*, *20*). In the alkaline phosphatase preparations, some uteri have pronounced activity at the surface of the luminal epithelial cells and the gland cells. Two variations from this pattern may be observed. In one there is somewhat reduced activity in the basal portions of the glands, and in the other there is a relative absence to activity in the intermediate segment. In the polysaccharide preparations, variation can be seen in both the diastase-resistant polysaccharides and glycogen. One or two animals had abundant glycogen in both the basal and the distal portions of the luminal epithelial cells and scattered glycogen throughout the glands. Several animals had glycogen in the basal portions of the luminal epithelial cells and a few granules of glycogen in the basal portions of the glands. The remaining animals had very little glycogen except for a few granules in the basal portions of the glands. Diastase-resistant polysaccharides were abundant in one animal. In all animals there was a very faint diastase-resistant PAS-positive fringe along the luminal and glandular epithelium. In a number of endometria, portions of the basal, and sometimes the intermediate, region of the gland contain PAS-positive material throughout the apical portions of the cells.

It was occasionally possible to discern a very fine granulation in the distal end of some of the gland cells. This granulation appeared to be mildly PAS-positive and diastase-resistant and was absent from some of the late-delay and from all early-implantation animals. In electron micrographs distinct granules are present in many of the glandular epithelial cells (Enders, Enders, and Schlafke, 1963). These granules occupy the same position as the mildly PAS-positive granules and are probably the same structures. Because of the small size of the granules (less than 0.5 μ) they can be studied more aptly by electron microscopy.

An extreme example of variations revealed by histochemical methods is seen in the presence or absence of lipid. As previously reported by A. C. Enders (1961), lipid is uncommon in the endometrium during delayed implantation. However, one animal had large quantities of phospholipid present throughout the luminal epithelium and glands. Two other animals had lipid droplets present distal and sometimes basal to the nuclei of the luminal epithelial cells but very little lipid elsewhere. Preliminary observations with the electron microscope indicate, however, that there is usually more lipid present in the luminal epithelium than we were able to demonstrate with Sudan black coloration of formalin-fixed or Elftman's fixed material or with Flemming's fixative. Succinic dehydrogenase activity was uniformly high in all the epithelial cells of the endometrium and showed very little variation.

The variation in the endometria reported above might be attributed to differences in individual animals, but it is also possible, indeed it seems more likely, that the endometrium is different at different times within the same animal. Diastase-resistant polysaccharides are accumulated at an inconstant rate. The phosphatase activity also varies. It is therefore probable that the blastocysts are presented with a somewhat different environment at different times throughout the delay period.

At the time of implantation, the uterus undergoes a number of changes. As in the cat (Dawson and Kosters, 1944), the endometrium becomes more dentate, with the inclusion of the junctional zone of the glands into the surface epithelium. In addition, the glands become somewhat more coiled. Once again, little lipid is present at this stage, nor is there much demonstrable glycogen. Most of the diastase-resistant PAS-positive material is situated within the lumina of the glands. The alkaline phosphatase activity is relatively high, with activity being demonstrable in both the luminal and all the glandular epithelium. The cytological changes that occur in gland cells at implantation are marked and form the basis of a separate study (Enders, Enders, and Schlafke, 1963).

Summary and Conclusions

The mink is unique among animals exhibiting delay of implantation in that both breeding and fertilization may occur during the delay period. As might be expected, considerable variation in structure of the female reproductive tract is found during the delay period. Contrary to previous reports, it is found that the corpora lutea luteinize but that the cells do not hypertrophy until implantation. The variation in structure of the reproductive tract may be summarized in regard to follicular or luteal ascendancy (Table 1). However, a regular cycle during delay cannot be discerned.

TABLE 1

	FOLLICULAR PHASE	DELAY			LUTEAL PHASE
	PRE-OVULATION	FOLLICULAR ASCENDANCY	LUTEAL ASCENDANCY	LATE DELAY	POST-IMPLANTATION
OVARIES					
FOLLICLES	many, small	large	small	large	
CORPORA LUTEA	none	small	luteinizing	luteinizing	luteinized
ENDOMETRIUM					
HISTOLOGY	low columnar	columnar	columnar	tall columnar vacuolated	palisade
GLYCOGEN	high, esp. gland. ep.	moderate	low	high, esp. lum. ep.	low
ALKALINE PHOSPHATASE	lumen mouth	lumen mouth base	lumen mouth neck base	lumen mouth neck base	heavy throughout
LIPID	little, lum. ep.	little, lum. ep. some neck	lum. ep.	decreased	slight
VAGINA	cornified	highly cornified	thin cornified	cornified	progressively mucified

The reported differences in the uterus observed indicate that the environment of the blastocysts varies considerably during the delay period. The ability of the mink blastocyst to withstand altered environmental conditions has been demonstrated in vitro by R. K. Enders and Pearson (1946). This appears to be another instance in which the requirements for continued existence of the blastocyst are less restrictive than those for continued development.

The variation in condition of the reproductive tract during the delay period makes the administration of exogenous hormones of doubtful usefulness in interpreting the hormonal basis of delayed implantation in this species. This variation may help to explain the negative results obtained by Hammond (1951) with progesterone and by Cochrane and Shackelford (1962) with estrogen and progesterone in attempting to induce implantation in the intact mink.

References

Caulfield, J. B. 1957. Effects of varying the vehicle for OsO_4 in tissue fixation. J. Biophys. & Biochem. Cytol., **3**:827.

Cochrane, R. L., and R. M. Shackelford. 1962. Effects of exogenous estrogen alone and in combination with progesterone on pregnancy in the intact mink. J. Endocrin., **25**:101–6.

Dawson, A. B., and B. A. Kosters. 1944. Pre-implantation changes in the uterine mucosa of the cat. Am. J. Anat., **75**:1–35.

Enders, A. C. 1961. Comparative studies on the endometrium of delayed implantation. Anat. Rec., **139**:483–97.

———. 1962. Observations on the fine structure of lutein cells. J. Cell Biol., **12**:101–13.

Enders, A. C., R. K. Enders, and S. J. Schlafke. 1963. An electron microscope study of the gland cells of the mink endometrium. *Ibid.*, Vol. **18.**

Enders, R. K. 1939. Reproductive phenomena in the mink (*Mustela vison*). Anat. Rec., **75**:122 (suppl.).

———. 1952. Reproduction in the mink (*Mustela vison*). Proc. Am. Phil. Soc., **96**:691–755.

———. 1956. Delayed implantation in mammals. In C. A. Villee (ed.), Gestation: Trans., 2d Conf. New York: Josiah Macy, Jr., Foundation.

Enders, R. K., and A. K. Pearson. 1946. Mink blastocysts *in vitro*. Anat. Rec., **96**:570.

Hammond, J., Jr. 1951. Failure of progesterone treatment to affect delayed implantation in the mink. J. Endocrin., **7**:330–34.

Hansson, A. 1947. The physiology of reproduction in the mink (*Mustela vison*), with special reference to delayed implantation. Acta Zool., **28**:1–136.

Johansson, I., and O. Venge. 1951. Relation of the mating interval to the occurrence of superfetation in the mink. Acta Zool., **32**:255–58.

Kirk, R. J. 1962. Effect of darkness on the mink reproductive cycle. Am. Fur Breeder, **35**:20–21.

Shackelford, R. M. 1948. Reproduction in the mink. The Honker (yearbook of the mink industry), pp. 163–64.

———. 1950. Genetics of the Ranch Mink. New York: Pillsbury Pub., Inc.

Discussion was deferred until after Dr. Orsini's paper.

U. B. BAEVSKY

The Effect of Embryonic Diapause on the Nuclei and Mitotic Activity of Mink and Rat Blastocysts

THE LITERATURE on mammalian embryos at the diapause (delayed implantation) stage is extremely scanty (Bischoff, 1854; Keibel, 1902; Patterson, 1913; Fischer, 1932; Hamlett, 1932; R. Enders and Pearson, 1943, 1946; Hansson, 1947; Baevsky, 1955, 1960, 1961; A. Enders, 1962). This is apparently the principal reason for the lack of unanimity as to whether development is continued during the diapause (*viz.*, differentiation and cell division in particular) or is completely blocked. It is claimed by some authors that development is only slowed up (Keibel, 1902; Sakurai, 1906, Fischer, 1932; Baevsky, 1955, 1960, 1961; A. Enders, 1962), whereas, according to others (Bischoff, 1854; Hamlett, 1932, 1935; Brambell, 1937), it is stopped altogether. Hamlett (1935) has even coined the term "discontinuous" for such a kind of embryonic development. This controversy can be solved by following the changes in size of the embryo during diapause, as well as the orientation, migration, and division of the cells in the embryo and trophoblast. Of particular interest in this connection are the changes of cell nuclei of the embryo and of their activity. This problem is likewise controversial. According to Hamlett (1935), the mitoses recorded by Keibel (1902) and Sakurai (1906) in the cells of the early embryo of the roe deer preclude any true embryonic diapause in this animal. However, it is claimed by Fischer (1932) that mitoses and delayed cell division do occur in the embryo of the European badger *during* the embryonic diapause. Mitoses have likewise been noted in the cells of the armadillo blastocyst (A. Enders, 1962). In this connection the relationship of

DR. U. B. BAEVSKY is a candidate of biological science in the Laboratory of Vertebrate Embryology, A. N. Severtzov Institute of Animal Morphology, Academy of Sciences of the U.S.S.R., Moscow.

mitotic activity to increase in size of cell nuclei of the sable and mink blastocysts is of particular interest (Baevsky, 1960, 1961).

It is well known that the change in nuclear size is linked not only with the reproductive activity of the nuclei but also with their functional activity in cell specialization. This may be exemplified by diurnal changes in nuclear diameter in the cells of the renal tubules (Kolb, 1961). Hence it seemed worthwhile to elucidate the significance and range of this increase.

The solution of this problem could presumably be facilitated by a comparative study of the phenomenon in different species with a dissimilar type of embryonic diapause, namely, obligate diapause reappearing in each reproductive cycle, and the facultative one apparent only under definite conditions.

Obligate diapause was studied in embryos of two species (sable and mink) belonging to two different genera (*Martes* and *Mustela*) of the family Mustelidae. A comparison of both these species seemed of interest, since their relative genetic relationship is contrasted by a great difference in the length of the diapause. In the sable (*Martes zibellina*) the diapause begins soon after mating, which takes place in July or the beginning of August and is completed in March. The diapause therefore lasts 7–7.5 months. In the mink (*Mustela vison*) 8–10 days after mating (March) the blastocysts in more than 98 per cent of the animals enter the diapause stage, the length of which may range up to 45 days (Hansson, 1947; R. K. Enders, 1952).

Obligate embryonic diapause, first described in the roe deer (*Capreolus capreolus*) by Bischoff (1845), bears no relationship to either favorable or unfavorable conditions, whereas, facultative diapause becomes apparent only under definite conditions—coincidence of time of cleavage and blastocyst formation with suckling of a concurrent litter. Both facultative and obligate diapauses consist of an increase in the length of gestation accompanying a delay of implantation. Lengthening of gestation in lactating mice was reported in 1887 by Lataste, by King (1913) in the rat, and more recently by Sharman (1955*a*, 1955*b*, 1959) in marsupials. Delayed implantation in mice has been reported (Enzmann, Saphir, and Pincus, 1932) to be accompanied by embryonic diapause, and similar observations have been made in rats by Baevsky (1961). In the albino rat (*Rattus norvegicus albinus*), which is the object of the present study, facultative diapause lasts up to 10 days. Its length increases with the number of sucklings (King, 1913; Baevsky, 1961). Of particular advantage to this study is the fact that the length and variability of the rat diapause approaches that of the mink. It seemed of greatest interest to find out whether or not the increase in size of the cell nuclei of the embryos depends on type of the embryonic diapause.

Materials and Methods

Thirty-six sable blastocysts, 101 mink blastocysts, and 75 rat blastocysts have been studied. In order that the topographic changes and displacement of the cell material could be followed, whole preparations were made by gradual dehydration to preserve the shape of the embryo. The preparations were oriented, and the blastocysts were pasted to thin cellophane plate (1.5–2 mm.), by means of pink oil and chloroform, and imbedded in balsam after supporting glass capillaries had been fastened to the coverslip. The diameter of the capillaries exceeded the sum of the blastocyst diameter and the thickness of the cellophane plate by a value less than the focal distance of the 60× objective. In this way the blastocyst pole facing the coverslip could be examined by oil immersion without disturbing the intact state of the blastocyst.

For karyometric observations a series of Ehrlich hematoxylin-stained paraffin sections (5–6 μ) was prepared. The measurements were made along the maximal diameter and perpendicular to it at ×900 and ×1350 magnification.

Experimental Results

During the 7–7.5-month embryonic diapause the size of the sable blastocyst greatly increases (Baevsky, 1955), and a marked increase can be noted in the monthly diameter (in September, 554, 722 μ; in October, 757, 932 μ; in November, 750, 805, 850, 905, 910, 1050, 1160, 1175 μ). Along with the increase in size of the blastocyst a change was noted in the shape of the embryonic knot (Pl. I, *1*, *2*, *3*), which is flat in September (Pl. I, *1*) but becomes convex and stratified in February (Pl. I, *3*). No mitotic figures have been found in the whole preparations and sections of the sable blastocyst so far studied. The nuclei in the embryonic knots of the three blastocysts examined in September, November, and February showed a marked increase in diameter that was dissimilar in rate. In the interval between September and November the nuclei exhibit an appreciable tendency toward an increase as computed from the differences of their mean arithmetic values (0.6 ± 0.3). The Student's distribution method not only confirms this observation but also proves that the nuclear increase is real ($t = 2.76$; $P = 0.012$). The size differences were significantly greater (2.52 ± 0.33) from November to February. Similar changes were found in the blastocysts of the mink with a much shorter embryonic diapause—up to 33–45 days (Hansson, 1947; R. K. Enders, 1952).

As regards its steady reappearance in every reproductive cycle, the diapause in the mink does not seem to be markedly different from that of the sable. Yet several cases have been reported by Hansson (less than

2 per cent out of 324) in which implantation in the mink has started immediately after migration of the blastocysts from the oviducts to the uterine horns (8–10 days after mating).

Thus, it appears that the major differences in embryonic diapause of the mink and the sable are due to the shorter and more variable length of this stage in the mink rather than to the diapause's being less obligate. The variations in length of the diapause might be connected with ovarian activity, which is resumed at different times prior to diapause completion. The resumption of activity of the gonads is manifested in superfetation (Shackelford, 1952) and distinctly affects the pattern of the

TABLE 1

INCREASE IN DIAMETER OF MINK BLASTOCYSTS WITH INCREASE IN AGE

Age (Days)	Number	Diameter (μ)	Average Diameter (μ)
9–10.......	9	182.3, 140.3, 168.3, 175.3, 203.4, 203.4, 238.5, 166.3, 203.4	175.9
11..........	6	196.4, 161.4, 231.5, 133.3, 196.4, 140.3	176.5
12..........	1	133.2	133.2
13..........	7	294.6, 385.8, 315.6, 336.7, 280.6, 308.6, 322.6	280.6
14–9........	5	252.5, 308.6, 294.6, 315.6, 277.0	289.7
14–21.......	8	243.8, 237.5, 262.5, 275.0, 250.0, 301.6, 294.6, 294.6	269.9
15–22.......	6	322.7, 343.7, 322.7, 336.7, 357.8, 364.8	341.6
18–20.......	4	470.0, 434.9, 392.8, 441.9	434.9
19–26.......	1	543.4	543.4
20..........	5	448.9, 396.3, 498.0, 484.0, 470.0	459.4
24..........	5	533.1, 308.6, 1234.6, 1087.3, 1164.4	865.5
25..........	3	736.5, 610.3, 638.3	661.7

changes undergone by the embryo during diapause. It will appear from the evidence presented below that, for this reason, no conclusive answer can be given as to whether changes occur in mink that might indicate development during embryonic diapause. The blastocysts show distinct changes in appearance, increasing in size with age, which results in an increase, although not regular, of their average diameter (Table 1).

Because of considerable variability in cell numbers in embryos of similar age (Table 2), cell counts of mink blastocysts of different ages do not help in determining whether development is continued or blocked during the diapause.

It might appear from the cell counts that at the diapause stage mitoses are absent—a conclusion strengthened by various indications of cell-division derangement, which are apparent in some preparations and especially distinct in sections of a blastocyst 11 days after mating. In the presumptive Rauber's layer of this embryo, closely adjacent pairs of nuclei appeared, while in the inner cell mass (embryoblast) was noted a group of 5 closely adjacent nuclei, one of which was similar in appearance to a normal nucleus. In addition to cytotomy derangements in the cells of the embryonic knot of mink blastocysts of different ages, some fragments of disintegrated nuclei often occur (Pl. II, *4;* as in sable, Pl. I, *3*). It may be assumed that the destructive effect of the conditions of embryonic diapause is confined to definite nuclei, probably in the reduplication or early prophase stage, at the moment the diapause sets in. This is suggested by the fact that according to some authors this phase is quite susceptible to various agents (for a review see Prokofieva-Belgovskaya, 1960). In our preparations all cell nuclei of the blastocysts studied were in the interphase, which favors the suggestion made above.

It will be noted that such events in blastocysts as the change in shape of the embryonic knot, definite orientation, and translocation of cells

TABLE 2

CELL COUNTS OF MINK BLASTOCYSTS

References	Blastocyst Age (Days)	No. Blasto-cysts	No. Cells
R. K. ENDERS	11	8	251, 230, 219, 211, 194, 173, 172, 144, 274, 266, 220, 196, 190, 62
	13	6	274, 266, 220, 196, 190, 62
U. B. BAEVSKY	11	1	300
	12	1	280–300
	18–20	1	273
	20–21	1	363

(during separation of the embryonic knot and differentiation of an additional number of trophoblast cells) are indicative of a delayed differentiation during diapause corresponding quite closely to generally adopted criteria (Grobstein, 1959). This process, however, suggests only a physiological activity of the nuclei, since in both the sable and the mink during diapause no mitotic figures have been found. It might therefore be suggested that within a certain range no strict correlation exists between these processes and mitotic activity.

Nuclear measurements during embryonic diapause in mink blastocysts (Fig. 1) corroborate the increase in nuclear size as recorded in sable blastocysts. It will be noted that this concerns either all or most of the nuclei. Although the differences in nuclear size persist at all three stages studied (11–12, 14–21, and 24 hours following mating) the minima, median, and maxima of the variation curves (ordinate-*p*-frequency of occurrence, abscissa-nuclear size in μ) are markedly shifted to the right. This suggests a synchronous increase in interphase nuclei, which is the most conclusive evidence of changes in the diapause embryo. The presence of a statistically significant increase in nuclear size (the difference between the first and the second stage, 0.95 ± 0.13, and between the second and the third stage, 3.39 ± 0.10) can hardly be attributed to nuclear preparation for mitosis, since in mammals cleavage is known to be of an asynchronous type.

Nuclear measurements at the stage of resumption of mitotic activity (24 days after mating, see Fig. 1) indicate that the number of nuclei with a two- to sixfold increase in nuclear volume is 83 per cent (152

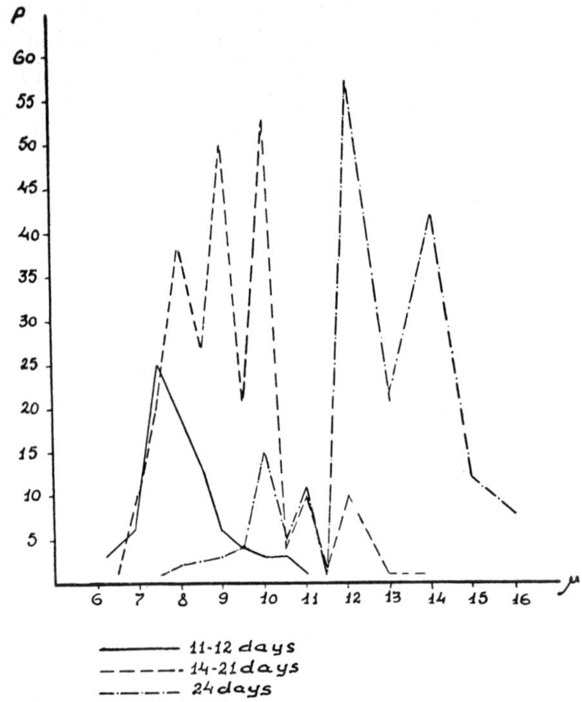

FIG. 1.—Curves of variation in nuclear size in mink blastocysts on days 11–12, 14–21, and 24 after mating (P = occurrence frequency).

nuclei out of 182) on the assumption that the minimal diameter of cell nucleus (immediately after division) is 8 μ (as a matter of fact, the minimum is even somewhat less; see Fig. 1).

The high percentage of large nuclei might have been accounted for by synchronization during diapause of the rhythm of mitotic activity. This assumption, however, does not prove valid if a comparison is made between the percentage of large nuclei (83 per cent) and that of dividing cells (2.8 per cent) as computed from the mitotic figures (4 per 144 cells of the embryonic disk of a 24-day blastocyst with Abercrombie's [1946] correction). It seems doubtful, therefore, that the increase in nuclear size mentioned above is linked only with preparation of the cells for mitotic activity. This conclusion complies with the resting state of the nuclei's (15–16 μ in diameter) attaining a sixfold increase in volume (20 per cent of the total number at the stage of resumed mitotic activity).

It will be of interest to note that the general pattern of cell-division blockade and of increase in nuclear size closely resembles that found by Brachet (1960) in the frog morula developing after in vitro treatment with ribonuclease. Obviously, no conclusions can as yet be made from this analogy, although the morphological and cytophysiological similarity of the end result is certainly interesting. At least, mass increase of nuclear size is by no means pathological, since mitotic activity is resumed at a stage when the nuclei, as evidenced from statistical treatment, are particularly large.

The sable and mink blastocysts are very similar, as seen from a study of their embryonic diapause. In both animals the size of the blastocyst increases (mostly because of an increase in the cavity of the embryo and extension of the trophoblast cells); the cells of the embryonic knot separate; they undergo partial differentiation, as manifested in orientation and displacement of the cells from the embryoblast into the trophoblast; and, finally, nuclear size increases. The stage of resumption of mitotic activity in both kinds of embryo is characterized by differentiation of the embryonic knot into ecto- and endoderm (Baevsky, 1955, 1961).

The results obtained with the *Martes* and *Mustela* blastocysts with obligate diapause have been compared with those found in the blastocysts of the albino rat. Diapause in the rat, although facultative, approaches in length and variability that of the mink. During embryonic diapause the diameter of the rat blastocyst markedly increases. The average length of 33 blastocysts at the 5-day stage is 94.3 μ, and that of 42 blastocysts of the 10–15-day stage is 105.6 μ. The effect of the conditions under which the diapause becomes manifest is quite apparent by the time of blastocyst formation. Unlike the blastocyst of similar age developing at the conventional rate, no regular cell orientation is to be noted in the embryoblast of a 5-day blastocyst in the diapause state or any cell differentiation into ecto- and endoderm (Pl. II, *5*, *6*). The influence of these conditions might also be revealed at an earlier stage, such as formation of the blastocyst cavity, or even in the course of cleavage of the ovum.

The increase in blastocyst size during diapause is accompanied by an extremely slow differentiation of the embryoblast as manifested in a gradual orientation of its cells parallel to the long axis of the blastocyst. As with sable and mink embryos, the rat embryoblast differentiates, upon completion of the diapause, into ecto- and endoderm (Baevsky,

1961). It will be noted that in the rat blastocyst, as in that of the mink, binucleate cells can be found, indicating a derangement of the cytotomic processes.

In view of the similarity between the initial and the final stage of diapause and of the changes undergone by the embryos during this period, it might have been assumed that nuclear changes are likewise similar. However, the results of karyometric observations proved quite unexpected. In fact, the cell nuclei did not change in size either at the onset or throughout the embryonic diapause. Moreover, nuclear size was similar in 5-day embryos either developing at the usual rate or in the diapause state (Fig. 2). Statistical treatment of the figures obtained

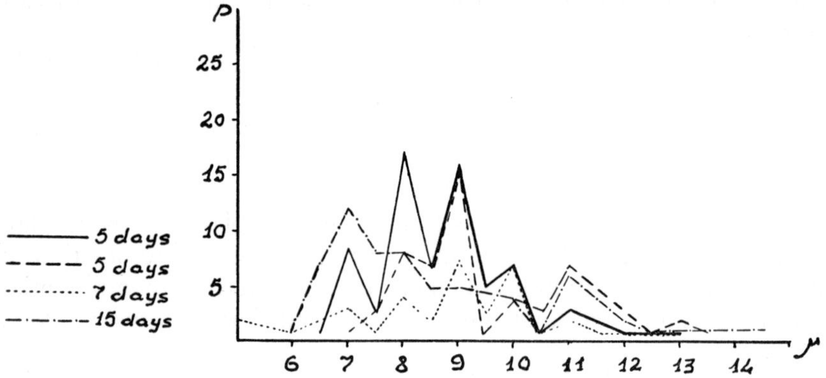

FIG. 2.—Curves of variation in nuclear size in rat blastocysts on day 5 (*solid line*) of development without diapause and on days 5, 7, and 15 after mating (diapause state).

confirmed these observations. The differences in nuclear size of the 5-day blastocyst in the diapause and in the non-diapause state proved non-significant (0.958 ± 0.542). A tendency toward an increase in nuclear size is apparent from a comparison of nuclei of diapause embryos 5 and 7 days after mating (0.760 ± 0.362). The differences in nuclear diameter on days 7 and 15 of diapause also proved non-significant (0.570 ± 0.377). The greatest differences were found between nuclei of trophoblast cells of diapause blastocysts and of those developing at the usual rate (0.760 ± 0.277). This tendency, however, was connected with a change in nuclear shape, which becomes more flattened with increase in the size of the blastocyst cavity.

This question might be answered more conclusively by measuring nuclear volumes. Yet it will be noted that experts in statistical treatment of biological data admit three degrees of accuracy in estimating statistical significance (Plokhinsky, 1961). It is assumed, indeed, that a twofold ratio of the difference to the error will suffice to acknowledge the first degree of significance. From this point of view the difference in nuclear size in 5- and 7-day diapause should be regarded as the first degree of significance with a probability of faithful judgment 0.9545. It is worth mentioning that the difference in nuclear state during obligate and facultative diapause becomes particularly distinct if one compares the variation curves of the mink (Fig. 1) and the rat (Fig. 2). Figure 2 illustrates the curves of nuclear size for 5-day development at the normal rate and for diapause blastocysts 5, 7, and 15 days after mating. The characteristic difference between the variation curves of the mink and the rat consists in the fact that in the mink the minima, median, and maxima are shifted to the right in accordance with the stage (age of the embryo), whereas in the rat no such shifts can be recorded. Here an almost perfect coincidence is noted between the frequency peaks of nuclei of a definite size in all four stages studied.

Discussion

The foregoing evidence indicates an appreciable increase in nuclear size with age in the sable and mink embryos, that is, in species with an obligate type of diapause, whereas nuclei of rat blastocysts exhibit only a certain tendency toward an increase in diameter. This is confirmed by statistical treatment, which shows that, in the embryos that undergo a diapause of the facultative type, the increase in nuclear size is statistically insignificant at three stages.

The significance of the increase (two- to sixfold) in nuclear volume during the embryonic diapause of the obligate type remains obscure and most probably cannot be conceived of as only a process that leads to preparation of mitotic divisions. This conclusion is based on the following: (1) mass (almost synchronous) increase in nuclear size toward the end of the diapause (in no less than 83 per cent of the total number) in animals that are known to have an asynchronous type of cleavage and (2) low mitotic activity (index = 2.8 per cent) after completion of the diapause. This indicates lack of actual synchronization of the mitotic rhythm, which might have been attributed to embryonic diapause.

The statistically insignificant increase in nuclear size in the rat embryo contradicts the notion that the phenomenon at issue is appropriate to diapauses of different types. And yet, the study of the sable, mink, and rat blastocyst in a state of profound inhibition has revealed some fundamentally similar characters as well. The time from blastocyst arrival in the uterine horns and up to implantation consists, in these species, of two distinct periods: (1) stoppage of mitotic activity and (2) resumption of that activity—disappearance of the Rauber's layer and beginning of differentiation of the embryoblast into ecto- and endoderm. Embryonic diapause coincides in time with the first period, and hence resumption of mitotic activity should be regarded as the time of completion of the diapause. If stoppage of mitotic activity and the time of its resumption (which are similar at the respective stages in all the species studied) are regarded as substantial features of diapause, it may be assumed that during this period no complete stoppage of development occurs. Symptoms of delayed differentiation are apparent from the orientation and displacement of cells, with the resulting separation of the embryonic knot, a change in its shape, and formation in the course of increase of the blastocyst cavity of an additional number of trophoblast cells. In the rat the second period is shorter than in the mink and sable, and resumption of mitotic activity is followed rapidly by implantation.

The problem at issue as to the limits of embryonic diapause is closely connected with the nature of this phenomenon, and it would be of interest to elucidate the connection between the increase in nuclear size noted above and the nature of inhibition (obligate diapause). Of particular interest is the active part played in the processes underlying diapause by the embryo itself.

Until recently, most students of the unusually long gestation period regarded the attachment of the embryo as the function of the maternal organism only (King, 1913; Kirkham, 1918; Mirskaia and Crew, 1930; Hain, 1934, 1935*a*, 1935*b*; Kirsch, 1938; Weichert, 1940, 1942; Shackelford, 1952; Courrier and Marois, 1954; A. Enders and Buchanan, 1959; Canivenc and Laffargue, 1958; Canivenc, Blanquet, and Bonnin-Laffargue, 1960; Ruffié, Bonnin-Laffargue, and Canivenc, 1961; Bonnin-Laffargue and Canivenc, 1961), although a quite opposite concept has also been advanced (Brambell, 1937). Even if Brambell's viewpoint cannot be accepted as a whole, it apparently implies that the active state and development processes in the embryo are not indifferent to the implantation process. This concept is corroborated by the fact that, under the conditions of superfetation involving changes in hormonal interrelations, the embryos of earlier ovulations either remain in the state of embryonic diapause or succumb. This point of view is strengthened by the persistence of a minimal length of the embryonic diapause (3 weeks) in the nine-banded armadillo in spite of ovariectomy. And yet, on the whole, the length of the embryonic diapause is greatly decreased by this experimental procedure (A. Enders and Buchanan, 1959)—from 14 to 18 weeks (Hamlett, 1932) to the minimum given above. Mention of the appreciable resistance of the sable embryonic diapause to light manipulation is also pertinent (Beliaev, Pereldik, and Portnova, 1951).

In this connection the comparison of nuclear size of blastocysts in species with a completely obligate diapause (sable), almost complete obligate diapause (mink), and a facultative diapause (rat) suggests the

PLATE I

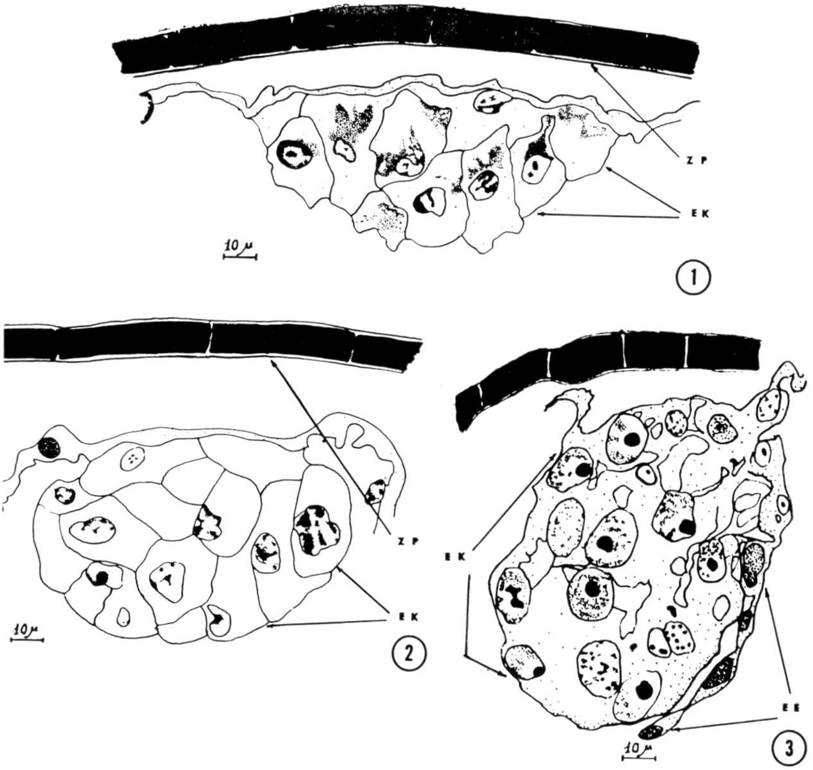

1, Section through embryonic knot of September sable blastocyst; *zp*, zona pellucida; *ek*, embryonic knot.

2, Section through embryonic knot of November sable blastocyst; *zp*, zona pellucida; *ek*, embryonic knot.

3, Section through embryonic knot of February sable blastocyst; *ek*, embryonic knot; *ee*, embryonic endoderm.

PLATE 2

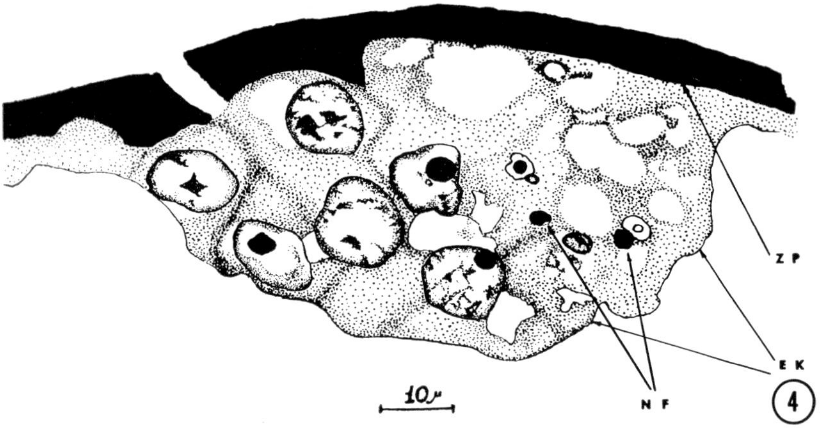

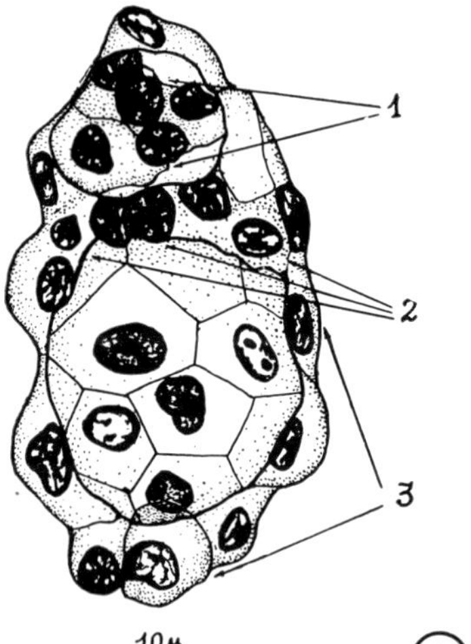

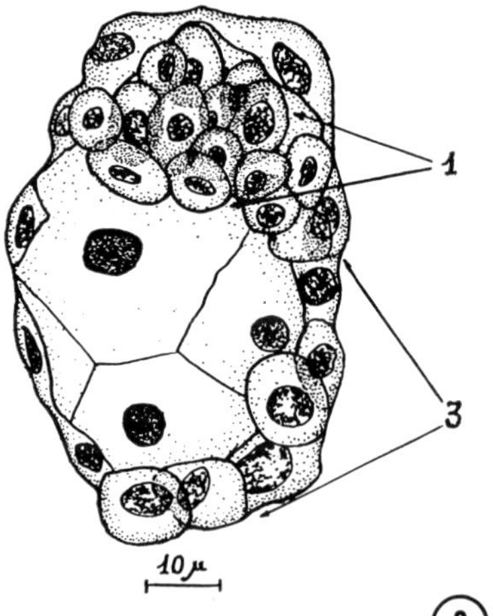

4, Section through embryonic knot of mink blastocyst (15 days after mating); *zp*, zona pellucida; *ek*, embryonic knot; *nf*, nuclear fragments.

5, Rat blastocyst (5 days after mating), development without diapause; *1*, ectoderm; *2*, endoderm; *3*, trophoblast.

6, Rat blastocyst (5 days after mating), diapause; *1*, embryoblast; *3*, trophoblast.

existence of some species with nuclear changes intermediate between both animal groups (with a facultative and an obligate diapause). Perhaps different ranges of nuclear changes can correspond to a different rate of obligate diapause. This might be manifest in a varying percentage of individuals with obligate diapause within a given species. Species with the so-called alternative gestation period, such as the roe deer (Prell, 1938; Stieve, 1950) and ermine (Deanesly, 1943; Watzka, 1940), might represent a link leading to the diapause of the mink type. From this point of view a series of animals with an increasing rate of obligate embryonic diapause could be listed that might be of genetic interest.

Summary

1. During obligate embryonic diapause in the sable (*Martes zibelina*) and mink (*Mustela vison*) an appreciable, statistically significant increase is noted in nuclear volume (in the mink a two- to sixfold one).

2. This nuclear increase is of mass (almost synchronous) character (not less than 83 per cent of the total number of nuclei) in animals with an asynchronous type of cleavage.

3. In the rat (*Rattus norvegicus albinus*) only a tendency toward an increase in nuclear volume is noted during facultative embryonic diapause. The increase is statistically insignificant.

4. During diapause of the facultative and obligate type at comparable stages of development no mitotic activity is apparent, although some symptoms of delayed differentiation of the embryoblast (inner cell mass) can be distinguished.

References

Abercrombie, M. 1946. Estimation of nuclear population from microtome sections. Anat. Rec., **94**:239.

Baevsky, U. B. 1955. On embryonic diapause in the sable. Doklady Akad. Nauk SSSR, **105**:866.

———. 1960*a*. Observations on changes in the blastocyst of albino rats during "lactation" diapause. Arkh. Anat. Histol. Embryol., **41**:14.

———. 1960*b*. Observations on some stages of intrauterine development of the sable. Trudy Inst. Morph. Jiv., **30**:246.

———. 1961. Some peculiarities of embryonic diapause in the mink (*Mustela vison* Schreb). Doklady Akad. Nauk SSSR, **139**:499.

Beliaev, D. K., N. S. Pereldik, and N. T. Portnova. 1951. Experimental reduction of the period of embryonic development in the sable. J. Obs. Biol., **12**:260.

Bischoff, T. L. W. 1854. Entwicklungsgeschichte des Rehes. Giessen, Germany.

Bonnin-Laffargue, M., and R. Canivenc. 1961. Étude de l'activité du blaireau européen *Meles meles* L. Mammalia, **25**:476.

BRACHET, J. 1960. The Biological Role of Ribonucleic Acids. New York: Academic Press.

BRAMBELL, F. W. R. 1937. The influence of lactation on the implantation of mammalian embryo. Am. J. Obstet. & Gynec., **33**:942.

CANIVENC, R., J. CROIZET, P. BLANQUET, and M. BONNIN-LAFFARGUE. 1960. Mesure de l'activité journalière du blaireau européen *Meles meles* L. Acad. Sci., **250**:1915–17.

CANIVENC, R., and M. LAFFARGUE. 1958. Action de différents équilibres hormonaux sur la phase de vie libre de l'œuf fécondé chez le blaireau européen (*Meles meles* L.). C.R. Soc. Biol., **152**:58.

COURRIER, R., and M. MAROIS. 1954. Retard de la nidation et du développement fœtal chez la ratte en hypothermy. Ann. Endocrin., **15**:738.

DANIEL, I. F. 1910. Observation on the period of gestation in white mice. J. Exp. Zool., **9**:865.

DEANESLY, R. 1943. Delayed implantation in the stoat (*Mustela erminea*). Nature, **151**:365.

ENDERS, A. C. 1961. Comparative studies on the endometrium of delayed implantation. Anat. Rec., **139**:483.

———. 1962. The structure of the armadillo blastocyst. J. Anat., **96**:39.

ENDERS, A. C., and G. D. BUCHANAN. 1959. Some effects of ovariectomy and injection of ovarian hormones in the armadillo. J. Endocrin., **19**:251.

ENDERS, R. K. 1952. Reproduction in the mink (*Mustela vison*). Proc. Am. Phil. Soc., **96**:691.

ENDERS, R. K., and O. P. PEARSON 1943. The blastocyst of the fisher. Anat. Rec., **85**:285.

ENZMANN, E. V., N. R. SAPHIR, and G. PINCUS. 1932. Delayed pregnancy in mice. Anat. Rec., **54**:325.

FISCHER, E. 1931. Die Entwicklungsgeschichte des Dachses und die Frage der Zwillingsbildung. Verh. Anat. Ges. Jena, **40**:22.

GROBSTEIN, C. 1959. Differentiation of vertebrate cells. In J. BRACHET and A. MIRSKY (eds.), The Cell. New York: Academic Press.

HAIN, A. M. 1934. The effect of suckling on the duration of pregnancy in the rat (Wistar albino). J. Exp. Biol., **2**:279.

———. 1935*a*. The effect (*a*) of litter-size on growth and (*b*) of estrone administered during lactation (rat). Quart. J. Exp. Physiol., **25**:303.

———. 1935*b*. The physiology of pregnancy in the rat, a hormonal investigation into the mechanism of parturition: Effect on the female rat of the ante-natal administration of estrin to the mother. *Ibid.*, p. 131.

HAMLETT, G. W. D. 1932. Observation on the embryology of badger. Anat. Rec., **53**:283.

———. 1935. Delayed implantation and discontinuous development in the mammals. Quart. Rev. Biol., **10**:432.

HANSSON, A. 1947. The physiology of reproduction in mink (*Mustela vison* Schreb) with special reference to delayed implantation. Acta Zool., **28**:1.

KEIBEL, F. 1902. Die Entwicklung des Rehes bis zur Anlage des Mesoblast. Arch. Anat. u. Physiol. Abt., **24**:293–314.

KING, J. L. 1913. Some anomalies in the gestation of albino rat. Biol. Bull., **24**:377.

———. 1938. Influence on the duration of gestation of injection of pregnancy urine extract in the rat before and after implantation. Am. J. Physiol., **122**: 455.

KIRKHAM, W. B. 1918. Observation on the relation between suckling and the rate of embryonic development in mice. J. Exp. Zool., **27**:49.

KIRSCH, R. E. 1938. A study on the control of length of gestation in rat with note on maintenance and termination of gestation. Am. J. Physiol., **122**:86.

KOLB, I. 1961. Karyometrische Untersuchungen zur Histophysiologie der Niere. V. Mitteilung Tagesrhythmische Anderungen der Kerngrossen in der Nierenepithelie der Ratte. Anat. Anz., **110**:270.

LATASTE, F. 1887. Recherches de zooéthique sur les mammifères de l'ordre des rongeurs. Act. Soc. Linn. Bordeaux, **40**:202.

MIRSKAIA, L., and F. A. E. CREW. 1931. On the pregnancy rate in the lactating mouse and the effect of suckling on the duration of pregnancy. Proc. Roy. Soc. Edinburgh, **51**:1.

PATTERSON, J. T. 1913. Polyembryonic development in *Tatusia novemcincta*. J. Morphol., **24**:559.

PLOKHINSKY, N. A. 1961. Biometry. Novosibirsk: Izd. SO AN SSSR.

PRELL, H. L. 1938. Die Tragzeit des Rehes: Ein historischer Ruckblick.

PROKOFIEVA-BELGOVSKAYA, A. A. 1960. Ionizing radiation and heredity: The structure of the chromosome. In The Résumés of Science. Biol. Sciences, **3**:7.

RUFFIÉ, A., M. BONNIN-LAFFARGUE, and R. CANIVENC. 1961. Les taux du prégnandiol urinaire au cours de la grossesse chez le blaireau européen, *Meles meles* L. C. R. Soc. Biol., **155**:759.

SAKURAI, T. 1906. Normentafel zur Entwicklungsgeschichte des Rehes. In Normentaf. zur Entwicklungsgeschichte der Wirbeltiere, No. 6.

SHACKELFORD, R. M. 1952. Superfetation in the ranch mink. Am. Naturalist, **86**:311.

SHARMAN, G. B. 1955*a*. Studies on marsupial reproduction. 3. Normal and delayed pregnancy in *Setonix brachyurus*. Aust. J. Zool., **3**:56.

———. 1955*b*. Studies on marsupial reproduction. 4. Delayed birth in *Protemnodon eugenii*. *Ibid*., p. 156.

———. 1959. Marsupial reproduction. Monog. Biol., **8**:332.

STIEVE, H. 1950. Anatomische-biologische Untersuchungen über die Fortpflanzungstatigkeit des europaischen Rehes. Ztschr. Mikro-anat. Forsch., **55**:427.

WATZKA, M. 1940. Mikroskopisch-anatomische Untersuchungen über Ranzeit und Tragdauer des Hermelins (*Putorius ermineus*). Ztschr. Mikro-anat. Forsch., **48**:359.

WEICHERT, C. K. 1940. The experimental shortening of delayed pregnancy in the albino rat. Anat. Rec., **77**:31.

———. 1942. The experimental control of prolonged pregnancy in the lactating rat by means of estrogen. *Ibid*., **83**:1.

———. 1943. Effect of environmental stilbestrol in shortening prolonged gestation in the lactating rat. Proc. Soc. Exp. Biol. & Med., **53**:203.

Dr. Baevsky was unable to be present at the symposium. A summary of his paper was read, but no discussion was held.

MARGARET WARD ORSINI

Morphological Evidence on the Intrauterine Career of the Ovum

THE PRESENT experiments on the hamster demonstrate a relatively precise and consistent correlation between morphological events and postfertilization age. This presentation describes the morphological correlates of the late preimplantation period, early and late implantation, and development up to vascularization of the chorioallantoic placenta.

In our previous work with the hamster (Orsini and Meyer, 1959; Prasad, Orsini, and Meyer, 1960; Orsini and Meyer, 1962) we have shown that progesterone alone is the necessary and sufficient ovarian contribution for normal implantation. Exogenous progesterone is adequate for the normal succession of these events in females ovariectomized, ovariectomized and adrenalectomized, or hypophysectomized. No delay in implantation has ever been indicated. Evidence has only recently been obtained, however, of the role of progesterone in the preimplantation period, and these experiments form a part of the present presentation.

Development of the benzyl-benzoate clearing technique has provided a useful tool for visualization of the morphology of both normal and abnormal development. The biochemical nature and fine structure of the opaque areas characterizing the conceptual sites seen in the cleared uteri will be discussed.

Additional information is presented on the period of first contact of the ovum with the uterus. Study of this immediate preimplantation period has been stimulated by the work of Alexandre Psychoyos (1960*a*, 1960*b*, 1961), who, by injection of Geigy blue into the blood stream, demonstrated discretely spaced sites of increased capillary permeability in the rat uterus prior to decidualization. He believed this extravasation of dye to be the first indication of nidation, claiming that it first appears

DR. MARGARET WARD ORSINI is a research associate in the Department of Anatomy, the University of Wisconsin, Madison.

when the rat blastocyst is free of the zona pellucida but unattached to the uterine epithelium.

Although the hamster is my main experimental animal, observations from comparable periods in mouse, rabbit, and rat will be cited when pertinent.

Material and Methods

All hamsters used were of known reproductive history. The age of development of all ova is given in terms of developmental age determined by the relation of the time of mating to the time of ovulation. When mating occurs prior to ovulation, developmental and ovulation age coincide. All material for the present study is from matings *prior* to ovulation, since matings after ovulation are known to result in low fertility (Ward, 1946, 1948*a*, 1948*b*).

Our hamsters are maintained in two separate colonies in air-conditioned rooms. The normal colony quarters receive outside light. Here estrus begins in the late afternoon or evening prior to the postestrous discharge, the peak of ovulatory activity is approximately at 1:00 A.M. of the day of the postestrous discharge, and implantation begins on day 5 subsequent to mating, or at 4 days and 4–6 hours developmental age. Parturition occurs on day 16 following mating.

In the LD colony (reversed light and dark, with light from 10:00 P.M. to 10:00 A.M.), estrus occurs from 9:00 A.M. on. Ovulation is occurring by 5:00 P.M., and developmental age is calculated from this time. Implantation begins at approximately 5:00–8:00 P.M. on day 4 following mating, that is, at 4 days and 0–4 hours developmental age.

All females of breeding age are checked daily for the vaginal phenomena characterizing the estrous cycle, pregnancy, etc. (Orsini, 1961). Only females that have displayed at least two normal cycles and weigh 80 gm. or more are mated. Weights are recorded daily of pregnant, lactating, experimental, and all cycling animals in postestrum. Females are placed with males, and matings are observed in the LD colony, usually beginning at 9:00–10:00 A.M. The females in the normal colony are put with males in the late afternoon or evening for observed copulation. All matings are checked by sperm smears.

At autopsy the animal is exsanguinated; the reproductive tract is cleared by the benzyl-benzoate technique and studied by oblique illumination. This technique has been described in detail in the *Journal of Reproduction and Fertility* (Orsini, 1962*a*, 1962*b*).

To reveal the localized regions of increased capillary permeability, $\frac{1}{4}$ cc. of 1 per cent Pontamine Blue in saline is injected into the femoral vein of an anesthetized hamster 15 minutes prior to autopsy.

Uteri are flushed with physiological saline, using a 1-cc. hypodermic syringe with a 27-gage needle. Repeated flushings are necessary in later stages. Ovariectomies are performed by the dorsal approach using a ×5 magnifying head loop. A small hemostat is placed on the ovarian blood vessels, the surface of the bursa is opened and pulled back, and the remaining bursa, ovary, and immediately surrounding fat are cut out. No vascular ligations are made.

Observations

PREIMPLANTATION

Because of their large size, rabbit blastocysts may be followed through oviduct and uterus in cleared material. (All rabbit tracts were dated from the time of artificial insemination; the previous mating history was unknown.) At 4 days and 6 hours the ova are clumped in the upper portion of the uterus, visible only under a dissecting microscope. By 5 days they are distributing along the uterus, and by 5 days and 22 hours they are "spaced" (Pl. I, *1*). Evidence of the high preimplantation loss of conceptuses is apparent, indicated by differences in size between littermate blastocysts in these early stages (Pl. I, *3*) and by resorption sites later (Pl. I, *2*; Table 1).

In the mouse (material furnished by H. M. Bruce of the National Institute for Medical Research, Mill Hill, England) preimplantation blastocysts are frequently visible within the cleared uteri. They appear as minute, slightly refractile bodies within the lumen of the uterus, detectable only by use of the dissecting microscope; these are extremely difficult to photograph. A cleared uterus from a mouse killed at 10:30 A.M. on day 4 after a copulation plug was discovered shows such an unimplanted ovum (Pl. I, *5*).

Plate II, 7, shows sections from mouse C77, killed at 11:30 A.M. on day 4 after a morning parturition—mating had already taken place by the time the litter was discovered. Two clumps of refractile bodies were visible in the gross specimen; sections of this portion of the uterus reveal seven blastocysts in two separate clumps. Obviously, spacing had not yet taken place. Note that no uterine response to the presence of these unimplanted blastocysts is visible.

Up to this time, it has proved impossible to detect the unimplanted ova in guinea pigs, rats, and hamsters. Probably preimplantation blastocysts are recognizable only when the uterus is delicate and thin, as in the mouse, or in forms like the rabbit, subject to marked preimplantation growth of the blastocyst.

Stimulated by the work of Psychoyos, an attempt was made to determine the time of loss of the zona pellucida from ova in four different physiological states: normal pregnant hamsters, hamsters made pseudopregnant by mating with vasectomized males, normally cycling unbred hamsters, and pregnant hamsters castrated on day 2 after pregnancy but given *no* exogenous hormone. The data indicating the presence or absence of the zona pellucida surrounding the flushed ova are shown in Table 2. The zona is seen to be lost *late* on day 3 or early on day 4 in normal pregnancy and in pseudopregnancy. It is *not lost* from ova of cycling unbred females or of females castrated on day 2 after mating. Development of morulae and blastocysts was observed in the ova of the castrate animals. Two of the twenty-three hamsters in the castrate group were castrated on day 3 after mating; here, too, the zona was retained.

TABLE 1

RABBIT MATERIAL AVAILABLE FOR STUDY OF UTERINE DEVELOPMENT

Age (Post-artificial Insemination)	Gross Appearance of Uterine Horns	Observations in Cleared Uterus
4 days and 6 hours	0	0.1–0.4-mm. diam., 11 ova, clustered at ovarian end of uterus; ova difficult to see
5 days	0	8 ova—spacing along uterus; difficult to see
5 days and 22 hours	0	9 ova—one 1-mm., rest 3-mm. diam.; apparently "spaced"; now visible to naked eye in cleared specimen
6 days and 1 hour	0	10 ova
6 days and 21 hours	3	3 in one horn
	0	1 in other
7 days and 1 hour	1	2 in one horn, 4 in other
	0	4 variation in development
7 days and 22 hours	3	3 in one horn
	4	4 in other
8 days and 2 hours	3	3 plus 1 degenerating site
	4	4 plus 3 degenerating sites
9 days	6	6—heart visible; all normal
	4	4

All stages of "dissolution" of the zona were encountered in the first two groups (normal pregnant and pseudopregnant females), including expansion and thinning with the assumption of an irregular shape, then breaking of the expanded zona. No indication of such changes was encountered in the castrate or cycling groups. The foregoing data indicate that loss of the zona pellucida from the hamster ovum may well be progesterone dependent.

Another point of interest in the flushing experiments was the great difference in ease of recovery of ova, dependent upon their developmental age. Late on day 3 and very early on day 4, all ova recovered were found within the first milliliter of flushing fluid, and usually within the first drop. The number of ova recovered closely paralleled the number of corpora (the ease of counting corpora lutea varies among animals). Then, suddenly, at approximately the middle of day 4 (at 3 days and 10 hours developmental age) it becomes almost impossible to recover ova, even by flushing four times. The number of ova recovered drops sharply. The time of appearance of this refractory period varies among individuals; I have obtained blastocysts as late as 3 days and 19 hours from the LD colony, approximately 94 hours postcoitus, and at

TABLE 2

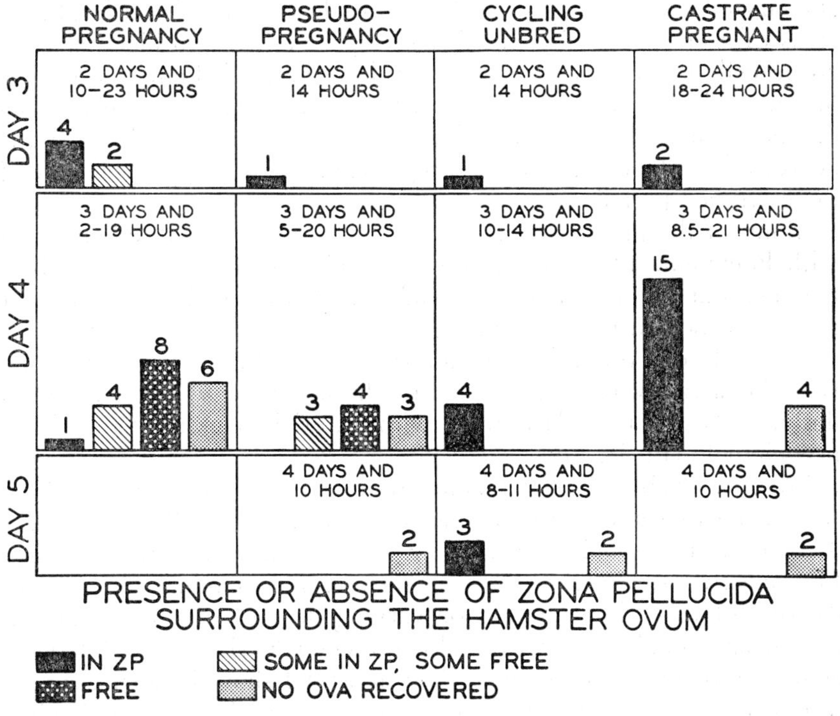

3 days and 13 hours from the normal colony. Hamilton and Samuel (1956) stated that they were unable to flush out uterine blastocysts after 88.5 hours postcoitus. This refractory state may indicate the period of initial contact between blastocyst and uterus.

An experimental approach to this question would be to establish the effect of castration without any exogenous progesterone at this time. One pilot study has been made. Five animals were castrated between 3 days and 9.5–16.5 hours and autopsied 24 hours later. Four of the five did show luminal changes (Orsini, 1962) indicative of early implantation; three of these showed minute abnormal opacities within these conceptual regions displaying luminal changes. Only one such area from one animal has been sectioned to date. Here the blastocyst is in superficial contact with the uterine epithelium (Pl. II, 7). Development of the blastocyst has progressed to the clear delineation of enlarged giant cells at the abembryonic pole; these are filled with phagocytosed material. The number of giant cells is not comparable to the number found in the normal site at comparable autopsy age, and the inner cell mass is necrotic.

The area of decidua present is slightly less than that of the normal at comparable autopsy age, and the *stage* of development is earlier. Large areas of necrosis are obvious. A large space filled with blood and necrotic cells is obvious immediately below the epithelium; the uterine lumen is filled with blood. No real implantation has taken place, and degeneration is obvious in both blastocyst and uterus, although the degree of development of both is representative of a stage well beyond the castration period.

Many of the previously mentioned flushed series had been injected with Pontamine Blue. No castrate or cycling tract ever showed blue regions; four of the 12 injected pseudopregnant tracts did. No pregnant tract ever showed Pontamine Blue–positive regions prior to 3 days and 17 hours. In one tract, from an animal killed at 3 days and 18.5 hours, two blue areas were apparent in each horn (Pl. II, 9). One horn, on flushing, showed two blastocysts, with material adherent to the abembryonic pole (Pl. II, *10*).

Presence or absence of Pontamine Blue areas and uterine morphology were compared among thirty-nine pregnant animals killed between 3 days and 17 hours and 4 days. Twenty-six animals did show Pontamine Blue–positive regions; in each of such regions luminal changes indicative of early implantation or varying degrees of opacity indicative of later implantation were also present (Pl. III, *11* and *14*). Four animals showing no Pontamine Blue areas did show luminal changes. Variation in stage of development was observed among individual animals mated and killed at identical times; variation within individual animals is also indicated by different degrees of development of opacity within the blue regions.

The intensity of the Pontamine Blue varies with the stage of implantation; it is extremely pale in the early stages and becomes more obvious and prominent in advanced stages of implantation. It is retained throughout the clearing process. It does tend to obscure the fine morphology of the uterus in the earliest stages but is extremely valuable in enabling the observer to obtain desired areas for special techniques.

IMPLANTATION

The earliest morphological indication of implantation is the appearance of distinct localized luminal changes within the uterus. If one views such a uterus from its *lateral* aspect, distinct "conceptual" regions of relatively clear endometrium are clearly distinguishable from the intergestational areas marked by prominent undulation of the uterine lumen (Pl. II, *9*; Pl. III, *13*). In such clear "conceptual" areas the uterine lumen may be seen as a fine straight line passing through the clear chamber; it is most easily observed from the antimesometrial aspect.

Then, at the center of the clear conceptual region, at a point corresponding to the antimesometrial surface of the endometrium, an extremely fine refractile series of granules or vesicles appears. These resemble those marking the site of the blastocyst in the preimplantation stage in the mouse, but they are now encircled by a changed, clear endometrium. These fine particles correspond in size to dust particles, and it is only by careful focusing up and down that the observer can determine that these minute specks lie within the endometrium.

From their first appearance the specks enlarge, and a slight cloudiness may be seen to extend into the adjacent endometrium. The specks fuse into a slightly opaque dot (Pl. III, *14*); viewing it from its antimesometrial or mesometrial aspect one can see that this is made up of two parts —one on each lateral aspect of the lumen (Pl. III, *13*). As this slight opacity continues to enlarge, it gradually becomes more and more opaque. By 4 days and 12–14 hours it is a small, pale shield, slightly concave at its mesometrial surface, which apparently borders on the lumen (Pl. IV, *17*).

Now, what histological stages of development are correlated with these implantation stages?

Tracts with luminal changes (Pl. II, *9*; Pl. III, *11*) indicating conceptual areas show young blastocysts in contact with the uterine epithelium (Pl. II, *8*; Pl. III, *12*). The intimacy of this contact varies from entirely superficial to those with penetration of abembryonic cell processes between the epithelial cells. Vascular engorgement is present in the subepithelial region, slight enlargement of the immediate subepithelial connective-tissue cells foreshadows decidual changes, but no true decidua is present. Some of these tracts had shown positive Pontamine Blue regions, so Pontamine Blue does indicate conceptual areas prior to decidualization.

When opacity appears in the gross cleared uterus, decidualization appears histologically. The contact of the blastocyst is now more extensive, and the development of the blastocyst itself has advanced (Pl. III, *14*, *15*, *16*).

Among the hamster tracts collected for these early periods of implantation, there is variation in degree of development among animals mated and killed at the same time, and even within individual tracts. The same variation is paralleled by intensity of Pontamine Blue as well. In subsequent development the opacity marking the conceptual regions increases in intensity and follows a definite morphological pattern, which makes it possible to distinguish between these days of early development. By 5 days and 12 hours (Pl. IV, *18*) the opacity is whiter and the mesometrial surface becomes convex toward the mesometrium. Slight uterine swelling is now grossly visible at the conceptual areas. By 6 days and 12 hours (Pl. IV, *19*) the opacity fills almost all the conceptual swelling, leaving a narrow non-opaque rim. It is obviously hollow at the center and has a pattern of dense antimesometrial wings within the opacity itself. By 7 days and 12 hours (Pl. IV, *20*) the antimesometrial portion begins to clear, and by 8 days and 12 hours (Pl. IV, *21*) the antimesometrial half of the conceptual swelling is clear. Body form is now being established in the embryo, and the fetus is clearly distinguishable within the greatly enlarging extraembryonic cavity. In the latter part of this day the chorioallantoic circulation is established, and at this time opacity begins to appear within the heart.

The foregoing presents a survey of the normal development and also of controls for experimental work.

This last summer, investigation of the biochemistry and fine structure of the opacities was begun. Association with decidua was suggested by the developmental pattern; association with glycogen was suspected because of similar opacity in the muscularis of the uterus and in the developing fetal heart (Pl. V, *26;* Pl. VI, *27*) and liver. It is relatively easy to dissect out the opaque mass marking the conceptual region from the rest of the uterus during days 6 and 7. Biochemical analyses of such pooled opacities versus the remainder of the uterus were carried out by Mr. George Foster and Dr. Frank Strong, of the Department of Biochemistry at the University of Wisconsin, and revealed that the amount of glycogen per gram of tissue in the opacities is thirty times that in the uterus, phospholipids are in the ratio of 6 to 1 and protein content is identical; both are negative for pentoses.

Dr. David Slautterback, of the Anatomy Department, studied with the electron microscope opacities from pregnant females and deciduomata with developmental ages of 5 days and 17 hours and 6 days and 12 hours. He reports the presence in both of masses of particulate glycogen—so judged by the appearance of 350 A unit particles of irregular shape and high density, which stain preferentially with lead.

Parallel stages of developmental morphology are found in the rat (Pl.

V, *22–26*), mouse (Pl. III, *13*), and guinea pig (Pl. VI, *27*), but the opacity follows a slightly different pattern in each species.

In experimental studies of early implantation, use of primiparous animals is highly desirable. Pigmentation resulting from previous pregnancies (Pl. IV, *20*) tends to obscure detail in multiparous animals. Besides the prominent placental scars at the uterine-mesometrial junction, diffuse pigment is present throughout the endometrium, and at most previous conceptual sites a fine circumferential ring of pigment marks the region of the decidua parietalis. This pigment *does* seem to affect the site of subsequent litters; in all parous stages studied the "implantation-placentation" site is always between the prominent placental scars; and, although by late gestation such scars may appear above the conceptual swelling, the main vascular supply never coincides with a previous scar.

The presence of such pigment in concentrated zones within tracts of experimental primiparous animals indicates attempted implantation. In the material used to determine the effect of varying levels of progesterone on implantation in castrate hamsters, all stages of implantation from normal sites through resorptions appearing as small white opacities of abnormal pattern to such discrete masses of pigment were encountered at the .0625 level (Pl. I, *4*; Pl. VI, *28*).

Stages of resorption are also encountered in tracts of normally pregnant animals (Pl. IV, *19* and *21*). Such stages are often not visible grossly but are obvious in the cleared specimen.

Now what is the effect of castration at various stages of gestation? From previous work (Prasad, Orsini, and Meyer, 1960; Orsini and Meyer, 1959; Orsini and Meyer, 1962) we know that castration in the preimplantation period with 2–4 mg. or less of progesterone daily allows normal implantation. I have been asked whether such animals could carry their litters to term. Of thirteen animals, castrated during day 2 of pregnancy and given 4 mg. of progesterone daily, ten had living young at autopsy approximately 24 hours prior to expected parturition, two were not pregnant, one died with a ruptured uterus on day 15, and one of the ten living had living young ruptured into the peritoneal cavity.

Three others were castrated at this same period and were given 2 mg. of progesterone daily. One was not pregnant, one had five living young 24 hours prior to parturition, and the third showed resorption of the entire litter.

Nine hamsters were castrated at periods varying from 9 days and 13 hours to 11 days and 12 hours. All had some living young on day 15.

Castration at 4 days and 19–20 hours in three animals (two given 4 mg. and one given 2 mg.) resulted in no survival, although development continued for some time.

Two were castrated during day 6; one at 5 days and 13 hours given 2 mg. daily showed complete resorption, the other castrated at 5 days and 18 hours and given 4 mg. daily had ten living young on day 15. Castration at 6 days and 12 hours with 2 mg. of progesterone resulted in abortion on days 12–13 (1 case). Castration at 8 days and 14 hours with 4 mg. progesterone resulted in abortion on day 13.

Additional material will be required to elucidate these findings, but it does appear that pregnancy can be maintained by progesterone alone after castration in the preimplantation period or in the second half of gestation. This is opposed to the earlier findings of Klein (1938), who stated that estrogen as well as progesterone was required to maintain pregnancy. This preliminary data also suggests varying needs during gestation, or perhaps critical developmental periods, during which the resistance to any "stress" may be lowered.

Castration of pregnant females without exogenous progesterone results in almost immediate external vaginal bleeding. Tracts from such animals show obvious abnormalities on clearing and dark areas at autopsy. The opacities of early implantation, 24–48 hours after castration at 4 days and 12 hours are pale, and the shape is obviously abnormal (Pl. VI, *29* and *30*). In later stages of gestation by 24 hours after castration the conceptual area appears to be sloughing off from the endometrium.

SUMMARY

1. Unattached uterine blastocysts are visible within the cleared uteri of mouse and rabbit.

2. Loss of the zona pellucida from the hamster ova is associated with the presence of progesterone.

3. Exact correlation with developmental age of presence or absence of the zona pellucida, Pontamine Blue reaction, first "attachment" of the blastocyst, and uterine histology is definitely suggested. Free morulae and blastocysts can be flushed from the uterus in the early part of day 4 of gestation, prior to appearance of Pontamine Blue regions. Difficulty in recovery of ova by flushing develops at 3 days and 10–12 hours. The first Pontamine Blue–positive uteri are recovered at 3 days and 17 hours. Luminal changes indicate conceptual areas at the same time as does the reaction to Pontamine Blue. Histological sections from such uteri show contact between the young blastocyst and the uterine epithelium. No decidua is present in these early stages.

4. Later stages of implantation appear as opaque conceptual areas in the cleared uteri. Decidual development accompanies and parallels the development of opacity. The pattern of the conceptual opacity follows a definite continued development, which characterizes the stages of pregnancy of days 5–9. Abnormalities in the opacity are associated with

degeneration histologically. Biochemical and electron microscope studies of the conceptual opaque regions of days 6 and 7 of gestation do indicate association with high glycogen content.

5. Use of the physiological technique of Pontamine Blue injection and of the benzyl-benzoate clearing techniques provides visualization of normal and abnormal implantation sites. The clearing technique is also of value in teratological studies and in experimental studies dealing with presence or absence of nidation.

ACKNOWLEDGMENTS

This research was supported by the National Institutes of Health (H-4202) and by the NIH General Research Support Grant of the University of Wisconsin.

The author is indebted to Dr. Harland W. Mossman, of the Department of Anatomy, University of Wisconsin, for editorial criticism in the preparation of the manuscript and to Mrs. Ruth Zevnik and Miss Jo Jennings for technical aid in preparation of the material.

REFERENCES

HAMILTON, W. J., and D. M. SAMUEL. 1956. The early development of the golden hamster (*Cricetus auratus*). J. Anat., **90**:395–416.

KLEIN, M. 1938. Relation between the uterus and the ovaries in the pregnant hamster. Proc. Roy. Soc. London, B, **125**:348–64.

ORSINI, M. W. 1961. The external vaginal phenomena characterizing the stages of the estrous cycle, pregnancy, pseudopregnancy, lactation, and the anestrous hamster, *Mesocricetus auratus* Waterhouse. Proc. Animal Care Panel, **11**:193–206.

———. 1962*a*. Technique of preparation, study and photography of benzyl-benzoate cleared material for embryological studies. J. Reprod. & Fertil., **3**:283–87.

———. 1962*b*. Study of ova-implantation in the hamster, rat, mouse, guinea pig and rabbit in cleared uterine tracts. J. Reprod. & Steril., **3**:278–93.

ORSINI, M. W., and R. K. MEYER. 1959. Implantation of the castrate hamster in the absence of exogenous estrogen. Anat. Rec., **134**:619–20.

———. 1962. Effect of varying doses of progesterone on implantation in the ovariectomized hamster. Proc. Soc. Exp. Biol. & Med., **110**:713–15.

PRASAD, M. R. N., M. W. ORSINI, and R. K. MEYER. 1960. Nidation in progesterone-treated, estrogen-deficient hamsters, *Mesocricetus auratus* (Waterhouse). Proc. Soc. Exp. Biol. & Med., **104**:48–51.

PSYCHOYOS, A. 1960*a*. La réaction déciduale est précédée de modifications précoces de la perméabilité capillaire de l'utérus. Comp. rend. Séances Soc. Biol., **154**:1384.

———. 1960*b*. Nouvelle contribution à l'étude de la nidation de l'œuf chez la ratte. Compt. rend. Séances Acad. Sci., **251**:3073–75.

———. 1961. Perméabilité capillaire et décidualization utérine. *Ibid.*, **252**:1515.

WARD, M. C. 1946. A study of the estrous cycle and the breeding of the golden hamster, *Cricetus auratus*. Anat. Rec., **94**:139.

———. 1948. The early development and implantation of the golden hamster, *Cricetus auratus*, and the associated endometrial changes. Am. J. Anat., **82**: 231–76.

DISCUSSION (*Chairman:* E. W. DEMPSEY)

KREHBIEL: Dr. Orsini stated that she got the Pontamine Blue reaction in pseudopregnant uteri.

ORSINI: I have injected, with Pontamine Blue, many pseudopregnant hamsters that had been stimulated for decidualization; such tracts are evenly positive at the decidual regions. However, I was extremely surprised when I found that 4 of the 12 pseudopregnant animals injected with Pontamine Blue showed a positive reaction when they had received no stimulus for decidualization. I serially sectioned one of the blue regions from such an animal killed at 3 days and 11 hours; I had flushed the other horn, which also showed three blue regions, and recovered three nude ova. The sections showed one ova, free of its zona, in a region of the uterus. It looked as though it were attempting to implant. The male had been vasectomized many months prior to this mating, had been used to induce pseudopregnancy in a number of females, and was not fertile. I do not believe that this ovum would have "induced" further changes. I do believe it had "induced" luminal changes and the Pontamine Blue reaction. I think that it would have degenerated, but the very close similarity to early attachment is startling. This is the only sectioned area from the four animals. I must section more before any conclusions can be made.

SHARMAN: How many days postovulation?

ORSINI: Three days and 11 hours postovulation.

ALDEN: You mentioned the appearance of pseudopregnancy. Was the zona disappearing? Are you willing to relate this to the appearance of abembryonic trophoblast cells?

ORSINI: I simply flushed the blastocysts free from the uterus. Those which I flushed free at the time when Pontamine Blue showed, 3 days and 18.5 hours, had a ragged abembryonic edge.

ALDEN: I wonder whether you have added to your earlier work the disappearance of zona pellucida in relationship to Pontamine Blue. Does the Pontamine Blue reaction precede the disappearance of the zona?

ORSINI: I never found Pontamine Blue areas before the disappearance of the zona pellucida.

NOYES: Would fixation dissolve the zona?

ORSINI: The zona preserves well. I do not think the zona will come

PLATE I

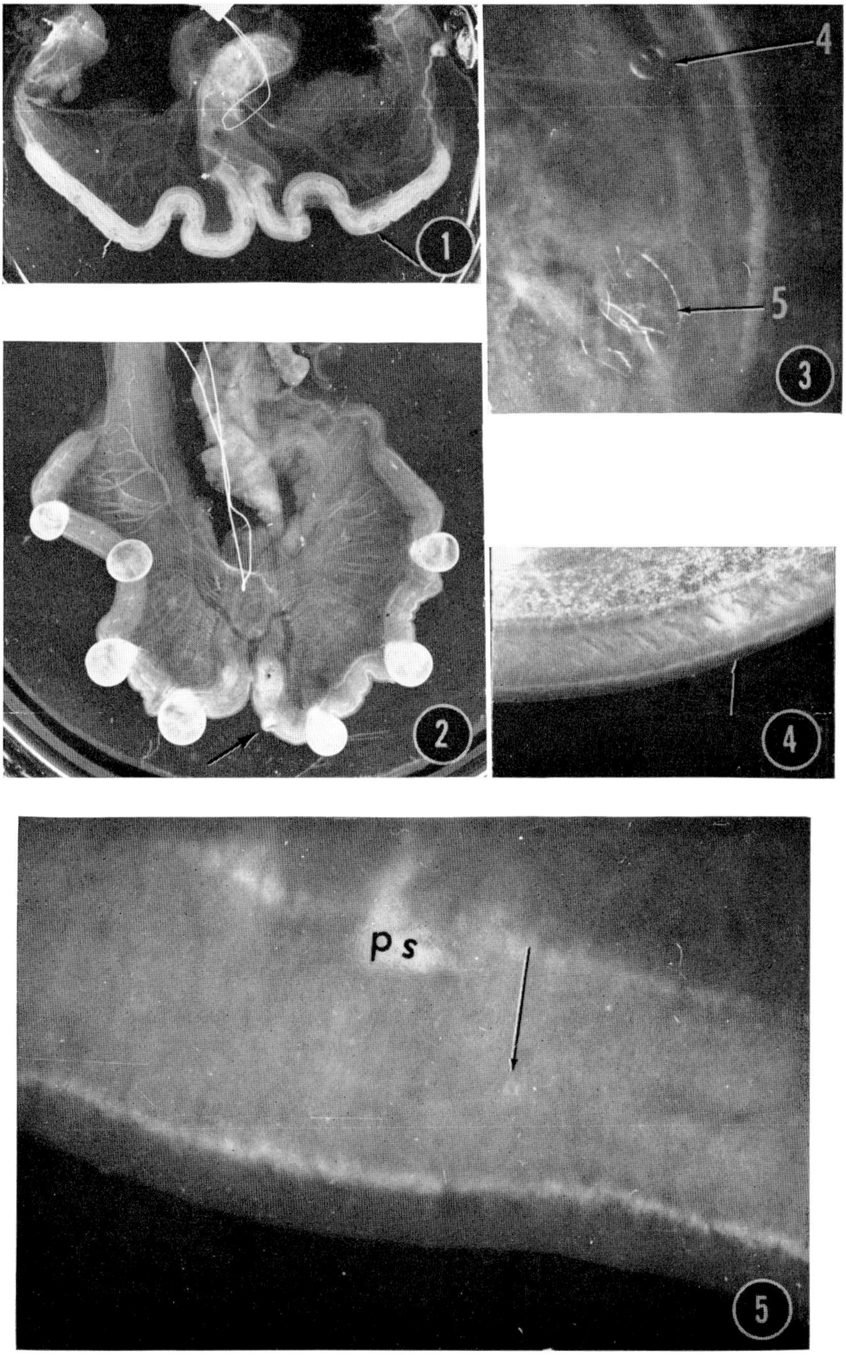

PLATE I

Plates I–VI, except *10*, are of material cleared through the benzyl-benzoate technique. All sectioned material is at 7–8 μ. All other figures are *optical* sections of gross uteri photographed with oblique illumination. In all figures the orientation is such that the mesometrium is toward the top of the plate.

1, Cleared rabbit tract at 5 days and 22 hours after artificial insemination. With oblique light, clear zones reveal the location of the blastocysts. Two arrows indicate two of the seven such clear zones showing. $\times \frac{1}{2}$.

2, Cleared rabbit tract at 8 days and 2 hours. Note degenerating fourth conceptus (*arrow*) near cervix on one uterine horn. $\times \frac{1}{2}$.

3, Photograph of one portion of rabbit uterus shown in *1* showing fourth and fifth blastocysts of one horn (indicated by numbers). The fourth is an extremely small disc denoting possible early degeneration, while the fifth is typical of all the others, resembling crushed cellophane. $\times$10.

4, Cleared hamster uterus from series castrated second day after observed mating, given 0.0625 mg. of progesterone daily and autopsied at 6 days and 12 hours. Hemosiderin pigment granules are apparent in a delicate ring (*arrow*) about the uterine horn, indicating site of resorption of attempted nidation. This animal had had no previous mating. $\times$3.

5, Cleared tract of mouse killed at 10:30 A.M. on day 4 after parturition. A circular refractile ring (*arrow*) denotes an unattached blastocyst within the uterine lumen. Slight opacity characterizes the muscularis of the uterus. *PS* marks site of placental scar. $\times$33.

PLATE II

6, Sections from mouse uterus that showed two distinct clumps of refractile bodies within the cleared uterus. Two groups of unattached and unspaced blastocysts were found, seven in area *A* and two in area *B*. $\times$22.

7, Section of uterus from hamster castrated at 3 days and 16.5 hours and autopsied at 4 days and 16 hours. No progesterone was given. Note decidua has developed but implantation is not taking place. The blastocyst (*arrow*) has a necrotic inner cell mass. Blood is apparent in the uterine lumen.

8, Sections from one of the conceptual regions of the uterus in *9* marked by Pontamine Blue and luminal changes. A naked blastocyst is shown, contact with the uterine epithelium in this and all sections is only superficial. No real decidua is present. $\times$75.

9, Cleared uterus of hamster killed at 3 days and 18.5 hours. This hamster had been injected with Pontamine Blue, and two blue areas were present in each uterine horn. Luminal changes are visible in the two clear regions (*arrows*) of this *unflushed* horn. $\times$7.

10, Two blastocysts flushed from other horn of uterus shown in *9*. This hamster had been given Pontamine Blue and showed two blue areas in each horn at autopsy at 3 days and 18.5 hours. Both blastocysts appear to have material adherent to the abembryonic pole. $\times$75.

PLATE II

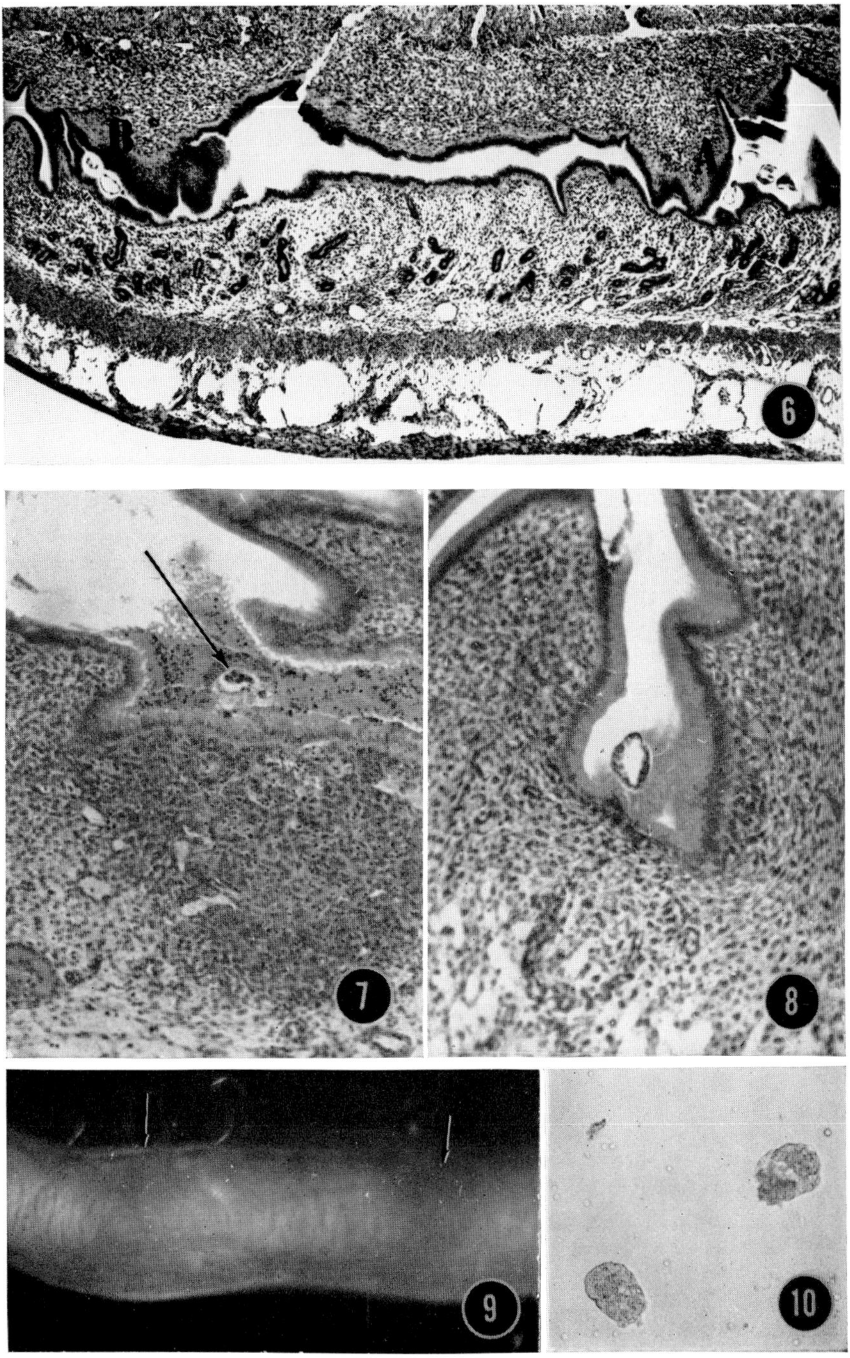

PLATE III

11, Luminal changes and Pontamine Blue areas in a cleared hamster tract autopsied at 4 days and 10 minutes. Two conceptual regions are shown in one horn, seven in the other. ×1.2.

12, Sections of the second conceptual site on the horn with two shown in *11*. The abembryonic cells of this blastocyst are just penetrating between the epithelial cells. Edema is marked. ×75.

13, Cleared mouse uterus (4 days plus some hours after detection of copulation plug) viewed from the antimesometrial surface to demonstrate the bilateral nature of first opaque ring. Site of opacity is indicated by arrow. Note straight character of uterine lumen in conceptual region and undulating character at each side. ×11.

14, Early opacity in conceptual region of cleared hamster uterus at 4 days and 8 hours. ×7.

15, Blastocyst from hamster tract at 4 days and 6.5 hours. The gross, cleared conceptual areas showed slight opaque dots. Giant-cell processes have penetrated through the uterine epithelium, and decidual cords are apparent. ×75.

16, Sections from conceptual area shown in *14*. Decidua is more extensive. ×75.

PLATE III

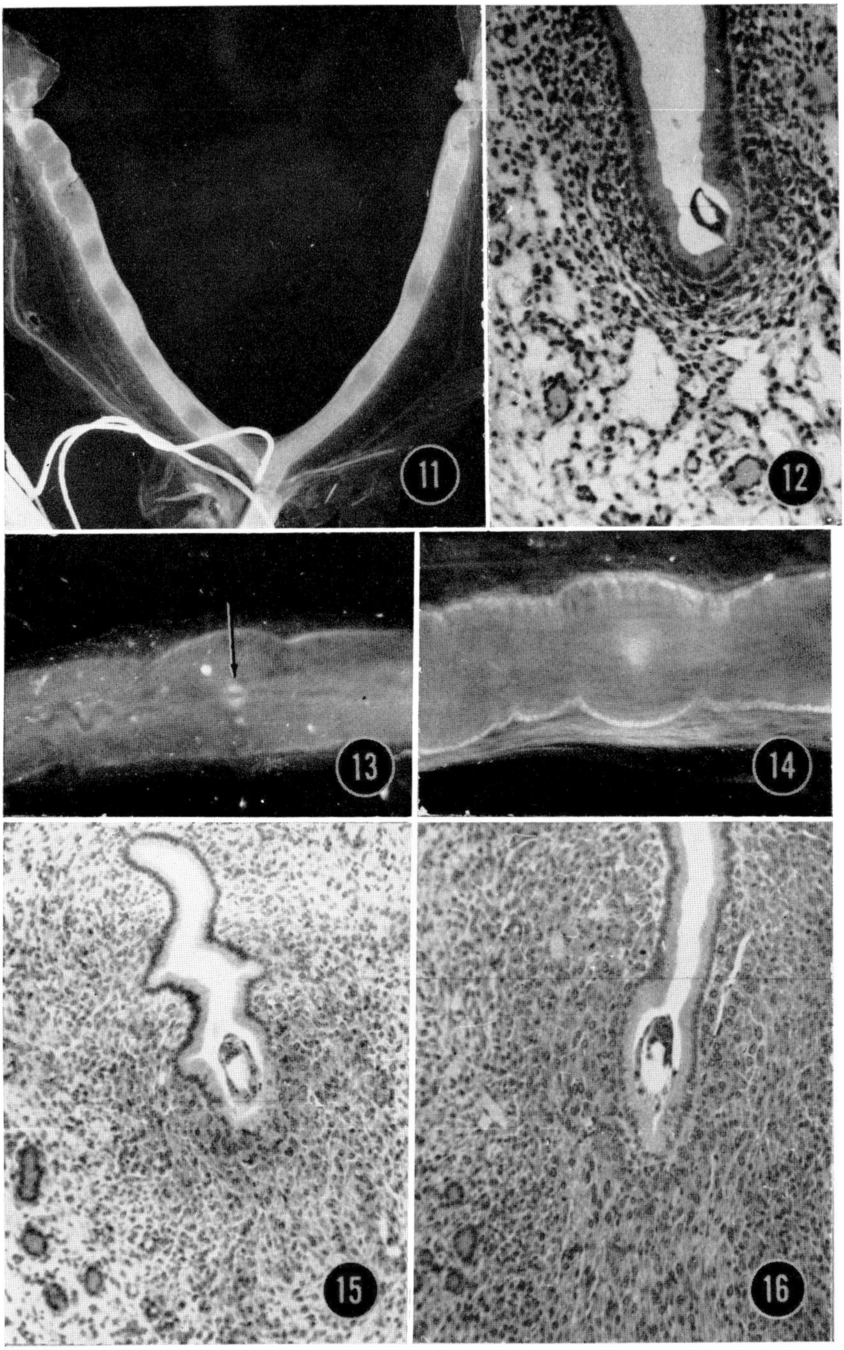

PLATE IV

17, Portion of a cleared hamster uterus at 4 days and 12 hours. Four opacities are visible; second from the right is much smaller and barely visible. ×2.2.

18, Cleared hamster uterus at 5 days and 12 hours. Five opacities are visible. Note that second from left is slightly smaller than other four. Note characteristic shield-like configuration. ×2.2.

19, Cleared hamster uterus at 6 days and 12 hours. Note tiny opacity at extreme left indicating resorption. Opacity is at height of development at this time. The second and third conceptual swellings at left are superficially fused. ×2.2.

20, Three hamster conceptual areas at 7 days and 12 hours. Note that the opacity is regressing from the antimesometrial side, and within this region the inverted yolk sac is visible. This tract is from a parous animal, and two placental scars are visible at the mesometro-uterine junction. ×2.2.

21, Portion of a cleared hamster uterus at 8 days and 12 hours. Note enlargement of clear antimesometrial area. With higher magnification, body form can be distinguished. The conceptual swelling at the right is in early resorption. ×2.2.

PLATE IV

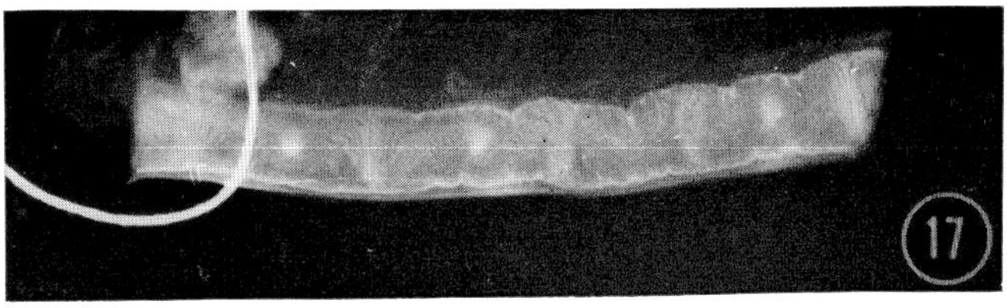

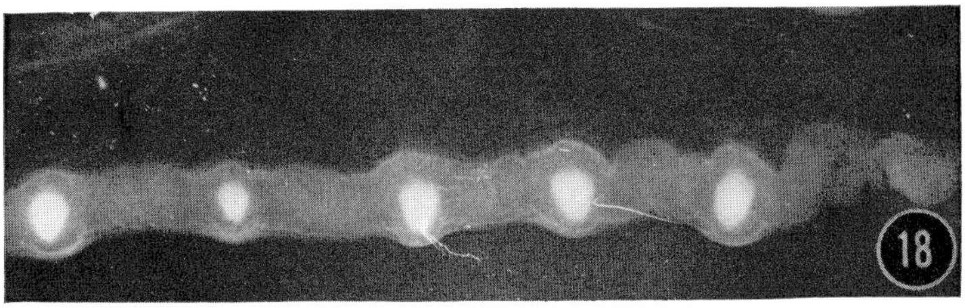

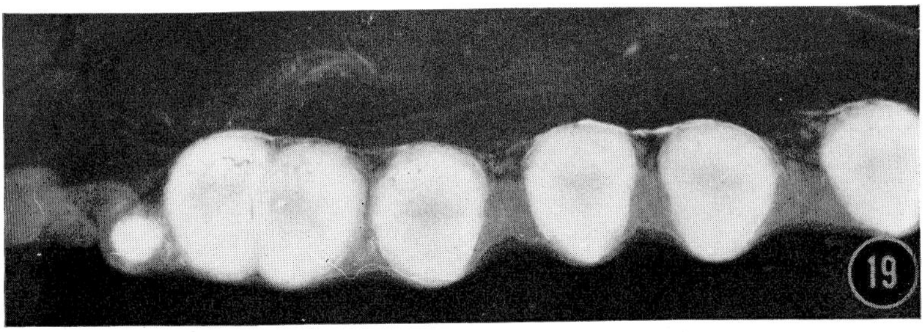

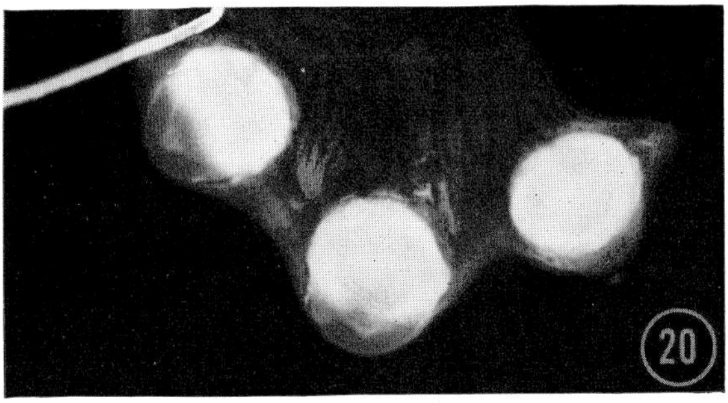

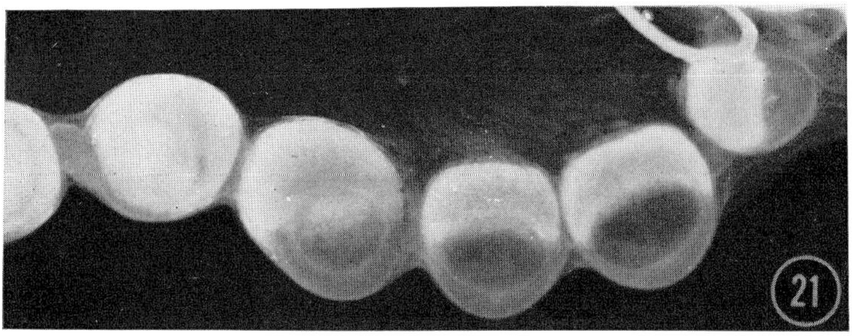

PLATE V

22, Portion of a cleared rat uterus autopsied at 5 days and 9 hours. One conceptual area is shown at the center (*arrow*); another is at far left. Note luminal changes indicative of implantation, with prominent undulations of uterine lumen in intergestational regions and slight displacement of lumen toward the mesometrium in the conceptual region. No external swelling is visible as yet. A blastocyst in superficial contact with the epithelium was found on sectioning this conceptual region. ×4.

23, Portion of a cleared rat uterus at 6 days and 12 hours. Note that external swelling and localized opacity are now visible. ×1.7.

24, Portion of a cleared rat uterus at 7 days and 12 hours. Note intense opacity of pronounced mesometrial swellings. ×1.7.

25, Portion of cleared rat uterus at 8 days and 12 hours. Conceptus has been peeled out of central gestational swelling. ×1.7.

26, Four cleared conceptual swellings in rat uterus at 13 days and 12 hours. Body form is now obvious, and sharp opacity marks the site of the fetal heart (*arrow*). ×1.7.

PLATE V

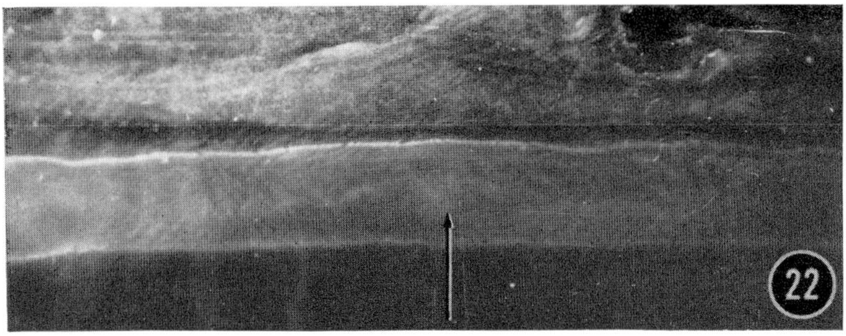

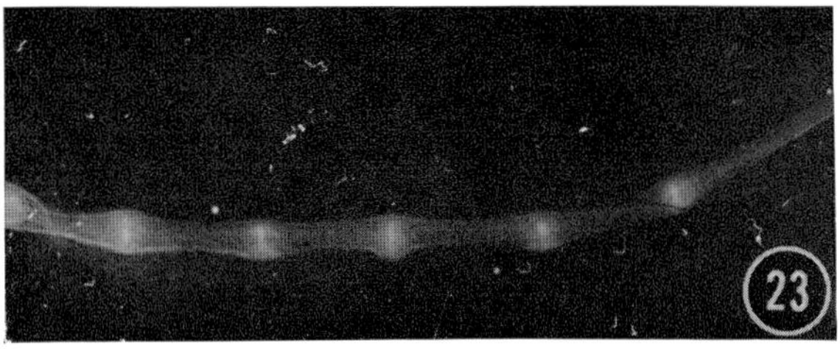

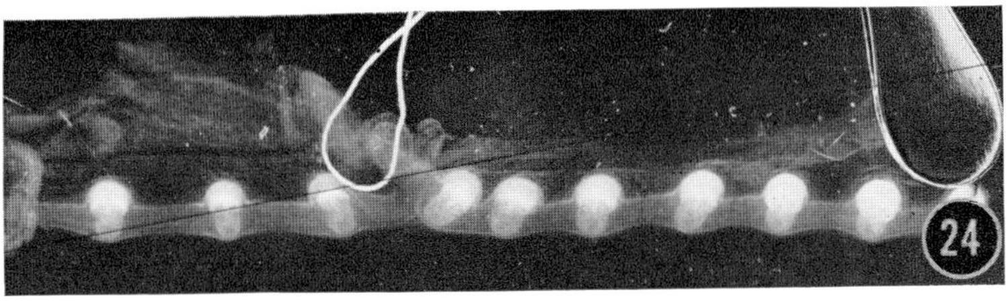

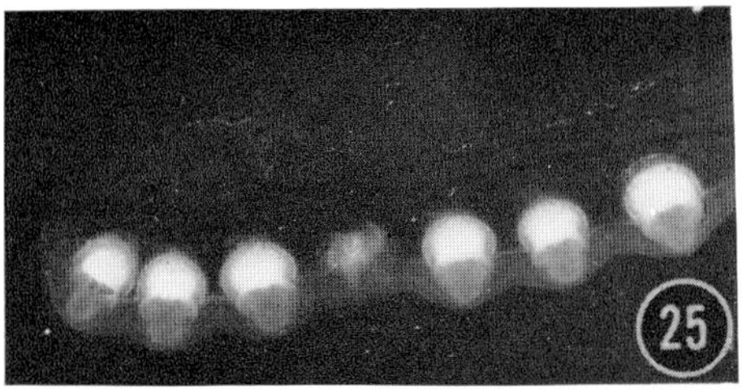

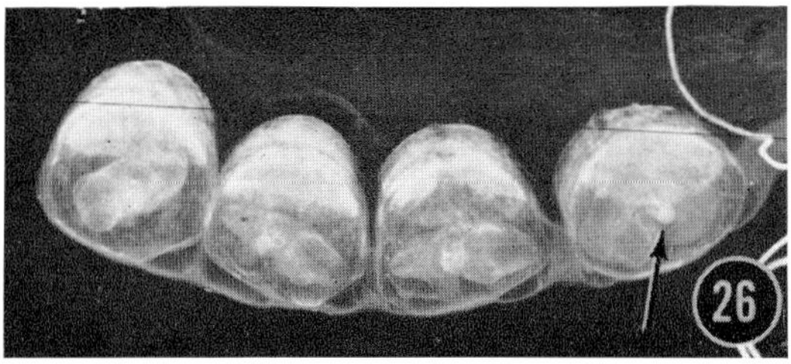

PLATE VI

27, Cleared guinea-pig conceptual swelling at day 16 showing pattern of opacity. Opacity characterizes mesometrial (basal) decidua and heart. ×7.

28, Portions of two cleared tracts from hamsters castrated on second day after mating, given 0.0625 mg. of progesterone daily, and autopsied at 6 days and 12 hours. One normal conceptus is shown in one horn; three stages of resorption. ×1.

29, Portion of cleared uterus from hamster castrated at 4 days and 12 hours and autopsied at 5 days and 12 hours; no progesterone given. Note abnormalities in pattern and in opacity at the four conceptual regions shown. ×7.5.

30, Cleared uterus at 5 days and 12 hours showing normal conditions at same magnification as *29*. ×7.5.

PLATE VI

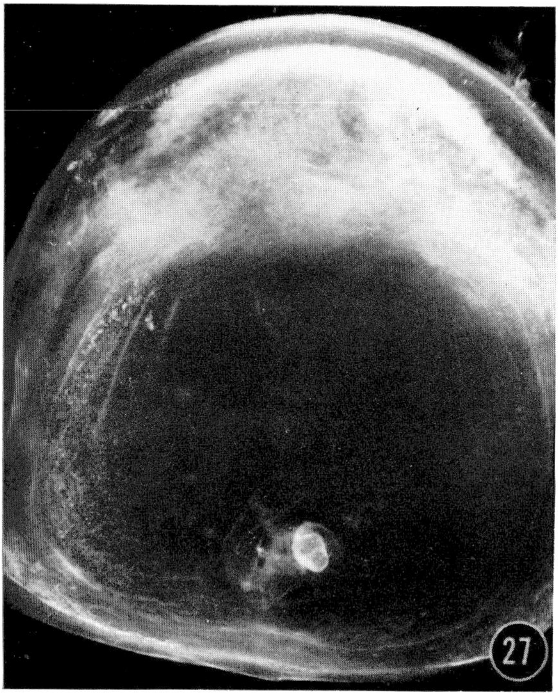

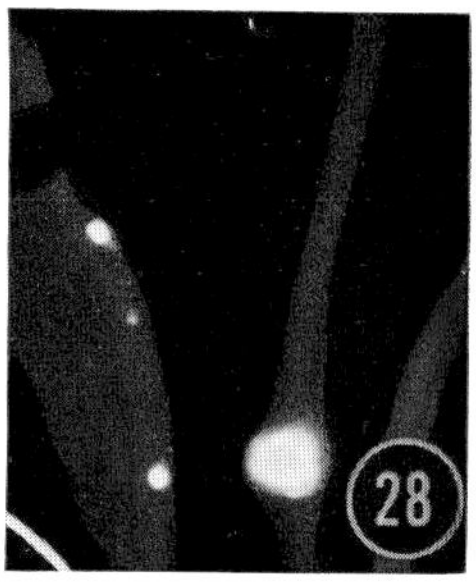

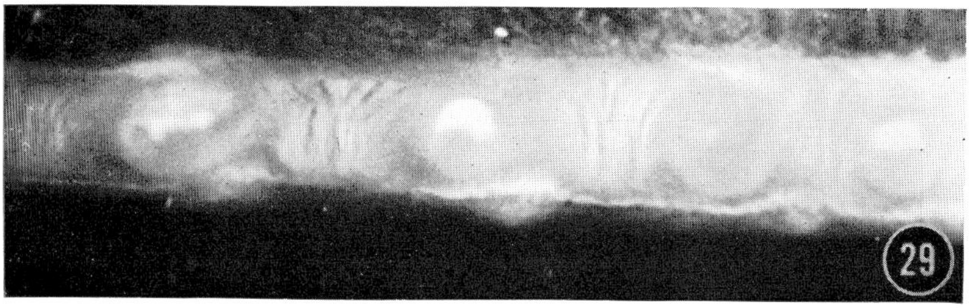

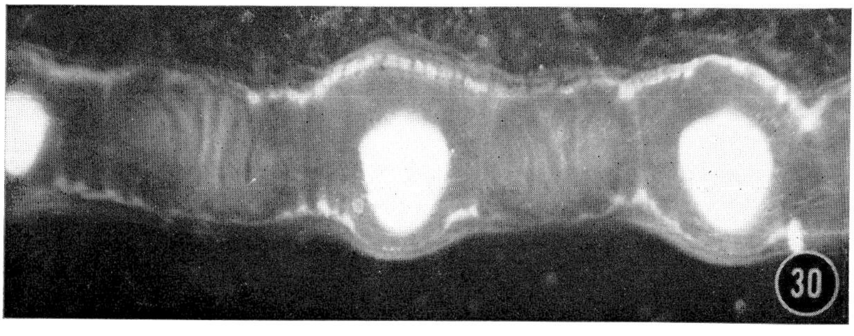

away that easily. I find all stages of dissolution; the zona enlarges at the same time the blastocyst enlarges, and finally the zona breaks.

NOYES: You found an unfertilized egg without the zona?

ORSINI: Yes, in the other horn also there were ova (three) which were not fertilized. Only in the pseudopregnant animal or pregnant animal will unfertilized ova shed the zona. I believe this suggests that progesterone from the corpus luteum is important. In castrates without progesterone (castrated at 1 day and 12 hours) the zona persists.

DEMPSEY: Were there any observations indicating whether the zona eroded from the outside or from the inside?

ORSINI: Developmental age is important—degeneration is correlated with this. I flushed four groups. In the first two groups, consisting of animals from normal pregnancy and psuedopregnancy, the zona came off very late on day 3 or early on day 4 (2 days and 21 hours up to about 3 days and 7–9 hours). In the third group, consisting of cycling females killed at the stage of the postestrous discharge, the ova were always in the zona; it never came off, and the egg degenerated within it. In the fourth group, consisting of females ovariectomized at 1 day and 12–17 hours, development proceeded from the uncleaved eggs to morulae and blastocysts, but always in the zona.

R. ENDERS: We have kept mink blastocysts alive for about six months in vitro. We offered all kinds of insults to them to induce growth of the blastocyst. Nothing we could do would free the blastocyst from the zona pellucida or induce the blastocyst to grow.

HARTMAN: Marsupials have had eons of time learning to get rid of the zona pellucida. In marsupials, the ovum is provided with three envelopes: zona, thick layer of mucus, as in the Lagomorpha (rabbits and hares), and a shell membrane, as in the Sauropsida. The tubal passage in the opossum is accomplished in 24 hours, as compared with about $2\frac{1}{2}$ days in the Eutheria from mouse to cow. The rapid passage of the opossum egg I attributed to the large number of corpora lutea—22 ova to the average batch. At one time R. K. Enders and I produced in a single opossum female a total of 400 corpora lutea, which was quite a task for Bob to count. As all three envelopes stretch 100–200-fold or more in utero as the vesicle grows, all three envelopes thin out greatly, resulting, I imagine, from molecular changes under enzymatic influences. I have never seen the envelopes in opossum vesicles burst. However, you will recall that, as seen in Lewis and Gregory's motion picture of developing rabbit eggs in vitro, at the ninety-sixth hour the zona burst and development ended. In the opossum, by the ninth day the envelopes have disappeared and the yolk sac lies in direct contact with the greatly modified uterine epithelium.

SHARMAN: The tubal journey is also short in marsupials with only one egg, as in Setonix, so the presence of numerous corpora lutea cannot be an explanation in this species.

BIGGERS: I was interested in Dr. Orsini's remarks on force breeding. There is good evidence that this occurs in the mouse. We were interested in determining the total number of young that a female mouse can produce. After the litters were born, the embyros were removed and the females bred at the postpartum estrus. This was tried both in intact females and in those with one ovary removed. In mice with two ovaries, 7 pregnancies are normal, then the litter size falls off. After 15 times the females are sterile. With one ovary, 5 pregnancies occur, then litter size falls off until after 10 pregnancies they are sterile. The mice with one ovary produce one-half as many young as those with two ovaries. Because mice have two independent uteri, the single uterine horn used is exhausted in those with one ovary. After sterility, we find ova in ovaries plus resorptions. My mice breed for two years, similar to what you described for the hamster.

DEANESLY: If a female is permitted to lactate, the placental sites in the uterus would be more regressed than if mating took place immediately postpartum in the absence of suckling young.

DEMPSEY: You showed two corpora lutea side by side in the same mink ovary. Could you elaborate a little on this? What are your thoughts as to the capability of these two corpora? Is one older than the other? Does one occur precociously as a result of the first mating and the other from the second mating? Does one acquire dominance over the other?

R. ENDERS: These are probably from a single mating. The follicles ruptured within three hours of each other. There may be 5–8 corpora in a single ovary.

DEMPSEY: The mink has a large amount of interstitial tissue. In delay, the vagina is cornified. Might not the interstitial tissue be a source of estrogen?

R. ENDERS: Smears were taken every four hours for three weeks from 12 mink; this induced ovulation. One smear daily did not induce ovulation in the majority of 65 mink. We found no correlation between follicular development and the vaginal smear. As soon as large follicles disappeared from the ovary, mucus appeared in the smear.

DEMPSEY: Had you reached the stage of implantation?

R. ENDERS: They will not breed once the large follicles are gone. I believe the estrogen does it. The interstitial tissue seems to develop more after the end of lactation than at any other time.

DEMPSEY: I am interested in the importance of the interstitial tissue in rabbit reproduction. It seems to have estrogenic effects. I have the feeling that the interstitial tissue has been commented on many times, but relatively little functional significance has ever been ascribed to it.

WRIGHT: I should like to ask Dr. Enders whether he has any idea as to how the particular type of delay in the mink evolved. A mink already pregnant can come into heat again. It does not seem to make sense. Do you have any idea of the origin of this?

R. ENDERS: No, I do not.

DEANESLY: I seem to recall an explanation by a naturalist that the male mink travels around during the breeding season, visiting the females.

R. ENDERS: Under normal conditions the female mink has a territory of twenty acres along streams. Males patrol up and down the streams. If the follicles persist until the females breed, there would be a certain advantage to having a variable time of mating but a restricted time of implantation.

By using mutations, we can assign each kit to a specific mating. But why does the last mating contribute up to 90 per cent of the litter? Yet, if a vasectomized male is used for the last mating, the litter is just as large as it would have been if the last mating had not taken place.

DEANESLY: A second estrus might expel the eggs from the first ovulation by muscular contractions. After sterile mating, no fertilized eggs passed into the uterus.

T. W. GLENISTER

Observations on Mammalian Blastocysts Implanting in Organ Culture

THE AIM in developing the tissue culture approach to the study of implantation has been to establish a method that would permit the investigation of the processes of implantation and the factors controlling the differentiation, invasiveness, and functions of trophoblast in an extracorporeal environment. This would provide conditions more readily controllable than those obtainable in an experimental animal.

The mutual relationship of trophoblast and endometrium during implantation would seem to be such that neither is solely responsible for the process, nor is either entirely passive (Eckstein, Shelesnyak, and Amoroso, 1959). It is also generally accepted that successful implantation is the result of a balanced interaction of systemic, uterine, and blastocyst factors. However, the proceedings of previous symposia on implantation (Symposia, 1959, 1960), and the contributions to the present symposium, all bear witness to the diversity of opinion regarding the relative importance of the various factors.

The study of embryo-endometrial relationships during implantation, in organ culture (Glenister, 1960, 1961*a*, 1961*b*, 1962), is a fairly obvious method of eliminating systemic factors and such uterine factors as the effect of the myometrium or the effect of circulation through endometrial blood vessels. Thus the possibilities of developing such a method had already been considered by Amoroso (1959), Meunier (1959), and Mayer (1960).

The rabbit has been selected for these experiments. This has proved to be an eminently satisfactory choice because, not only do these animals breed reliably and produce blastocysts that are large and relatively easy to manipulate, but the processes of implantation in the intact animal have been studied extensively. The study of implantation in the intact

DR. T. W. GLENISTER is a reader in anatomy in the University of London, at Charing Cross Hospital Medical School, England.

rabbit has been carried out notably by Böving (1959*a*, 1959*b*, 1959*c*, 1962), and more recently Larsen (1961) has studied the ultrastructural basis of the process.

Material and Methods

The details of the methods have been described previously (Glenister, 1960, 1961*a*, 1961*b*, 1962), but the basis of these methods consists of culturing blastocysts in contact with explants of endometrium (Pl. I, *1*). The blastocysts are explanted 6.5 days after the doe has been mated and the zona pellucida, which still surrounds the blastocyst at this stage, has been dissected off.

The endometrial explants are placed either on (1) a solid base of agar containing chick embryo extract and albumin, with a dozen drops of rabbit serum pipetted onto the explant to support the blastocyst; (2) a solid base of agar containing albumin only, with a dozen drops of the chemically defined 199 medium to support the blastocyst; or (3) a wire-mesh platform that is placed in 199 medium as in the method described by Trowell (1959). These last two methods have been applied to endometrial explants obtained from adult virgin animals. Steroid hormones have been added to the 199 medium in the proportion of 1 μg/ml of medium for estrogens and 2 μg/ml for progesterone.

Of the previously published results, the earlier ones (Glenister, 1960, 1961*a*, 1961*b*) refer to experiments in which the cultures were incubated in air. More recently (Glenister, 1962), the method has been improved considerably by incubating the explants in 95 per cent oxygen and 5 per cent carbon dioxide, as first suggested by Trowell (1959). To achieve this, the explants are incubated in a McIntosh and Fildes jar filled with the gaseous mixture, the lids of the Petri dishes containing the cultures being kept slightly raised by wire clips (Grover, 1961; Glenister, 1962).

The combined explants are fixed in Bouin's fluid on day 3 or day 6, serially sectioned and stained with hematoxylin and eosin.

Results and Discussion

The series of over two hundred explantation experiments, maintained in organ culture for 6 days by method 1 in an atmosphere of air, demonstrated that more than three-quarters of the blastocysts explanted effected implantation.

The proportion of blastocysts becoming implanted and the degree of invasiveness shown by their trophoblast appeared to be of the same order in the following combinations.

a) Blastocyst and endometrium obtained from the same doe, with the supporting serum prepared from the maternal blood.

b) Blastocyst incubated on endometrium obtained from another doe at a corresponding stage of pregnancy, with the supporting serum prepared from blood obtained either from this pregnant doe or from the doe supplying the blastocyst.

c) Blastocyst and endometrium obtained from the same doe or from another doe at the same stage of pregnancy but with the supporting serum prepared from the blood of an adult virgin animal.

d) Blastocyst and supporting serum obtained from the same doe but with the endometrium obtained from an adult virgin animal.

e) Blastocysts incubated on endometrial explants of maternal origin but placed in the culture in such a way that the deep stromal aspect of the explant was uppermost. In this way the blastocyst was in direct contact with the stroma of the endometrium without any intervening uterine epithelium.

The only combination that has so far yielded any reduction in the incidence of implantation is one in which the blastocyst is incubated on endometrium obtained from an adult virgin animal, with the supporting serum prepared from blood from this adult virgin doe.

It was noticeable in this series that, despite the varied conditions under which these blastocysts became implanted, the invasion of the endometrium was effected by apparently primitive, pleomorphic, cellular trophoblast, which showed little tendency to differentiate into syncytium. This was irrespective of whether the embryonic, abembryonic, or equatorial aspects of the blastocyst surface were in contact with the endometrium. Although superficial attachment of the blastocyst to the endometrium might occur sooner, it took from 2 to 4 days after explantation for the trophoblast to start invading the endometrium.

Subsequently, a new series of experiments was instituted in which method 1 was used to incubate various combinations of blastocyst, endometrium, and serum either in a gaseous mixture of oxygen and carbon dioxide or as controls in air. The results are summarized in Table 1.

These results suggest that incubation in an atmosphere rich in oxygen favors the expansion of the explanted blastocysts and the differentiation of syncytium. This is of special interest because it has been stated that blastocysts are capable of anaerobic metabolism (see Vesterdal-Jørgensen, 1950, for discussion). However, the proportion of blastocysts becoming implanted and the degree of invasiveness shown by their trophoblast appear to be of the same order whether the explant is cultured in air or in oxygen and carbon dioxide.

With the use of oxygen and carbon dioxide it is also evident that, after a week in culture, the endometrial constituents of the explants show far fewer signs of tissue damage than do comparable explants incubated in air. The endometrium is devitalized only in the immediate vicinity of the attaching trophoblast, suggesting that it exerts a local destructive influence. Damage to the endometrial stroma is not, however, prerequisite before it can be invaded by trophoblast, and pleomorphic primitive trophoblast has been observed to insinuate itself between apparently undamaged stromal cells (Glenister, 1962) in a number of explants.

The experiments of Smithberg and Runner (1956, 1960) have shown that only very small quantities of steroid hormones are necessary to influence implantation in prepubertal animals. It was thought that, since the media used in the organ-culture experiments so far described consisted of biological fluids (which might or might not contain unknown

TABLE 1

	Incubated in Air (No.)	Incubated in O_2 and CO_2 (No.)
Blastocysts explanted	56	67
Blastocysts effecting implantation	41	49
Blastocysts expanding in culture and remaining expanded after 6 days	5	44
Experiments in which there was considerable invasion of endometrial stroma by pleomorphic trophoblast	21	28
Experiments in which there was any invasion of endometrial stroma by trophoblastic syncytium	1 doubtful	1 doubtful
Blastocysts forming syncytium	6	37
Blastocysts whose syncytium was formed by trophoblast related to well-differentiated mesenchyme	4	30
Blastocysts whose syncytium was formed by trophoblast related to poorly differentiated mesenchyme	2	7
Blastocysts possessing well-differentiated mesenchyme but the trophoblast of which failed to form syncytium	18	6

quantities of hormone), the method should be modified by the use of a chemically defined medium to replace the biological fluids used previously. It would then be possible to add known quantities of a hormone to the medium, which might make it possible to assess the role of such a hormone in implantation.

Methods 2 and 3 have been developed in connection with this approach to the problem. The concentrations of hormones used are the same as those shown by Everett (1962) to be effective in producing characteristic histological changes in guinea-pig endometrial explants. It has been confirmed that similar responses are obtained in rabbit endometrial explants when the same concentrations of hormones are used.

The preliminary results are disappointing, in that slightly more blastocysts implant when no estrogenic or progestational hormone is added to the medium than when such hormones are added. It should be pointed out that in these hormone-free control experiments an equivalent quantity of Tyrode solution containing the same concentration of ethanol was added to the medium. The results obtained so far are as follows:

a) *With the addition of estrone* (Pl. I, *5*), 11 out of 25 blastocysts became implanted; 15 out of 25 blastocysts remained expanded after six days in culture.

b) *With the addition of estradiol* (Pl. I, *6*), 6 out of 11 blastocysts became implanted; 3 out of 11 blastocysts remained expanded after six days in culture.

c) *With the addition of estrone and progesterone*, 13 out of 23 blastocysts became implanted; 10 out of 23 blastocysts remained expanded after six days in culture.

d) *With the addition of estradiol and progesterone*, 4 out of 11 blastocysts became implanted; 4 out of 11 blastocysts remained expanded after six days in culture.

e) *With the addition of progesterone* (Pl. I, *4*), 15 out of 24 blastocysts became implanted; 11 out of 24 blastocysts remained expanded after six days in culture.

f) *With no addition of hormone* (Pl. I, *3*), 17 out of 23 blastocysts became implanted; 13 out of 23 blastocysts remained expanded after six days in culture.

The histological examination of these specimens has not yet been completed, so no information can as yet be given about possible differences in histodifferentiation or of the degree of invasion of the endometrium by the trophoblast in explants cultured in different media.

The results presented so far suggest that, at any rate in organ culture using rabbit material, implantation is possible without the aid of the "muscular phase" of attachment described by Böving in the intact animal (1959*a*), since the endometrial explants are devoid of myometrium. The circulatory factors described by the same author are also non-operative in organ culture. The fact that blastocysts implanted quite satisfactorily in endometrium obtained from virgin animals showing no histological evidence of decidualization indicates that the induction of a decidual reaction (Shelesnyak, 1957, 1959, 1960; Shelesnyak and Kraicer, 1960) is not an obvious preliminary requirement for implantation in this set of circumstances. However, it should be noted that the epithelial and glandular components of endometrial explants obtained from virgin animals often show signs of a local growth-stimulating effect in the immediate vicinity of the explanted blastocyst (Pl. I, *2*). Also, all the evidence so far gleaned from these organ-culture experiments suggests that the role of hormones may not be as distinct, with regard to the control of trophoblastic attachment to, and invasion of, endometrium, as has been generally assumed.

The question naturally arises whether experiments that involve observing implantation in such an "unnatural" environment as organ culture can provide results that shed any light on the problem of implantation in the intact animal. In fact, in a recent publication Larsen (1962) suggests that the observations reported by this author (Glenister, 1961*b*) "could be called more correctly an ingrowth of trophoblastic tissue into a non-specific tissue *in vitro*." He adds that these explant experiments fail to imitate the processes by which the blastocyst becomes attached to the endometrium in the intact animal.

The first point that needs to be made is that, in addition to the environment being patently abnormal, an important factor in normal implantation has been discounted by artificial removal of the zona pellucida, thereby possibly "liberating" the trophoblast and abnormally favoring its activity. Another clear indication that the development of the blastocyst is not normal in organ culture is that the embryonic pole, although giving rise to well-differentiated embryonic structures, such as heart and neural tube, does not give rise to an organized embryo (Glenister, 1961*b*, 1962).

Although these facts all point to the essential "abnormality" of blastocyst implantation in culture, it is relevant to describe those features which show an essential similarity to the processes observed in intact animals.

The explanted blastocysts expand to a degree that, though not as great as that attained in the intact animal, indicates that they are capable of maintaining an osmotic gradient. As to the histological features, the uterine epithelium is converted to symplasma where the trophoblast of the explanted blastocyst comes in contact with it, just as occurs in relation to normally implanting rabbit blastocysts. In the cultured specimens this conversion to symplasma has been observed in relation to both primitive pleomorphic and syncytial trophoblast. However, it needs to be reiterated that, although syncytium has been observed over the free surface of the blastocyst, imbedded in cellular debris, extending into glandular crypts, or fusing with endometrial symplasma, further invasion into the endometrial stroma has been effected by primitive, pleomorphic, mainly cellular trophoblast.

The ultrastructure of explants cultured by method 1 has been examined to ascertain whether their ultramicroscopic details are in any way comparable to those described by Larsen (1961) in the intact animal. After three days in culture, parts of the blastocyst wall show some signs of disorganization (Glenister, 1962) that are not observable with the light microscope. After six days in culture there is no further deterioration. At attachment sites, both cellular trophoblast and syncytium have been observed to attach themselves to endometrial epithelium or, in other cases, to symplasma (Pl. II, *7*, *8*, *9*, *10*, *11*). At sites where trophoblastic syncytium fuses with endometrial symplasma, the appearances are strictly comparable to those observed by Larsen (1961) in intact animals, the embryonic and maternal cytoplasms fusing as a result of the disappearance of intervening cell membranes.

It should also be noted that the merging and fusion of the embryonic and maternal epithelia is associated with a preliminary loss of microvilli on both the surfaces that become apposed to one another (Pl. II, *9*). It has also been confirmed with the electron microscope that the trophoblast infiltrating the endometrial stroma in these specimens is cellular and not syncytial in structure (Pl. II, *12*), there being well-defined cell membranes separating the cells from one another.

Conclusions

Organ culture affords a means of studying the implantation of mammalian blastocysts in circumstances in which the effects of the myometrium, of intrauterine tension, of blastocyst turgidity, as well as endometrial vascular considerations (Böving, 1959*a*, 1959*b*, 1959*c*, 1962), can be discounted, as can any general systemic factors. The importance of the decidual reaction (Shelesnyak, 1957, 1959, 1960; Shelesnyak and Kraicer, 1960) in these explantation experiments is difficult to assess. On the one hand, it has not been necessary to modify the histological structure of endometrial explants obtained from virgin animals by adding hormones to the culture medium; on the other, there is evidence suggesting that in some cases blastocysts have had a growth-promoting effect on the epithelial components of the endometrium at implantation sites. Trophoblast is certainly capable of converting uterine epithelium to symplasma, and in certain instances it has had a local destructive influence on the endometrium at the site of attachment.

The results presented suggest that, at any rate in organ culture, invasion by trophoblast is effected by the primitive pleomorphic type, consisting of cellular trophoblast showing mitoses, giant cells with large single nuclei, and occasional multinucleated cells. Trophoblast differentiates into well-organized cellular and syncytial layers, apparently in relation to fetal mesenchyme, at sites where absorption or fusion with maternal epithelium rather than infiltration is required.

It is debatable whether results obtained in such abnormal conditions are applicable to the problem of implantation in an intact animal. It may well be that the absence of well-differentiated syncytium at sites of trophoblastic invasion in the endometrium is due to an insufficiency of oxygen reaching the invading trophoblast by diffusion through the endometrium, which is devoid of circulation in culture. Comparison of the differentiation of trophoblast in cultures incubated in air with those incubated in a raised concentration of oxygen has demonstrated clearly that the latter environment favors the differentiation of syncytium.

Although the abnormality of the environment and of some of the developmental features of the explanted blastocysts is manifest, enough similarities to the process of implantation in the intact animal have been observed at the macroscopic, microscopic, and ultramicroscopic levels to make perseverance with the method worthwhile.

ACKNOWLEDGMENTS

This project has been supported by grants initially from the British Empire Cancer Campaign and, more recently, from the Medical Research Council, which are gratefully acknowledged. I am indebted to Miss Janet Everett for her skilful and zealous assistance, to Mr. K. Iles for the photography, and to Mr. J. T. Syrett for the electron micrographs. I also wish to thank Dr. W. J. Tindall for organizing the supply of hormones from Organon Laboratories Ltd.

REFERENCES

AMOROSO, E. C. 1959. The attachment cone of the guinea-pig blastocyst as observed under time-lapse phase-contrast cinematography. In P. ECKSTEIN (ed.), Implantation of Ova, pp. 50–53. Mem. Soc. Endocrin., No. 6. Cambridge: Cambridge University Press.

BÖVING, B. G. 1959*a*. Implantation. Ann. N.Y. Acad. Sci., **75**:700–725.

———. 1959*b*. The biology of trophoblast. *Ibid*., **80**:21–43.

———. 1959*c*. Endocrine influences on implantation. In C. W. LLOYD (ed.), Recent Progress in Endocrinology of Reproduction, pp. 205–26. New York: Academic Press.

———. 1962. Anatomical analysis of rabbit trophoblast invasion. Carnegie Inst. Contrib. Embryol., **37**:33–55.

ECKSTEIN, P., M. C. SHELESNYAK, and E. C. AMOROSO, 1959. A survey of the physiology of ovum implantation in mammals. In P. ECKSTEIN (ed.), Implantation of Ova, pp. 3–12. Mem. Soc. Endocrin., No. 6. Cambridge: Cambridge University Press.

EVERETT, JANET. 1962. The influence of oestriol and progesterone on the endometrium of the guinea-pig *in vitro*. J. Endocrin., **24**:491–96.

GLENISTER, T. W. 1960. Experimental nidation of blastocysts in organ culture. Bull. Soc. Roy. Belg. Gynéc. Obstét., **30**:635–40.

———. 1961*a*. Organ culture as a new method for studying the implantation of mammalian blastocysts. Proc. Roy. Soc., B, **154**:428–41.

———. 1961*b*. Observations on the behaviour in organ culture of rabbit trophoblast from implanting blastocysts and early placentae. J. Anat., **95**:474–84.

———. 1962. Embryo-endometrial relationships during nidation in organ culture. J. Obstet. & Gynec. Brit. Comm., **69**:809–14.

GROVER, J. W. 1961. The enzymatic dissociation and reproducible reaggregation *in vitro* of 11-day embryonic chick lung. Devel. Biol., **3**:555–68.

LARSEN, J. F. 1961. Electron microscopy of the implantation site in the rabbit. Am. J. Anat., **109**:319–34.

———. 1962. Electron microscopy of the uterine epithelium in the rabbit. J. Cell Biol., **14**:49–64.

MAYER, G. 1960. Morphologie et physiologie comparées de l'ovo-implantation —résultats et problèmes. In G. MASSON (ed.), Les fonctions de nidation utérine et leurs troubles, pp. 1–32. Paris: Masson & Cie.

MEUNIER, J. M. 1959. Culture *in vitro* de fragments d'endomètre de lapin. C.R. Acad. Sci. Paris, **248**:304–7.

SHELESNYAK, M. C. 1957. Experimental studies on the role of histamin in implantation of the fertilized ovum. Bull. Soc. Roy. Belg. Gynéc. Obstét., **27**:521–37.

———. 1959. Histamine and nidation of the ovum. In P. ECKSTEIN (ed.), *Implantation of Ova*, pp. 84–88. Mem. Soc. Endocrin., No. 6. Cambridge: Cambridge University Press.

———. 1960. Nidation of the fertilized ovum. Endeavour, **19**:81–86.

SHELESNYAK, M. C., and KRAICER, P. F. 1960. Décidualisation: Une étude expérimentale. In G. MASSON (ed.), Les fonctions de nidation utérine et leurs troubles, pp. 87–101. Paris: Masson & Cie.

SMITHBERG, M., and M. N. RUNNER. 1960. Retention of blastocysts in non-progestational uteri of mice. J. Exp. Zool., **143**:21–31.

SYMPOSIUM ON IMPLANTATION. 1959. (Conference held in November, 1957.) P. ECKSTEIN (ed.), Implantation of Ova. Mem. Soc. Endocrin., No. 6. Cambridge: Cambridge University Press.

SYMPOSIUM ON IMPLANTATION. 1960. (Conference held in June, 1960.) G. MASSON (ed.), Les fonctions de la nidation utérine et leurs troubles: Colloque de la Société Nationale pour l'Étude de la Stérilité et de la Fécondité. Paris: Masson & Cie.

TROWELL, O. A. 1959. The culture of mature organs in a synthetic medium. Exp. Cell Res., **16**:118–47.

VESTERDAL-JØRGENSEN, J. 1950. The cytology of uterine epithelia. In K. BOWES (ed.), Modern Trends in Obstetrics and Gynaecology, pp. 486–505. London: Butterworth.

DISCUSSION (*Chairman:* E. W. DEMPSEY)

DEMPSEY: With respect to delayed implantation, it would seem that all you have to do is remove the zona. Also, I was interested in your statement that the trophoblast influences the endometrium in front of it. Wislocki, Heuser, and Streeter studied the placenta of the macaque in 1938. As the abembryonic pole of the trophoblast approached the opposite side of the uterus, there was a transformation of endometrium before contact was established.

HARTMAN: In the rhesus monkey, which has a double discoidal placenta (primary and secondary, with rich anastomosis from the former to the latter), both uterine surfaces, dorsal and ventral, react to the trophoblast. In man there has been described the occurrence, on the non-pregnant surface, of a fleeting reaction, where the epithelium appears "stung" by the trophoblast.

Many workers have compared the trophoblastic invasion to cancer. One would like to know what factors operate to call a halt to the invasion in normal pregnancy, in contrast, for example, to chorioepitheliomata. I am reminded of two opossum vesicles among many hundreds of normal ones in which cell division has "gone wild," every other cell being in mitosis (cf. Hartman, Figs. 14 and 18, in *Mammalian Germ Cells; Ciba Foundation Symposium, 1953*). I have found a few references to similar abnormal proliferations in very early embryos in higher mammals.

DAVIS: When you said that you could use endometrium from virgin rabbits, did you mean a mature rabbit in estrus or an immature one?

GLENISTER: I think that they would have to be called mature rabbits.

DAVIS: Is serum essential in the preparation in order to obtain growth?

GLENISTER: These last specimens were incubated in 119 medium with no serum factor at all.

DEMPSEY: It seems to me that syncytium develops normally in contact with maternal blood. Serum or blood might aid in its formation if added to the medium.

NELSON: I was interested in the fact that you were able to reverse the uterine explant and secure attachment of the blastocyst on the myometrial side of the explant. Have you used other tissues as explants, for example, omentum or intestinal tract, which are sites of attachment in some instances of ectopic implantation? I hasten to say that I do not regard either omentum or gut as having magic properites for blastocyst attachment, but they are examples of extrauterine tissue.

GLENISTER: Dr. Silver and I, working at the Middlesex Hospital Medical School, obtained an attachment to the chorioallantois of the chick and to the midbrain vesicle without too much difficulty.

NELSON: You have not used other tissues for explants?

GLENISTER: No.

ORSINI: I notice that you were cautious about mentioning giant cells and that you have giant cells present with high oxygen. I have reported on invasion of giant cells in arterial vessels, possibly correlated with high oxygen content. Is there a chemical factor in this instance? Were these cells in cellular spaces?

GLENISTER: They extend into the stroma and distribute themselves in the intercellular substance.

DAVIES: Larsen has studied implantation in the rabbit with the electron microscope. He also raised the problem of non-specific attachment in Dr. Glenister's work. The story involved in the rabbit is very complex. There was cytoplasmic fusion of the syncytiotrophoblast and the symplasma derived from the uterine epithelium. There was a disappearance of the cell membranes between the uterus and the trophoblast. There was a mingling of nuclei, and he speculated on the possible genetic significance of this. He showed the extreme resistance of the basement membrane to syncytial invasion. The trophoblast put out processes that broke and invaded the basement membrane of the uterine epithelium and spread widely in the connective tissue. Finally, the vessels were invaded and the endothelium replaced by syncytiotrophoblast.

SHARMAN: You said that you did not get the blastocyst to do anything while it still had the zona on it. Did you add hormones to try to break down the zona, or were these blastocysts on culture media without added hormone?

GLENISTER: No. They were incubated for long periods in serum from pregnant animals. The blastocyst did not implant. It tends to roll off the endometrium. We will have to go back and try again.

CLEWE: It should be pointed out that the layer which Dr. Glenister, with proper caution, called the "zona pellucida," for want of a better name, is not in fact composed principally of the zona pellucida of ovarian origin common to all mammals but is principally a pellucid layer acquired by the rabbit ovum after ovulation.

GLENISTER: I think that you will find a sufficient amount of disagreement. It is more than just mucin.

CLEWE: I agree that there is a visible layer present that can be stripped off. It represents principally the mucin layer (formerly called "albumin layer") laid down on the rabbit ovum by the oviduct and probably also the "gloiolemma" described by Böving (1954, Cold Spring Harbor Symposia on Quantitative Biology, **19**:9–28), which is added in the uterus. I do not doubt that the zona pellucida of ovarian origin is still present, but it is a very small portion of the layer surrounding the blastocyst. If one assumes that the volume of the zona pellucida of ovarian origin does not change and calculates its thickness when stretched over the surface of a 3-mm. blastocyst, it will be found to be on the order of 0.02 microns thick. The layer observed is much thicker than this.

GLASSER: At what pressures do you gas your 199 medium with air and with 95 per cent O_2/5 per cent CO_2? Assuming that the gassing pressures are equal, how much more O_2 is dissolved in the 199 medium when you use the O_2/CO_2 mixture in place of air? What is the effect on your organ cultures if the gassing pressures are increased by one, by two atmospheres?

GLENISTER: Mr. McDougle has been trying different atmospheres. Adult tissues do better if the oxygen tension is increased. But I suggest that fetal tissues do far worse. They are sensitive to oxygen poison.

MAYER: How can we explain the fact that the blastocyst in the uterine lumen is so sensitive to its environment, as indicated by the hormonal requirements, and that it can attach to an unprepared endometrium in vitro?

LUTWAK-MANN: I believe that it is the endometrium and *its* metabolism that must be taken into consideration under experimental conditions like these. The effects upon the embryos would thus arise secondarily.

RUNNER: The nice work of Dr. Glenister in vitro has analogy in the experiments of transplanting blastocyst to ectopic sites. The ectopic site may be in immature, castrate male or female hosts. Both show that the blastocyst is ready to go. Incidentally, in the rat and mouse it makes no difference if the zona is on or off at the time of transplantation. In the uterus of the castrated female mouse, by contrast, the blastocyst sits and does nothing. After it has sat for 18 days, one can inject progesterone and get implantation. This engima of behavior of blastocysts in the uterus, as compared to explant or transplant to ectopic sites, seems a highly significant one for understanding nidation. The intact uterine epithelium of the non-progestational uterus must have a positive effect that is holding back the blastocyst. Perhaps the approach of Dr. Glenister will enable us to assess the inhibitory factor or factors associated with delayed implantation.

SHELESNYAK: As far as we know, one cannot get rabbit blastocysts to delay. When Dr. Glenister transfers to rat and mouse, this will be pertinent.

NOYES: If you put cancer cells in the endometrium, do you get "implantation"?

GLENISTER: We have tried putting other tissues but not cancer cells.

PLATE I

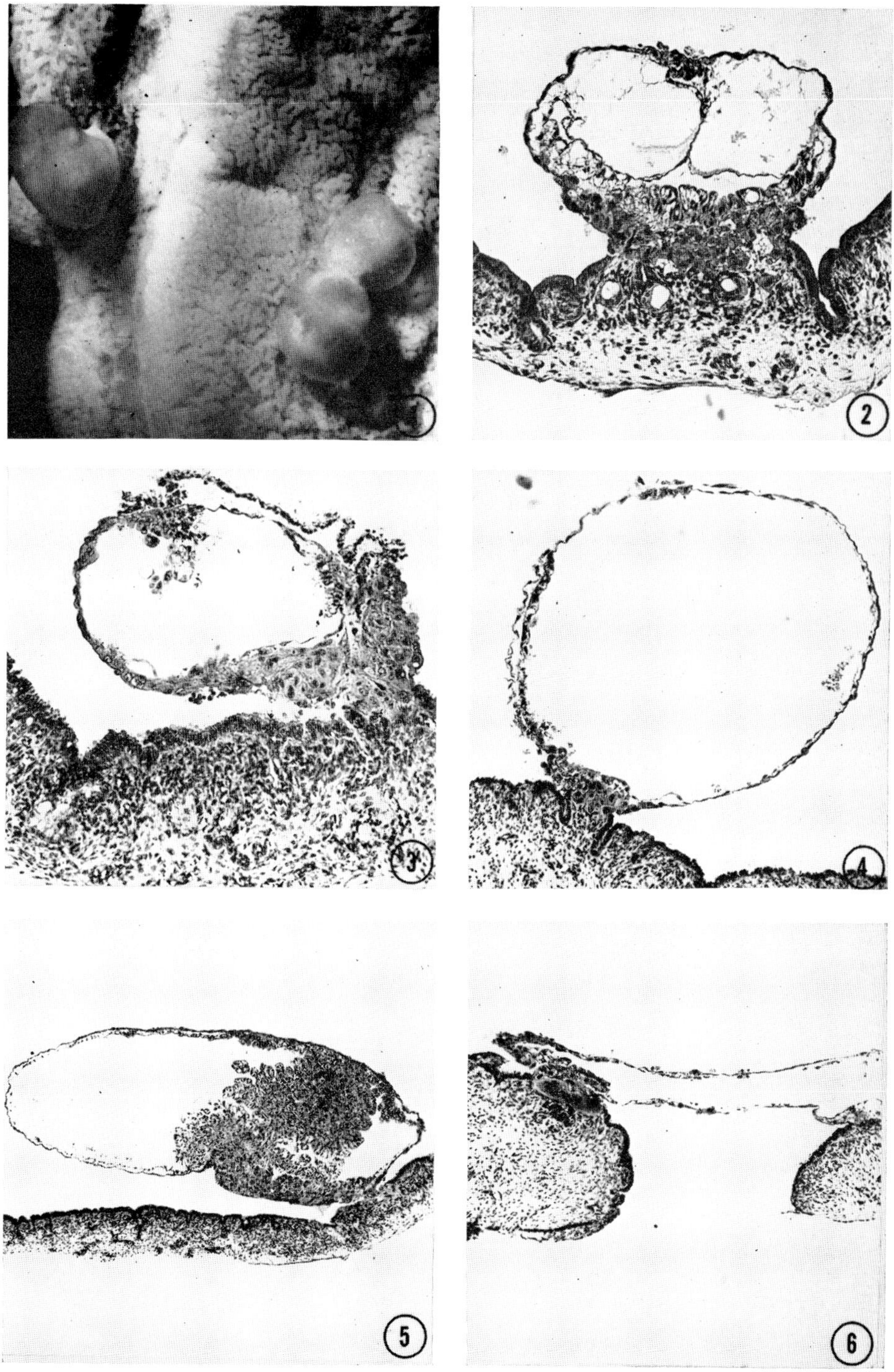

PLATE I

1, Photograph of three rabbit blastocysts attaching themselves to an explant of maternal endometrium 72 hours after explantation. ×10.7.

2, Photomicrograph of a section through an implanting blastocyst fixed 6 days after explantation on endometrium obtained from an adult virgin animal, with supporting serum prepared from blood obtained from this doe. The uterine epithelium is tall, and there has been proliferation of the uterine glands at the site of implantation. ×88.

3, Photomicrograph of a section through an implanting blastocyst fixed 6 days after explantation on endometrium obtained from a virgin doe and incubated in 199 medium to which no hormones were added. ×88.

4, Photomicrograph of a section through an implanting blastocyst fixed 6 days after explantation on endometrium obtained from a virgin doe and incubated in 199 medium to which progesterone had been added. ×79.

5, Photomicrograph of a section through an implanting blastocyst fixed 6 days after explantation on endometrium obtained from a virgin doe and incubated in 199 medium to which estrone had been added. ×36.

6, Photomicrograph of a section through an implanting blastocyst fixed 6 days after explantation on endometrium obtained from a virgin doe and incubated in 199 medium to which estradiol had been added. ×70.

PLATE II

7, Electron micrograph showing a trophoblastic giant cell (*TC*), the nucleus of which (*TN*) contains two nucleoli, effecting attachment to the epithelium (*ME*) of a maternal endometrial explant. ×3,000.

8, Electron micrograph of same specimen as shown in 7 but seen at a higher magnification. The cytoplasm of the trophoblastic giant cell (*TC*) appears to be merging with the cytoplasm of the epithelium (*ME*) of the maternal endometrial explant at the site marked by an arrow. ×12,000.

9, Electron micrograph showing part of the nucleus (*TN*) and a portion of the cytoplasm of a trophoblastic giant cell (*TC*) merging with the epithelial symplasma (*MS*) of a maternal endometrial explant. On the left, where the trophoblast is not in contact with the symplasma, the free uterine surface possesses microvilli (*MV*). The remains of the cell membranes, separating the trophoblastic cytoplasm from that of the uterine symplasma, are indicated by arrows. ×6,000.

10, Electron micrograph showing the site of attachment of a blastocyst to a maternal endometrial explant. Portions of cytotrophoblastic cells (*CT*) are seen at the top left. The cytoplasm of the trophoblastic syncytium (*TS*) is seen to be merging with the cytoplasm of the maternal epithelial symplasma (*MS*). The basement membrane (*BM*) of the maternal epithelium is seen at the lower right. ×1,100.

11, Electron micrograph of the site of attachment of a blastocyst to an explant of maternal endometrium showing an area of fusion between the cytoplasm of the trophoblastic syncytium (*TS*) and maternal epithelial symplasma (*MS*). ×3,000.

12, Electron micrograph of attachment site of a blastocyst to an explant of maternal endometrium showing two nuclei (*TN*) of trophoblastic cells separated by a cell boundary (*arrow*). These cells are seen to be infiltrating the endometrial stroma (*ES*). The base of a maternal epithelial cell (*ME*) is seen at the top left. ×3,000.

PLATE II

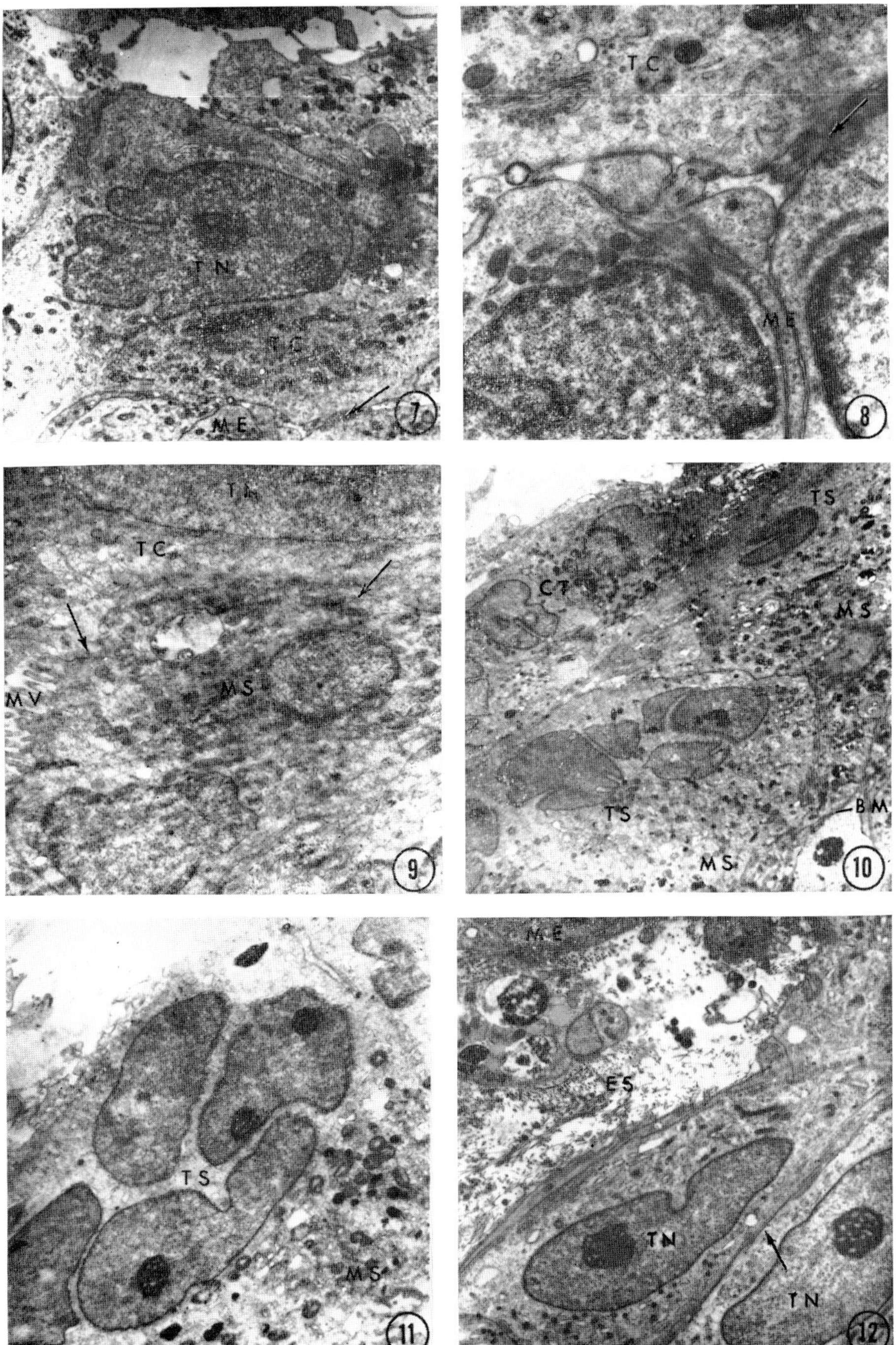

WARREN O. NELSON, OSCAR W. DAVIDSON,
AND KENRO WADA

Studies on Interference with Zygote Development and Implantation

THE ANTIFERTILITY effect of Ethamoxytriphetol (MER-25) in rats was correlated with damage to zygotes during their passage through the oviduct (Segal and Nelson, 1958). Similar action was shown with Chlomiphene (MRL-41) when used in the case of both normal (Segal and Nelson, 1961) and delayed (Segal and Davidson, 1962) implantation. Furthermore, antifertility effects occurred after implantation, when higher doses of MRL-41 were used (Barnes and Meyer, 1962). A diphenylinden derivative (U-11555A) had the same effect on fertility as the triphenyl derivatives of chlorotrianisene (Duncan, Stucki, Lyster, and Lednicer, 1962). The present report describes studies with U-11555A and with two diphenyldihydronaphthalenes, U-10520A and U-11100A, as well as some further observations on MRL-41.

MATERIAL AND METHODS

Holtzman strain rats fed on a standard diet were used. Virgin females in estrus were caged with males of proved fertility. Vaginal smears were taken daily. The day that sperm was found in the vagina was recorded as day 1 of pregnancy. All compounds were given orally by stomach tube.

1-(p-[β-diethylaminoethoxy] phenyl)-1,2-diphenyl-2-chloroethylene (Chlomiphene, MRL-41) was dissolved in chloroform and the solution suspended in warm olive oil. The other compounds, 2-(p-[6-methoxy-2-phenylinden-3yl]phenoxy)-triethylamine, hydrochloride (U-11555A); 2-(p-[3,4-dihydro-6-methoxy-2-phenyl-1-naphthyl]phenoxy)-triethyl-

DR. WARREN O. NELSON is medical director, the Population Council Laboratories, Rockefeller Institute, New York.

amine, hydrochloride (U-10520A); and 1-(2-[p-(3,4-dihydro-6-methoxy-2-phenyl-1-naphthyl)phenoxy]ethyl)-pyrrolidine, hydrochloride (U-11100A) were suspended in a 0.25 per cent solution of methylcellulose. Hereafter, the several compounds will be referred to by their respective code numbers, MRL-41, U-11555A, U-10520A, and U-11100A, respectively.

In all experiments with these compounds, treatment was given in either single or multiple administrations. Further details regarding treatment schedules are described in the results of individual experiments. Observations of effects on zygotes were made either by serial sections of fixed fallopian tubes or by flushing the tubes with saline. Delayed implantation studies were performed in rats mated while nursing litters of eight pups. In some experiments, laparotomies were performed between the tenth and fifteenth day of gestation. Uteri were examined for presence of implantation sites or number of embryos.

TABLE 1

RATS TREATED WITH MRL-41 0.3 MG/KG/DAY

Treatment Days of Pregnancy	No. Animals	No. Animals Implanted	No. Deliveries	Av. No. Pups
1– 4	10	0	0	....
5– 8	10	8	8	10.0
7–10	10	9	9	9.6
20–23	5	5	5	10.2
Controls	15	14	14	10.4

RESULTS

STUDIES WITH MRL-41

Table 1 shows results observed in animals treated at various stages of pregnancy with one 0.3 mg/kg dose of MRL-41 each day for four days. Animals treated during the first four days of pregnancy failed to deliver. When treatment was given after the fourth day, implantation of zygotes took place and pregnancy continued uneventfully. Number of fetuses delivered compared favorably with control animals.

The effect of MRL-41 administered in a total amount of 0.9 mg/kg, divided in three doses during a single day, is shown in Table 2. In this experiment groups of 10 animals each received treatment for one day and were sacrificed on day 12 of pregnancy. Treatment on any one of the first three days was 100 per cent effective in preventing pregnancy.

On day 4, implantation occurred in one instance. Treatment on day

5, 6, or 7 possibly affected several animals, but the few instances of implantation failures are probably those which might ordinarily be expected. It is generally recognized that only 80–90 per cent of normal matings in rats are fertile.

Since evidence showed that MRL-41 exerted its antifertility effect during the preimplantation stages of embryonic development, interest was aroused in investigating its action on blastocysts during naturally delayed implantation.

TABLE 2

RATS TREATED WITH MRL-41 0.3 MG/KG 3 TIMES, ONE DAY

Treatment Day of Pregnancy	No. Animals	No. Animals Implanted	Effect (Per Cent)
1	10	0	100
2	10	0	100
3	10	0	100
4	10	1	90
5	10	8	20
6	10	9	10
7	10	9	10
8	10	10	0

TABLE 3

RATS TREATED WITH MRL-41 0.3 MG/KG/DAY (Lactating ♀♀)

Treatment Days of Pregnancy	No. Animals	No. Animals Implanted	No. Deliveries	Length of Pregnancy (Days)	Av. No. Pups
7–10	18	2	2	22–23	7.5
9–12	21	7	5	26–29	6.0
10–13	14	4	3	22–25	6.4

In our colony the delay in implantation ranged between 3 and 12 days in females mated during postpartum estrus. Results of treatment in 53 of these females are shown in Table 3. Free, living blastocysts remained vulnerable to the compound, since pregnancy was inhibited in the majority of cases. Occasionally, blastocysts apparently became implanted before treatment began and consequently escaped destruction. This might be expected in an experiment in which it was not possible to predict the extent of implantation delay in a given case.

STUDIES WITH U-11555A

Table 4 shows observed results with U-11555A in different doses. When the compound was given during days 1–4 at a 0.5 mg/kg/day dose, it was completely effective in inhibiting fertility in 8 out of 25 animals. In 17 rats it was only partially effective. These 17 delivered an average of 3.5 pups each. Range of litters was 1–8.

Nearly all animals delivered 5 or fewer pups, indicating destruction of the majority of zygotes. Most of these animals were laparotomized on day 10 or 12, and the number of implantation sites was noted. Generally, the number of sites corresponded to the number of pups born. In some cases, however, fewer pups than sites were found, suggesting that some embryos were not viable.

TABLE 4

RATS TREATED WITH U-11555A ON DAYS 1–4 AND 1–6

Treatment Days of Pregnancy	Cases	Doses Mg/Kg/Day	Length of Pseudopregnancy (Days)	Length of Pregnancy (Days)	Av. No. Pups
1–4........	8	0.5	18	....	0
1–4........	17	0.5	....	25	3.5
1–6........	8	0.5	20	....	0
1–4........	15	1	22	....	0
1–4........	5	2	17	....	0

When 0.5 mg/kg/day was given through day 6, it was completely effective. The same was true of 1 and 2 mg/kg/day administered during days 1–4. Laparotomies showed that no implantation occurred in animals receiving 2 mg/kg/day; on 1 mg/kg/day, 2 animals showed 2 and 1 implantation sites, respectively.

Table 5 shows results observed in animals treated with 5 mg/kg of U-11555A on any one of the first seven days of pregnancy. This treatment proved completely effective on days 1, 2, and 3 and was also effective on day 4 in all but one animal. On days 5, 6, and 7 it apparently had no effect. The number of implanted animals was slightly less than the number of inseminations. This difference probably reflects the spontaneous failures that may be expected in normal matings.

STUDIES WITH U-10520A

Observations with U-10520A are summarized in Table 6. So far, experience with this compound has been confined to administration during days 1–4 with doses ranging from 0.1 to 0.5 mg/kg/day.

At the highest dose, U-10520A was completely effective in inhibiting fertility. At the 0.25 mg/kg/day dose, 13 of 15 animals failed to deliver litters; the remaining 2 had relatively small litters, indicating failure of most of the zygotes to develop. The lowest dose used, 0.1 mg/kg/day, was apparently effective in about half the animals. In

TABLE 5

RATS GIVEN ONE TREATMENT WITH 5.0 MG/KG U-11555A ON DIFFERENT DAYS OF PREGNANCY

Treatment Day of Pregnancy	No. Animals	No. Animals Implanted*
1	10	0
2	10	0
3	10	0
4	10	1
5	10	8
6	9	8
7	6	5

* Animals sacrificed on days 10–12 of pregnancy.

TABLE 6

RATS TREATED WITH U-10520A ON DAYS 1–4

Doses	Cases	Length of Pseudo-pregnancy (Days)	Length of Pregnancy (Days)	Av. No. Pups
0.5 mg/kg	11	16	....	....
0.25	13	16	....	....
0.25	2	....	26	2*
0.1	3	19	....	....
0.1	4	....	25.5	3.5
Controls	8	....	23.5	8.5

* One animal had 4 pups; the other had littered but ate pups before observation could be made. Her weight loss indicated that she probably had 3 or 4 pups.

animals delivering litters, the numbers of pups were much below the colony average, again indicating the inability of many zygotes to develop normally.

The 8 control cases for U-10520A were animals that previously had been treated with the compound during days 1–4 and had failed to deliver litters. However, when mated without treatment, normal pregnancies and deliveries occurred.

STUDIES WITH U-11100A

Studies with U-10520A and U-11100A were carried out at approximately the same time. The latter drug was apparently more potent; consequently, attention was centered upon its effectiveness when given on a single day.

Table 7 summarizes observations on U-11100A administered during days 1–4. In 35 cases, 0.3 mg/kg/day proved completely effective. The 10 controls were animals that had been treated successfully with 0.3 mg/kg during their previous pregnancies.

TABLE 7

RATS TREATED WITH U-11100A ON DAYS 1–4

Doses	Cases	Length of Pseudopregnancy (Days)	Length of Pregnancy (Days)	Av. No. Pups
0.3 mg/kg/day.......	35	14	....	....
Control.............	10	....	23.6	8.2
0.1 mg/kg/day.......	24	17	....	....
0.1 mg/kg/day.......	3	....	29	2.3
Control.............	7	....	23	8.5

TABLE 8

RATS TREATED WITH U-11100A ON DAY 1 OF PREGNANCY

Doses	Cases	Length of Pseudopregnancy (Days)	Length of Pregnancy (Days)	Av. No. Pups
0.3 mg/kg once on day 1............	18	18	....	....
Control..........................	6	....	23	9.5
0.3 mg/kg twice on day 1...........	17	16	....	....
Control..........................	7	....	23	10

On 0.1 mg/kg/day, treatment was effective in 24 of 27 animals. In the remaining 3, small litters (1, 2, and 4 pups) were delivered and pregnancies were markedly prolonged (27, 33, and 28 days, respectively). These results suggest that a few zygotes escaped destruction and were implanted several days later than usual. The seven controls listed here were animals that had been treated successfully with 0.1 mg/kg/day during their previous pregnancies.

Table 8 summarizes results in animals treated with 0.3 mg/kg once or twice on the first day of pregnancy. None of these animals delivered litters, nor were any implantation sites observed at laparotomy on days

10 and 12. Control animals in this experiment were some of those effectively treated in previous pregnancies.

As has been noted earlier, the effect of the various compounds upon the developing zygotes has been studied by the serial sectioning of the fallopian tubes or by flushing the tubes and studying the intact zygotes at various days following the initiation of treatment. As has been observed in earlier studies with MER-25 (Segal and Nelson, 1958) the compounds used in this study caused marked damage to the developing ovum. These effects were manifest in both the cytoplasm and the nucleus and resulted in ovum death. Since the details of these effects are to be reported in another place, no attempt will be made at this time to describe them in detail. It is worthy of note, however, that in animals treated on the first day of pregnancy cleavage rarely continued beyond the two-cell stage of development and that in animals treated on day 2 or 3 similar inhibitory effects were manifest. Fragmentation and separation of the blastomeres followed rapidly so that in animals that received an effective single dose intact zygotes were rarely seen two days after treatment.

Discussion

Each of the compounds examined in this study was effective in inhibiting fertility in the rat if given during days when the fertilized egg was in the oviduct. After the developing egg passes into the uterus and prepares to implant, it is apparently less vulnerable to the effects of these compounds.

It will be recalled (Table 1) that animals treated after the fourth day showed normal progression of gestation, and in no instance were abnormalities of pregnancies observed. These findings were not entirely in agreement with those reported by Barnes and Meyer (1962), who did observe fetal losses in animals treated during the postimplantation stages of pregnancy. However, the dose of MRL-41 used in their experiments was more than three times that employed in ours. Furthermore, single or multiple laparotomies in their animals may have contributed to the effects they observed.

In experiments to be reported elsewhere we have recently observed that animals receiving 0.3 mg/kg/day from day 8 to day 20 of pregnancy did show frequent evidence of fetal loss. It therefore appears that MRL-41, when given in larger doses or over a longer period of time, may have an effect beyond that already noted for the preimplantation period.

Although effects of MRL-41 apparently extend to later stages of pregnancy when high doses or extended treatment is given, it is reasonable to center primary interest on the effects of minimal doses. With such doses only the very young zygote is affected during its tubal passage. However, it is possible to prolong the period of effectiveness for at least ten days in the case of delayed implantation. Thus, vulnerability of the zygote is apparently related more closely to its stage of development than to its position in the genital tract. Consequently, as far as can now be determined, compounds of the type used in this study have their effect directly on the zygote. In this connection it is pertinent to recall the studies of Segal and Tyler (1958), who showed that MER-25 affects Arbacia eggs. Furthermore, if the treated fertilized eggs are washed, it is possible to remove the compound, and development is reinitiated. Chang's (1959) in vitro studies on fertilized rabbit eggs showed a similar effect for MER-25. In these studies the compound obviously must have acted directly on the zygotes and not through an alteration of the physiology of the oviduct.

Although the mechanism appears to be similar whereby all the compounds under discussion have been effective antifertility agents, some differences in the minimal effective doses was evident. Thus, the most effective compound appears to be U-11100A, which was shown to prevent pregnancies when given in a single dose of 0.3 mg/kg on any one of the days during which the fertilized eggs were passing through the oviducts. As noted, this compound is a diphenyldihydronaphthalene. The other diphenyldihydronaphthalene, U-10520A, showed much the same degree of effectiveness as MRL-41, which is a derivative of chlorotrianisene. For both these compounds a total dose of approximately 1 mg/kg distributed over the first four days of pregnancy produced complete or almost complete inhibition of fertility. In the case of MRL-41 it was shown that a total dose of 0.9 mg/kg given during a single day was completely effective. The fourth compound, U-11555A, which is a diphenylinden, was the least effective of the compounds studied. In this case a total dose of 3 mg/kg distributed over a period of six days was required to effect complete inhibition of fertility. A total dose of 5 mg/kg given during a single day was also completely effective.

It is not possible on the basis of the evidence we have secured to do more than make a rough comparison of the effectiveness of the various compounds, since in some instances the minimal effective dose was not actually established. However, it is clearly evident that three different kinds of chemical compounds have been shown to have the same qualitative effect on the very young embryo. It is likely that there are other compounds, perhaps totally different in structure, even more effective than those which have been studied.

Although the application of this method of fertility control to the human being has not yet been made, it seems reasonable to expect that such studies will be undertaken in the hope that it will be possible to develop a method of fertility control whereby the ingestion of a single pill on the day after coitus will effectively control fertility. If it can be shown that compounds used in this manner are without side effects, it would seem likely that this method of fertility regulation would have certain advantages over existing methods of oral contraception.

Summary

Studies were made on the antifertility effects of four compounds, MRL-41, a derivative of chlorotrianisene; U-11555A, a diphenylinden derivative; and two diphenyldihydronaphthalenes, U-10520A and U-11100A.

It was shown that administration of each of these compounds during the first four days of pregnancy in the rat completely inhibited fertility. At dose levels that were effective during the first four days no effect was observed when treatment was initiated on the fifth or some later day of pregnancy.

In cases of delayed implantation it was shown that effective treatment might be given as late as the twelfth day following mating. This would indicate that it is the stage of embryonic development that is vulnerable to the effect of the compounds.

Although the mechanism whereby these compounds is effective is not completely understood, it is believed that they exert their control of fertility by direct action on the very young embryo during its passage through the fallopian tube.

Acknowledgments

The authors wish to acknowledge the kindness of Dr. Gordon Duncan of the Upjohn Company, Kalamazoo, Michigan, in supplying U-10520A, U-11100A, and U-11555A, and of Dr. Dorsey Holtkamp of the Charles Merrell Company, Cincinatti, Ohio, for supplies of MER-41.

References

Barnes, L. E., and R. K. Meyer. 1962. Effects of ethamoxytriphetol, MRL-37, and chlomiphene on reproduction in rats. Fertil. & Steril., **13**:472–80.

Chang, M. C. 1959. Degeneration of ova in the rat and rabbit following oral administration of 1-(p-2-diethylaminoethoxyphenyl)-1-2-p-anisylethanal. Endocrinology, **65**:339–42.

Duncan, G. W., J. C. Stucki, S. C. Lyster, and D. Lednicer. 1962. An orally effective mammalian anti-fertility agent. Proc. Soc. Exp. Biol. & Med., **109**: 163–66.

Segal, S. J., and O. W. Davidson, 1962. Prolonged anti-fertility action of chlomiphene in delayed implantation. Anat. Rec., **142**:278.

SEGAL, S. J., and W. O. NELSON. 1958. An orally active compound with anti-fertility effects in rats. Proc. Soc. Exp. Biol. & Med., **98**:431–36.

———. 1961. Anti-fertility action of chloramiphene. Anat. Rec., **139**:273.

SEGAL, S. J., and A. TYLER. 1958. Inhibiting action of a triphenylethanal derivative on the development of eggs of *Arbacia punctulata* and on the fertilizing capacity of sperm. Biol. Bull., **115**:364.

DISCUSSION (*Chairman:* R. K. MEYER)

ORSINI: I probably missed something. By what criteria would you say these animals are pseudopregnant? Is not the pseudopregnancy prolonged a little bit?

NELSON: Yes, pseudopregnancy was prolonged. It was recognized by the occurrence of a continuous diestrous smear. With MER-25 we showed that at appropriate times we could bring about a decidual reaction in the uterus.

ORSINI: Could you explain the prolonged pseudopregnancy?

NELSON: Not entirely. All the compounds can be shown to be both estrogenic and antiestrogenic, depending on the particular circumstances. At doses higher than those employed for the experiments just described, they will inhibit secretion of gonadotrophin. Perhaps some combination of these several effects has been responsible for the longer periods of pseudopregnancy in some of the animals.

YOCHIM: Would you say that the factors you mentioned might be the cause of delayed or prolonged pregnancy in those rats that did carry fetuses?

NELSON: It is possible, but I am, of course, far from certain. In those cases in which treatment was not completely effective, the litters were very small, 2, 3, or 4 rather than the usual 8–12 or so. It would appear that the drug caused the death of the majority of zygotes but that some survived and eventually were able to implant. Perhaps either implantation was delayed or development was retarded, resulting in a somewhat prolonged gestation.

YOCHIM: What of the sensitivity of the uterus during pregnancy? Do you think that this had been delayed?

NELSON: Timing of embryonic development in relation to maturation of the endometrium is important, of course. You should remember that these compounds do have certain antiestrogenic properties. I do not think that these properties are related to their antizygotic activity, but they might have some effect on the endometrial pattern and consequently on embryonic implantation.

GREENWALD: In the normal-pregnancy animals these compounds have been effective only while the eggs were in the oviduct. However, in the case of your delayed-implanting rats, the eggs are obviously *in utero* at the time the drugs are administered. This seems to rule out the oviducal environment as the factor responsible for embryonic death and places the emphasis on the stage of embryonic development as the cause of death.

NELSON: Fertilized eggs in the rat appear to implant about 5 days after ovulation. Since tubal passage requires between 3 and 4 days, the zygotes are free in the uterus about 1 day. During this time they continue to be vulnerable to the effects of the drugs. It appears that it is the stage of development and not the position of the zygote in the reproductive tract that determines whether or not damage occurs.

SHELESNYAK: I should like to come back to an intriguing aspect of this. You did mention the fact that you did some laparotomies at day 12. Did you see any general decidual reaction other than at specific implantation sites? As has been demonstrated, the existence of decidual tissue will, of course, prolong the period of pseudopregnancy. One other point that gives weight to your argument—what degree of resistance to damage is shown by the zygote? In lower doses, which would be less damaging, the prolongation period is greater. As, for example, 0.5 mg. of U-10520A is 16 days, 0.1 mg. is 19 days; with U-11100A, 0.3 mg. gives 14 days, and 0.1 mg. gives 17 days, or two days beyond the normal range.

NELSON: You recall that in those cases in which laparotomies were performed on day 12 there was no indication that implantations had occurred. Consequently, there seems to have been no stimulus for a decidual reaction, and, indeed, none was seen. With less than completely effective doses, as was mentioned in answer to one of Dr. Yochim's questions, some zygotes do survive and proceed through normal development and delivery. Such zygotes seem to have been able to resist the damaging effects of the compound at the level of administration. I doubt very much that there is a valid or significant relationship between the duration of pseudopregnancy and the dosage. If a relationship does exist, I can suggest only that it may be due directly or indirectly to the estrogenic and antiestrogenic properties of the compounds.

DEANESLY: Is decidual tissue required to prolong pseudopregnancy? Was there a luteotrophic effect? Did you find the full complement of eggs, or were some expelled after the compound had been given?

NELSON: I have no direct experience that would enable me to relate the duration of pseudopregnancy to the occurrence of decidual tissue. Dr. Shelesnyak has suggested that such a relationship does exist. It is likely that some "luteotrophic" effect would be involved in such a relationship. I am not confident enough in our skill in recovering eggs by tubal flushing to answer your last question. We expect, however, to get the answer.

ALDEN: When you speculated about the use in man, you said a single pill taken the day after coitus could be effective. I presume that you mean the day after ovulation?

NELSON: If and when we are in the position of knowing the time of ovulation for a given woman during a given cycle, it would be practical to say that an effective antizygotic compound might be ingested on the day following ovulation only. At the present time, it is my opinion that such a compound would have to be used after each coitus to insure against a pregnancy. Of course, a woman who has made the effort to ascertain the variable extent of her menstrual cycles can calculate the period when she is likely to ovulate, but this demands too much of women who are less than highly motivated toward the control of conception.

ALDEN: You believe that it would be effective only while the ovum is in the tube?

NELSON: Yes, if the drugs have the same effect in man as they do in other animals.

NUTTING: Could the extended period of pseudopregnancy be explained on the basis of antiestrogenic properties of the compound?

NELSON: I have no reason, on the basis of any observations we have made, to believe that the life of the corpus luteum is prolonged by the relatively small doses that are used to demonstrate an antiestrogenic effect. When doses that are 100 per cent effective in preventing fertility are employed, the ovarian cycle seems to be unchanged. The vaginal cycle is atypical, in that the sharply defined stages characteristic of the normal cycle do not occur. Nevertheless, these animals will mate, ovulate, and conceive.

SHELESNYAK: I believe that there is a contradiction in data, if you were right. With a greater dose there is a shorter period of prolongation. If it is antiestrogenic, one would expect the opposite.

BIGGERS: I wish to comment on whether these compounds have a direct effect on the embryos. Before continuing, I wish to ask whether you remember the doses used by Chang and Segal in their in vitro studies?

NELSON: Our best guess is that these various compounds do act directly on the young embryo. I believe that Chang used doses of 25–50 mg/kg in his rabbit studies and that Segal and Tyler used doses of 10^{-4} M in their studies on sea-urchin eggs.

BIGGERS: We have examined the effect of MRL-41 (chlomiphene) on organ cultures of mouse fallopian tubes in which zygotes develop into blastocysts. We could only damage the embryos if a concentration of 10^{-3} M chlomiphene was incorporated in the medium. Unfortunately, it is very hard to compare experiments done in vitro with those done in vivo from a quantitative point of view. However, from the doses you give, we may estimate that roughly 0.06 mg. MRL-41 was being given to each rat per day. No one knows how much of this reaches each fallopian tube. If we arbitrarily assume that it is one-thousandth, then 0.06 μg. of the drug reaches the tube. If this quantity was incorporated in our organ culture system, the concentration of MRL-41 would be approximately 10^{-8} M, or about 10^{-4}–10^{-5} of the dose we find effective. This wide discrepancy, although based on a very speculative argument, makes me doubt whether embryos are in fact very sensitive to MRL-41. The dose that we find effective in vitro is also the concentration required to produce non-specific cellular poisoning by a great many drugs. Thus, I suggest that MRL-41 acts indirectly on some other system necessary to maintain the function of the fallopian tube or that some chemical derivative, which arises in its metabolism in a site remote from the oviduct, has the toxic effect on the embryos.

NELSON: While we think these various compounds have a direct effect on the young embryo, there is no reason to suppose that the effect may not be due to some substance that is formed as a result of metabolic conversion. This is an example of the recognized problem of drug effects. We know the nature of the compound that we administer, but we know relatively little about what happens to it after it has been administered.

GLENISTER: Would you not agree that it is misleading to refer to these substances as antifertility agents, when they are antizygotic and in effect procure the termination of an early pregnancy?

NELSON: If you are defining antifertility effects as anything that interferes with gametes, you could be correct in your objection. But I believe that it is a more general term. However, there are so many kinds of antifertility effects that I think we should be more specific in cases in which the evidence provides a basis for doing so.

DE FEO: How do you establish the termination of pseudopregnancy? Do you take the appearance of full vaginal cornification as the end point?

NELSON: Yes.

DE FEO: When pseudopregnancy in the rat is prolonged (for example, massive deciduoma formation or hysterectomy), one often finds a proestrous smear that is followed by *leucocytes* rather than cornification. Such a smear is followed by ovulation. Unless one considers this as an end point, the figures on the length of pseudopregnancy may be exaggerated by 4–6 days.

DEMPSEY: You mentioned that the drug was effective four days after mating; you also mentioned that cycling continued in animals given the drug without mating. Is there any evidence as to the possible effect on the ovarian egg and on polar body formation or early cleavage following ovulation? At what stage in the embryonic development is the drug effective, and what is the duration of the effect of a single dose?

NELSON: We have not dealt with doses of these compounds appreciably higher than the amount required to inhibit fertility, so I cannot say anything about what might occur when very large doses are given. In our experience the drugs could be given for at least two weeks prior to mating without interfering with mating, conception, and normal pregnancy if treatment was suspended no later than the day of mating. In some instances, the resultant litters were reduced in numbers, suggesting a residual effect of the drug, but in other cases litter numbers were normal. All this indicates that ovarian eggs are not influenced by the compounds and that minimal doses have a short period of effectivity. A single small dose probably would be effective for no more than one day.

HARTMAN: In the monkey, I have determined the day, in some cases almost the hour, of ovulation by rectal bimanual palpation of the ovaries. In the absence of knowledge of the exact day of ovulation in women, it has been calculated that in man 250–500 copulations are performed to one conception. Only in primates is sex designed by the Creator for both recreation and procreation. From every medical, social, and religious standpoint it is important that a readily determined (by the woman herself) sign of impending (not already consummated) ovulation be discovered. (Cf. Hartman, 1962, *Science and the Safe Period*). In such researches the Planned Parenthood Federation of America and Catholic scientists have in recent years joined hands.

R. W. NOYES, Z. DICKMANN,
L. L. DOYLE, AND A. H. GATES

Ovum Transfers, Synchronous and Asynchronous, in the Study of Implantation

DURING THE LAST five years we have used the technique of ovum transfer in rats and mice to study certain processes related to implantation. The purpose of the present paper is to review this work briefly. References to work of others and details of our techniques can be found in previous publications (see References).

For the purposes of this paper, the processes that precede implantation may be discussed under four headings: development of the fertilized ovum, tubal transport of the developing ovum into the uterus, trophoblastic penetration of the zona pellucida, and endometrial differentiation. Although much qualitative information is available in each of these individual areas, much remains to be learned about the quantitative relationships of each to implantation.

It is generally accepted that ova play an active role in implantation, but exactly how mature an ovum must be before it can adhere to the endometrial epithelium and elicit an endometrial response is unknown. Tubal transport results in the passage of the developing ovum into a favorable uterine environment prior to implantation, but exactly how much acceleration or deceleration of the tubal ovum is compatible with implantation is unknown. The zona pellucida is shed prior to implantation in rats and mice, but whether ova artificially denuded of the zona

DR. ROBERT W. NOYES is professor and chairman of the Department of Obstetrics and Gynecology, School of Medicine, Vanderbilt University, Nashville, Tennessee. The work reported here was carried out while the senior author was associate professor of obstetrics and gynecology at Stanford University School of Medicine, Palo Alto, California.

pellucida can implant at an earlier than normal stage of development or whether the zona plays a significant role in implantation is unknown. Failure of endometrial development is held to be a cause of reproductive failure in women and animals, yet almost nothing is known about how widely endometrial development can deviate from "normal" without interfering with implantation.

Material and Methods

In our colony of *rats*, morulae entered the uterine horns on day 4 of pregnancy (day 1 being that on which a vaginal plug was found the morning following mating), and blastocysts implanted late on day 5. In our *mice*, ova entered the uterus on day 3 and implanted on day 4.

Recipient females were mated with vasectomized males, thus the recipients were pseudopregnant until developing ova were transferred into their uteri. Most transfers were done between 0900 and 1100 hours. The donors were killed, their uteri removed and flushed with tissue culture medium (Noyes and Dickmann, 1960), and the recovered ova transferred by means of a micropipette into the recipient's uterine horns. Each recipient received ova from two donors so that ova of one stage of development were transferred into one uterine horn and ova of a different stage of development were transferred to the other uterine horn of the same recipient. In most experiments the resulting fetuses in each uterine horn of the recipient animal were counted on day 18 of pregnancy.

A shorthand notation was adopted to describe the timing relationships of the transfer experiments. The notation $3 \rightarrow 4$ means that day-3 ova were transferred into the uterus of a recipient on day 4 of pseudopregnancy. All ova were transferred into the uterus. Ova that were in the earlier stages of development (rat, days 2 and 3; mouse, day 2) were recovered from the *oviduct* of the donor animal. For this reason, although $2 \rightarrow 2$, $3 \rightarrow 3$, and $4 \rightarrow 4$ will be referred to as *synchronous* transfers, the shorthand notation does not show that both rat and mouse day-2 ova, and rat day-3 ova, were transferred from the oviduct into the uterus.

Asynchronous transfers were of two types: ova less developed than the uterus, for example, $3 \rightarrow 4$, and ova more developed than the uterus, for example, $4 \rightarrow 3$. Our use of ovular age as the primary point of reference is arbitrary, and there is no intent to stress the importance of ovular development over endometrial development. In the examples given above, the reciprocal relationships may be read $3 \rightarrow 4$, the endometrium is one day more developed than the ova, and $4 \rightarrow 3$, the endometrium is one day less developed.

PLATE I

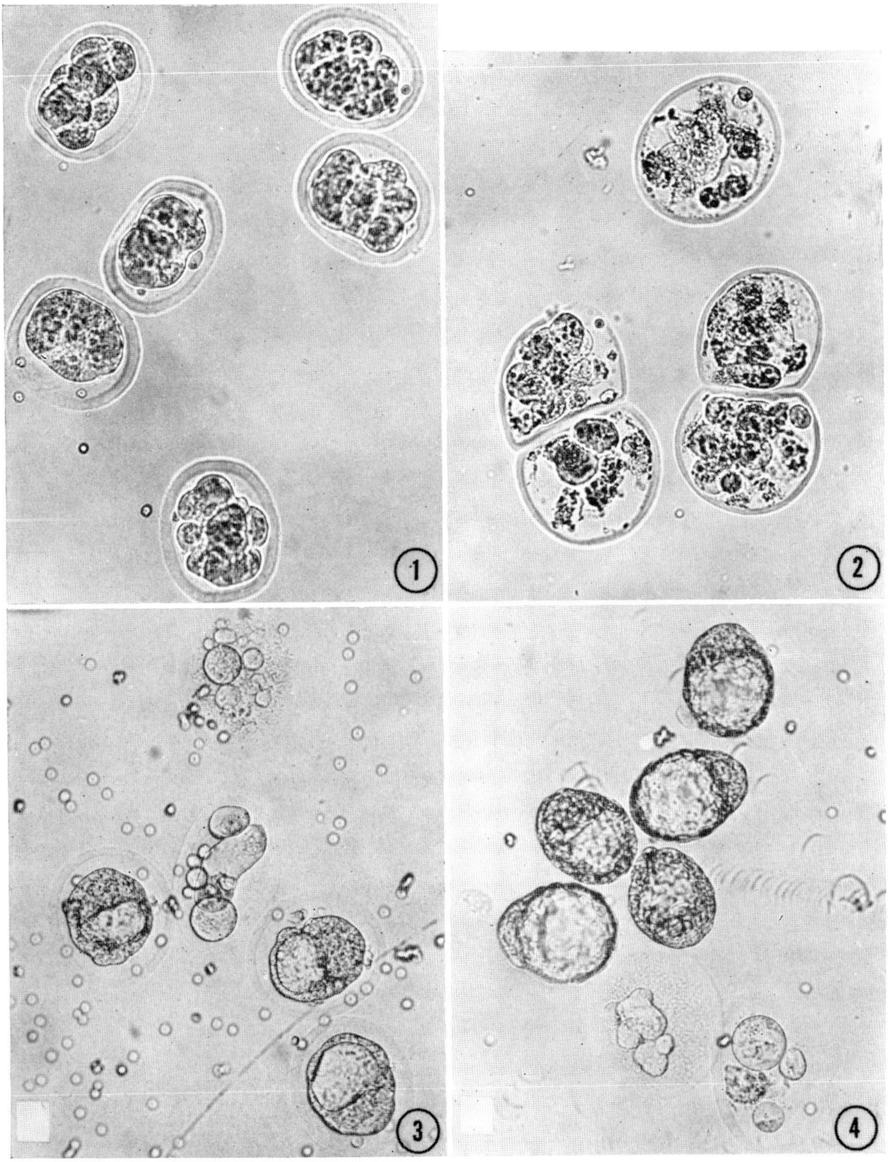

1, Six *rat* ova recovered from the uterus of a donor on day 4 of pregnancy (×180).

2, Five *rat* ova recovered 12 hours after transfer of day-4 ova into the uterus of a recipient on day 5 of pseudopregnancy (×180).

3, Two native and 3 donor *rat* ova recovered 1 day after the transfer of 4-day ova into the uterus of a recipient on day 4 of pseudopregnancy (×180).

4, Two native and 4 donor *rat* ova recovered 1 day after the transfer of day-5 ova into the opposite uterine horn of the same recipient as that in *3* (×180).

PLATE II

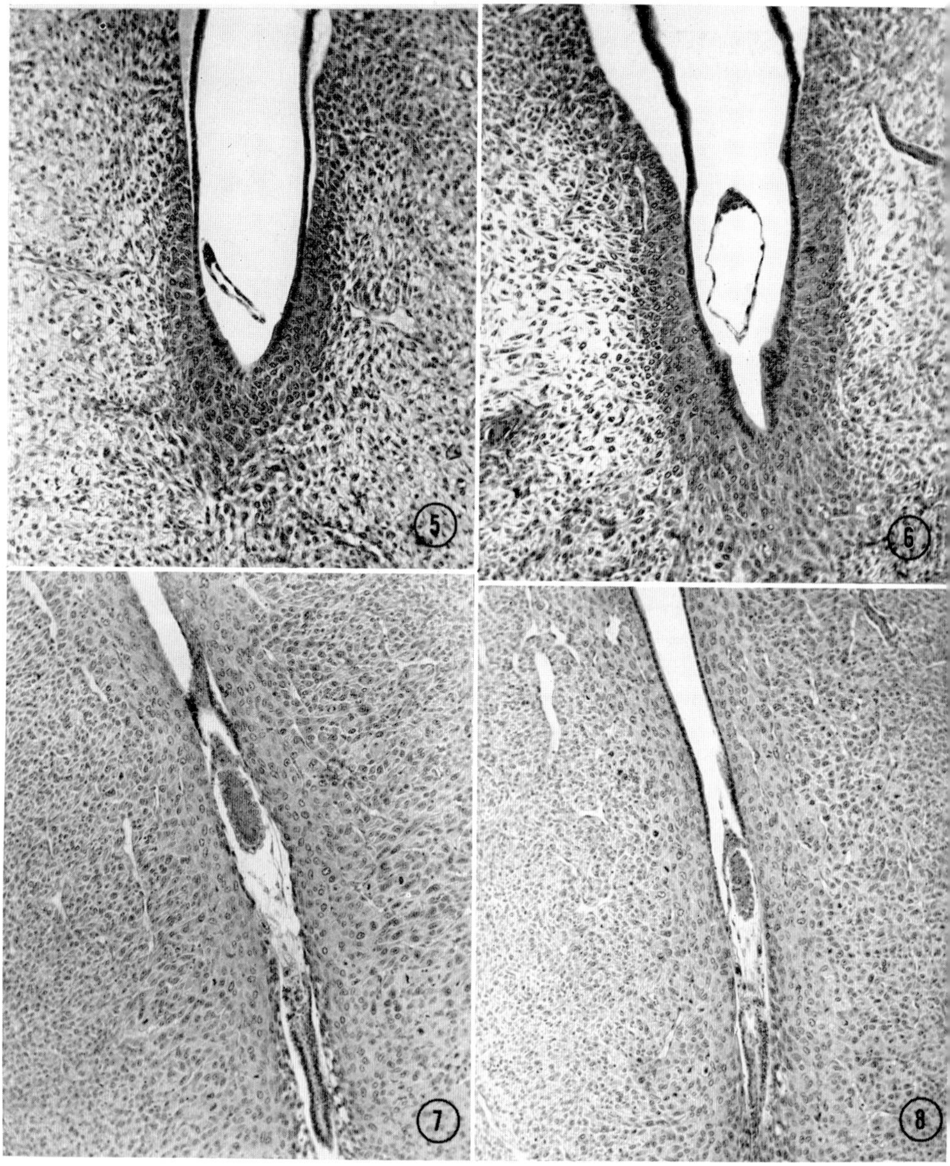

5, A *rat* ovum fixed 1 day after the transfer of day-5 ova to the uterus of a recipient on day 5 of pseudopregnancy (×180).

6, A *rat* ovum fixed 2 days after the transfer of day-5 ova to the uterus of a recipient on day 4 of pseudopregnancy (×180).

7, A *rat* ovum fixed 3 days after the transfer of day-4 ova into the uterus of a recipient on day 4 of pseudopregnancy (×180).

8, A *rat* ovum fixed 3 days after the transfer of day-5 ova into the uterus of a recipient on day 4 of pseudopregnancy (×180).

Results

SURVIVAL OF FETUSES TO TERM PREGNANCY

Figure 1 shows the percentage of *rat* ova that survived to term fetuses following transfer of 855 ova into the uterine horns of 60 recipients (Noyes and Dickmann, 1960). No ova survived transfer into the uterus on day 2, and relatively few survived on day 3. Synchronous 4 → 4 transfers resulted in the same high proportion of term fetuses as did 5 → 4 transfers; while 5 → 5 transfers were slightly less successful.

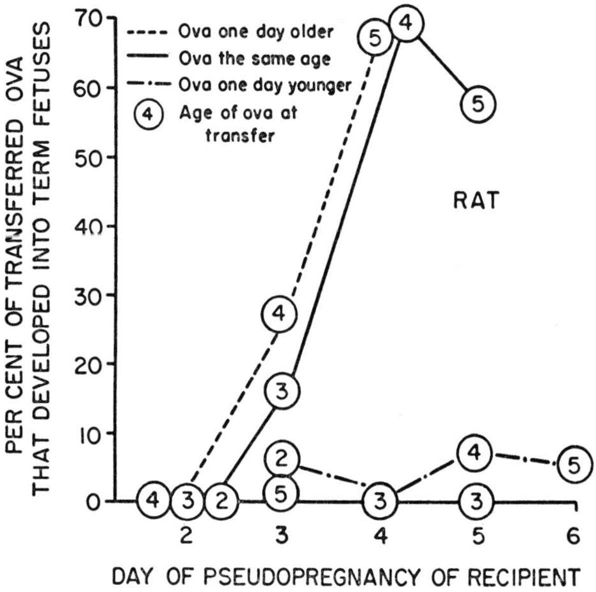

FIG. 1.—Percentage of 855 *rat* ova that survived to term pregnancy after transfer to the uterine horns of 60 pseudopregnant recipient rats.

Asynchronous transfers in which the ova were one day less developed than the uterus (3 → 4, 4 → 5, 5 → 6) were strikingly less successful than synchronous transfers or transfers in which the ovum was one day older than the uterus. Transfers two days out of synchrony (3 → 5, 5 → 3) were unsuccessful.

Figure 2 shows the proportions of 1,247 *mouse* ova that survived to term following their transfer to the uterine horns of 124 recipients (Doyle *et al.*, 1962). Qualitatively, the results were similar in mice and rats, but there were several quantitative differences. In mice 3 → 3 transfers were synchronous, since the ova were in the uterus by day 3. Thus about 40 per cent of ova yielded term fetuses following 3 → 3 and

4 → 3 transfers, and a similar yield was obtained following 4 → 4 transfers. Approximately the same percentage of day-5 ova survived whether they were transferred to uteri on day 3, 4, or 5. As in the rat, the transfer of mouse ova one day less developed than the uterus resulted in very few term fetuses.

In order to determine what had happened in cases in which the transferred ova failed to survive, the following experiments were carried out.

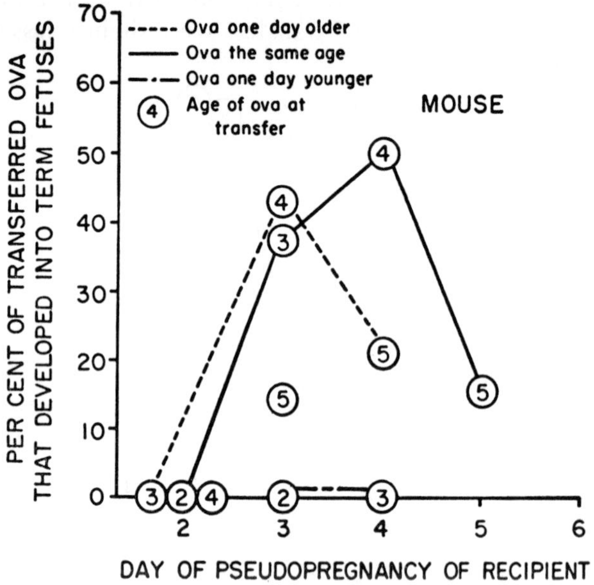

FIG. 2.—Percentage of 1,247 *mouse* ova that survived to term pregnancy after transfer to the uterine horns of 124 pseudopregnant recipient mice.

FATE OF ASYNCHRONOUSLY TRANSFERRED OVA

In these experiments, recipient females were mated one day before the donors. Table 1 shows that *in the rat*, when day-3 ova were recovered after 24 hours' residence in a day-4 uterus (or when day-2 ova were recovered after 48 hours in a day-3 uterus), the ova appeared to be normal (Dickmann and Noyes, 1960). But when day-4 ova were recovered after more than 9 hours' residence in a day-5 uterus, they were severely damaged (cf. Pl. I, *1* and *2*). It was concluded, therefore, that in the rat the endometrial environment, prior to implantation (days 3 and 4), permitted survival and development of relatively underdeveloped ova, then a sudden change, coinciding with the time of implantation (day 5), made the environment unfavorable for ovular survival.

Table 2 shows that *in the mouse* only about one-third of 1-day-younger ova could be recovered after 2–30 hours' residence in the uterus and that longer periods yielded even fewer ova (Doyle *et al.*, 1962). This low rate of recovery, plus the fact that the recovered ova appeared to be arrested in development and fragmented, suggested that the uterine environment of the mouse was incompatible with relatively underdeveloped ova. Unlike the rat, this incompatibility seemed to exist in the mouse throughout the early stages of pseudopregnancy.

TABLE 1

FATE OF DEVELOPING RAT OVA RECOVERED AFTER VARIOUS PERIODS OF TIME FOLLOWING TRANSFER TO RECIPIENT UTERUS, OVA BEING ONE DAY LESS DEVELOPED THAN UTERUS

Rat Ovular Development (Days)	Day of Pseudopregnancy of Recipient Rats	No. Hours Ova Left in Uterus	Hours Ova Subjected to Day-5 Uterine Conditions	Percentage Transferred Ova Recovered		Morphology
4 →	5	4– 6	4– 6	19/26	73	Good
		9	9	25/34	73	Variable
		12	12	11/17	64	Poor
		17–28	17–28	15/105	14	Poor
3 →	4	17–24	0	24/33	73	Good
		33–36	9–12	21/28	75	Variable
		41–48	17–24	0/20	0	Poor
2 →	3	16–18	0	9/19	47	Good
		24–25	0	4/19	21	Good
		32	0	1/10	10	Good
		48	0	4/8	50	Good
		57–59	9–11	1/26	4	Good

TABLE 2

FATE OF DEVELOPING MOUSE OVA RECOVERED AFTER VARIOUS PERIODS OF TIME FOLLOWING TRANSFER TO RECIPIENT UTERUS, OVA BEING ONE DAY LESS DEVELOPED THAN UTERUS

Mouse Ovular Development (Days)	Day of Pseudopregnancy of Recipient Mouse	No. Hours Ova Left in Uterus	Hours Ova Subjected to Day-4 Uterine Conditions	Percentage Transferred Ova Recovered	
4 →	5	4– 6	....	10/54	18
		7– 8	....	2/39	5
3 →	4	2– 6	2– 6	15/48	31
		18–19	18–19	1/25	4
		24–27	24–27	4/101	4
2 →	3	24	0	25/76	33
		30	6	8/23	35
		48	24	2/14	14

OVA 1 DAY OLDER THAN THE UTERUS

It was pointed out earlier that transfers of ova 1 day older than the uterus produced as many young as were produced by synchronous transfers, but two questions remained unanswered: Do these older ova implant sooner than ova that are the same stage as the uterus? Can older ova continue to develop in the uterus of the pseudopregnant animal without implanting?

In the rat, Table 3 shows that in the normal unoperated control the average number of ova that could be recovered by flushing the uterine horns decreased slightly between days 4 and 5, markedly between the morning and evening of day 5, and precipitously between the evening

TABLE 3

MEAN NUMBER OF OVA RECOVERED BY FLUSHING EACH UTERINE HORN OF UNOPERATED RATS ON DAYS 4–6 OF PREGNANCY AND OF RECIPIENT RATS ONE OR TWO DAYS FOLLOWING TRANSFER OF DAY-4 AND DAY-5 DONOR OVA INTO RECIPIENTS' UTERI ON DAY 4 OF PSEUDOPREGNANCY

Day (Hour) Ova Recovered	Mean No. Ova Recovered per Uterine Horn				
	Unoperated Controls	Synchronously Transferred		Asynchronously Transferred	
		Ova 1 Day *in Utero*	Ova 2 Days *in Utero*	Ova 1 Day *in Utero*	Ova 2 Days *in Utero*
4 (0900).......	4.2	....	....	....	....
5 (0900).......	4	5 (4→4)	....	5.5 (5→4)	....
5 (1900).......	3.2	....	....	....	....
6 (0900).......	1.5	1.5 (5→5)	2 (4→4)	....	2 (5→4)

of day 5 and the morning of day 6 (Dickmann and Noyes, 1960). This was also true of synchronously transferred ova. This suggested that implantation was occurring late on day 5 of pregnancy. When day-5 ova were asynchronously transferred to day-4 recipients and then the recipient uteri were flushed 1 day later, the recovery rate was good, but when the uteri were flushed 2 days later, the recovery rate was poor. It seemed, therefore, that the day-5 ova remained unattached and were 6 days old when they implanted, late on day 5 of pregnancy.

Histologic study suggested that the ova that were chronologically day 6 when they were implanted were developed further than the synchronously transferred controls (cf. Pl. II, *5* and *6*, also *7* and *8*) (Dickmann and Noyes, 1960). An effort was made to obtain a quantitative estimate of ovular development by counting the number of cells in the inner cell mass and also by estimating the volume of the trophoblast, but these methods did not establish significant differences between experimental results and controls.

In the mouse, synchronously and asynchronously transferred ova were flushed from the uterus at various times, the results being shown in Table 4. Statistical analysis showed that the point at which half the ova were recovered was 3 (1506) hours in the case of day-3 ova and 3 (1012) hours for day-4 ova. These values were not significantly different, and it was concluded that the older ova were implanting at about the same time as the controls. However, these points should not be taken as the median time for implantation because the proportion of ova that were not recovered included ova that were lost as well as ova that were too firmly implanted to be flushed from the uterus.

TABLE 4

NUMBER AND PERCENTAGE OF OVA RECOVERED FROM ONE OR MORE UTERINE HORNS OF 44 RECIPIENT MICE FOLLOWING TRANSFER OF DAY-3 AND DAY-4 OVA INTO RECIPIENTS' UTERI ON DAY 3 OF PSEUDOPREGNANCY

DAY (HOUR) OF PREGNANCY	NO. MOUSE UTERINE HORNS FLUSHED	SYNCHRONOUSLY TRANSFERRED 3-DAY MOUSE OVA		ASYNCHRONOUSLY TRANSFERRED 4-DAY MOUSE OVA	
		Ova Recovered/ Ova Transferred	Per Cent	Ova Recovered/ Ova Transferred	Per Cent
3 (0800)......	6	0/16	0	1/14	7
3 (0900)......	16	17/53	32	13/50	26
3 (1100)......	2	0/5	0	0/5	0
3 (1300)......	4	7/11	64	5/10	50
3 (1400)......	4	10/12	83	6/14	43
3 (1500)......	10	16/34	47	16/39	41
3 (1600)......	8	8/29	28	5/27	19
3 (1700)......	2	0/4	0	1/5	20
3 (2000)......	4	6/8	75	0/16	0
3 (2100)......	8	2/18	11	1/21	5
3 (2200)......	2	2/3	67	0/3	0
4 (0900)......	12	11/41	27	8/34	24
4 (1000)......	2	2/6	33	0/8	0
4 (1200)......	2	1/5	20	1/3	33
4 (1300)......	6	1/13	8	4/12	33

From the results described above, it is concluded that, in both rat and mouse, ova one day older than the uterus do not implant significantly earlier than synchronous controls. It is likely that the older ova continue to develop while waiting in a uterus that is relatively underdeveloped prior to the time of implantation, but further work is needed to establish this point.

THE DURATION OF ENDOMETRIAL SENSITIVITY

In the rat, deciduomata can be elicited by various stimuli on days 3–7 of pseudopregnancy. But the experiments reviewed above clearly show that neither synchronously transferred ova nor relatively underdeveloped ova implant before day 5. In order to test whether mature ova might be able to implant later than day 5, it was believed to be essential that ova of the same chronological stage as the uterus be used as test objects. Since intact ova cannot be obtained from the uterus on day 6 of pregnancy, indirect methods of obtaining chronologically day-6 ova were used. Rat ova were recovered from donors on day 5 and were transferred to day-4 recipients. After one day of "incubation," these day-6 ova were transferred into the uterus of a day-6 recipient. None of these blastocysts implanted.

TABLE 5

SURVIVAL OF "LATE" DAY-5 RAT OVA (1900 HOURS) TRANSFERRED INTO UTERUS LATE ON DAYS 5 AND 4 OF PSEUDOPREGNANCY, COMPARED WITH SURVIVAL OF "EARLY" DAY-5 RAT OVA (0900 HOURS) TRANSFERRRED INTO UTERUS EARLY ON DAYS 5 AND 4 OF PSEUDOPREGNANCY

Day (Hour) Rat Ova Recovered	Day (Hour) of Pseudopregnancy of Recipient Rat	Fetuses/ Ova Transferred	Per Cent
5 (1900)———	→5 (1900)	3/28	11
5 (1900)———	→4 (1900)	17/43	40
5 (0900)———	→5 (0900)	34/59	58
5 (0900)———	→4 (0900)	41/61	68

A point of incidental interest in the foregoing experiments was that no decidual reaction comparable to that normally seen on day 6 was noted on the day following 5 → 4 or 6 → 6 transfers. This, despite the fact that in both cases the endometrium was continuously subjected to the stimulus of blastocysts mature enough to implant. Perhaps the various artificial stimuli that have been used to elicit deciduomata are too gross to have much physiologic significance.

THE DURATION OF OVULAR COMPETENCE

As with the endometrium, the developing ovum might have a very limited period of optimal competence to implant. *In the rat*, Table 5 shows that only 11 per cent of "late" day-5 ova survived to term fetuses if they were placed in "late" day-5 uteri (Dickmann and Noyes, 1960). In order to distinguish whether ovular or endometrial factors were responsible for this low rate, late day-5 ova were transferred to late day-4 uteri, and 40 per cent survived to day 18 of pregnancy. This improvement indicated that late day-5 ova were capable of a much better implantation rate in the day-4 environment than they were able to achieve in a late day-5 endometrium. Experiments in which "early" day-5 ova were transferred early on days 5 and 4 (see Fig. 1) resulted in 58 per cent and 68 per cent survival, respectively, 70 per cent being optimal under our experimental conditions. It would seem that the ovum passes through a critical stage of maturation on day 5, and after this critical stage is passed the blastocyst rapidly loses its ability to implant even in optimal endometrial environment.

TABLE 6

NUMBER OF RAT OVA RECOVERED, NUMBER OF OVA PART WAY OUT OF ZONA PELLUCIDA, AND PERCENTAGE OF OVA FREE OF ZONA PELLUCIDA AT PROGRESSIVELY LATER TIMES ON DAY 5 OF PREGNANCY

Time on Day 5 Rat Ova Were Recovered	Average No. Ova Recovered per Uterine Horn	No. Ova with Blastocysts Part Way Out of Zona	Percentage of Ova Free of Zona
1000–1200	4.1	1	4
1300–1400	4.1	2	24
1900	4.1	2	77
1800–1900	3.1	0	88
2000	3	0	100

THE ZONA PELLUCIDA

Before the *rat ovum* attaches itself to the endometrium, the blastocyst separates itself from the zona pellucida. Table 6 shows that most ova are shedding their zonae between 1400 and 1900 on day 5 of pregnancy (Dickmann and Noyes, 1961). In only 5 of 715 day-5 ova the blastocysts were observed part way out of the zona, suggesting that in the individual ovum the shedding process is rapid.

Shedding of the zona depends on the maturity of the ovum and not on the changing uterine environment. Plate I, *3*, shows fertilized and unfertilized day-4 ova that have retained their zonae in the day-4 endometrium. Plate I, *4*, shows day-5 ova that have shed their zonae in the same day-4 environment. This experiment supports the findings of others, who have shown that the zona may be shed in the ligated oviduct and in the uterus during delayed implantation.

Forty-seven day-5 blastocysts were recovered from donors after they had shed their zonae, and 21 living fetuses were obtained when these ova were transferred to day-5 pseudopregnant recipients. This is conclusive evidence that in the rat the zona plays no vital role in implantation.

PREIMPLANTATION MATURATION OF THE OVUM AND FETAL DEVELOPMENT

In the first series of experiments, in which *rat ova* were transferred into the uteri of recipients on days 2–6 of pseudopregnancy, the fetuses were weighed in 3 recipients, and it was noted that the fetuses in one uterine horn were heavier than those in the other horn. Ova that were 1 day older than the corresponding stage of uterine development grew to be larger than the controls.

In order to check this preliminary observation more carefully, a series of experiments was carried out using both hybrid and backcross *mice* (Noyes *et al.*, 1961). Day-3 ova were transferred into one uterine horn, and day-4 ova into the other horn of mice on day 3 of pseudopregnancy.

TABLE 7

FACTORS CONTRIBUTING TO WEIGHT OF DAY-18 MOUSE FETUSES THAT SURVIVED IN BOTH UTERINE HORNS FOLLOWING TRANSFER OF DAY-3 AND DAY-4 OVA INTO UTERINE HORNS ON DAY 3 OF PSEUDOPREGNANCY

Factor Contributing to Mouse Fetal Weight	Estimates of Parameters (Mg.)	Standard Deviation of Estimate (Mg.)	Least Significant Differences (0.05) (Mg.)
Mean weight effect.........	814	35	69
Fetuses/uterine horn effect..	68*	27	54
Sex effect.................	32	46	92
Donor effect...............	− 34	24	48
Age effect.................	183*	23	46
Error term................	0	95	....

* Significant level 0.05.

The fetuses that survived to day 18 were removed from the uteri, weighed, and sexed. These data were punched on IBM cards and analyzed on a computer in such a way that an estimate was obtained for the contribution of several factors to fetal weight. An analysis of covariance was made for the following: weight of a particular fetus, mean weight of female fetuses resulting from day-3 hybrid ova, change in fetal weight because of varying numbers of fetuses within a given uterine horn, the difference in weight of male as against female fetuses, the difference in weight between fetuses resulting from backcross as against hybrid ova, and the difference in weight between fetuses resulting from day-4 as against day-3 ova.

Table 7 gives the factors obtained in 35 transfer experiments in which 158 ova resulted in 103 fetuses (Noyes *et al.*, 1961). Two results were significant: the decrease in weight of each fetus as the number of fetuses per uterine horn increased and the stage of maturation of the ovum relative to that of the uterus. Fetuses resulting from day-4 ova weighed 183 mg. more than did fetuses resulting from day-3 ova. This increase amounted to about one-quarter of the mean fetal weight and was equivalent to about two-thirds of the average gain in weight of mouse fetuses between days 18 and 19 of pregnancy. Evidently developmental processes within day-4 ova continue beyond the stage at which they are usually implanted, and this preimplantation development gives the older ova an advantage over the synchronously transferred control ova.

Discussion

The results of the foregoing experiments contributed to the following hypothesis. Implantation is the result of an interaction between the ovum and the endometrium, but the optimal interaction will take place only when the ovum and the endometrium have simultaneously reached specific stages in their development by the time they come in contact with each other. The processes that bring about these specific stages of ovular and endometrial development seem to be independent phenomena. Until at least day 5 of pregnancy in the rat, the ovum can mature and shed its zona pellucida either in the oviduct or in the uterus. The uterus develops under the control of the steroid hormones, independently of ovular influence, until late on day 5, when the endometrial environment suddenly changes, becoming detrimental to underdeveloped ova and stimulating developed and overdeveloped ova in such a way that they attach themselves to the endometrium and elicit the decidual reaction.

Beyond the critical late day-5 phase, both ova and endometrium rapidly lose their ability to participate in implantation. It as is though the ovum has a limited supply of "implantation material," and when this is used up the ovum can no longer participate in the interaction. This loss is not merely concomitant with increasing chronological age, because during delayed implantation no such rapid loss of implantability occurs. The loss of ability to implant takes place only in the particular environment of the late day-5 endometrium.

The endometrium also loses its capability of participating in the implantation interaction after late day 5. There is no gross evidence that ova elicit decidual reaction on day 4 or day 6 of pseudopregnancy the way less physiologic methods do. Thus, mature ova are possibly the only critical test objects for studying endometrial responsiveness to implantation.

The naturally occurring synchrony of development of ovum and endometrium is not optimal with respect to fetal weight at term. In both hybrid and backcross matings in mice, fetuses developing from ova that were one day overdeveloped in relation to the uterus weighed 25 per cent more than fetuses resulting from synchronous transfers. However, two days of overdevelopment relative to the uterus was detrimental to ovular survival.

It should be emphasized that ovular development and endometrial development were both normal in these experiments. In the asynchronous situation, endometrial development is always the reciprocal of ovular development. It is the relatively overdeveloped endometrium that is inhospitable to rat and mouse ova. One day of underdevelopment of the endometrium, relative to the ovum, favors survival of heavier fetuses than controls.

Although underdevelopment of the endometrium is believed to be a common cause of infertility and reproductive wastage in humans, the evidence to support this belief is equivocal. Presently available techniques do not permit a critical analysis of ovular-endometrial relationships in women, but we expect soon to undertake studies similar to those reported above in laboratory primates.

Conclusions

Synchronous and asynchronous ovum transfer experiments provided evidence that the implantation interaction between ovum and endometrium is a delicate balance between independent phenomena. The naturally occurring balance may not necessarily be the best one. Ova do not elicit gross decidual response over as wide a span of time as do less physiological stimuli. Further experiments, extended to other species, are needed to establish the general significance of this work.

Acknowledgments

This work was supported in part by grants RG5450 and RG7706 from the National Institutes of Health, U.S.P.H.S.; by grant G14355 from the National Science Foundation; by generous gifts from the Ortho Research Foundation (Dr. R. V. Chapple, director), the Ayerst Laboratories (Dr. J. B. Jewell, director), and the Squibb Institute for Medical Research (Dr. A. F. Langlykke, director); and by a private gift from Mrs. Lillian Howell.

We are grateful to Drs. D. L. Bentley and M. Klauber for statistical consultations and for major contributions to the experimental design and analysis. We acknowledge the assistance of Mr. W. Renner for photography, Drs. T. Clewe, F. Harrington, and S. Glasser for reading, and Mrs. I. Hays for preparing the manuscript.

References

Dickmann, Z., and R. W. Noyes. 1960. The fate of ova transferred into the uterus of the rat. J. Reprod. & Fertil., **1**:197–212.

———. 1961. The zona pellucida at the time of implantation. Fertil. & Steril., **12**:310–18.

DOYLE, L. L., A. H. GATES, R. W. NOYES, and M. KLAUBER. Asynchronous transfer of mouse ova. Fertil. & Steril. (In press.)
NOYES, R. W. 1959. The underdeveloped secretory endometrium. Am. J. Obstet. & Gynec., **77**:929–45.
NOYES, R. W., and Z. DICKMANN. 1960. Relationship of ovular age to endometrial development. J. Reprod. & Fertil., **1**:186–96.
———. 1961. Survival of ova transferred into the oviduct of the rat. Fertil. & Steril., **12**:67–79.
NOYES, R. W., L. L. DOYLE, and D. L. BENTLEY. 1961. Effect of preimplantation development on foetal weight in the rat. J. Reprod. & Fertil., **2**:238–45.
NOYES, R. W., L. L. DOYLE, A. H. GATES, and D. L. BENTLEY. 1961. Ovular maturation and fetal development. Fertil. & Steril., **12**:405–16.

DISCUSSION (*Chairman:* R. K. MEYER)

HAFEZ: In our work with the rabbit the percentage of implantation of old embryos to young endometrium did not exceed the controls (Hafez, 1963, J. Exp. Zool.). In other words, this may be interpreted to mean that the actual mechanical transfer of the embryo does not hinder the development of the embryos. In your experiments, was the percentage of implantation for the 4-day embryos transferred to 3-day endometrium better than that of 3-day embryos transferred to 3-day endometrium in both the rat and the mouse?

NOYES: Yes, but the implantation percentage was not statistically different.

HAFEZ: Your diagram on the release of the trophoblast from the zona pellucida may be interpreted as showing that the trophoblast squeezes itself through a cracked zona pellucida. Is that true, or does the zona pellucida split on the way to allow the trophoblast to come out without collapse? It would appear that in the rabbit the latter is true so that the blastocyst will not collapse prior to implantation.

DICKMANN: Our information to this point is as follows: On the fifth day of pregnancy, we find blastocysts that are no longer encased in a zona, and we also find empty zonae. These empty zonae do not seem to have a big crack.

HARTMAN: Apropos of Noyes's remarks about the escape of the blastocyst through a crack in the zona pellucida, may I say that in the opossum the zona grows over a hundred fold in area as the vesicle increases in size; the layer of mucus, and the shell membrane as well, stretch without bursting until they are absorbed altogether, leaving the yolk-sac membrane in direct contact with the uterine epithelium. One must presume that, under the influence of enzymes in the uterus, the egg membranes, under a chemical, change so as to permit their extreme attenuation and stretching. I am reminded of Lewis and Gregory's motion picture of the development of the rabbit egg in tissue culture, the zona bursting at hour 96 and the contents herniating out.

SHARMAN: I should like to refer to Dr. Hartman's earlier remarks about the fast tubal journey of *Didelphis* eggs, my own observations on the 24-hour tubal journey of the single egg of *Setonix* and *Trichosurus*, and Dr. Tyndale-Biscoe's experiments on transfer of *Setonix* embryos. I also recall a suggestion by Corner that the oviduct of eutherian mammals probably delays the egg in its tubal journey so that the uterus may be ready for its nidation when it arrives. Perhaps the marsupial uterus has a wider tolerance than that of eutherians so that there has been no need to evolve mechanisms to slow the egg in its tubal journey.

HAFEZ: I am concerned about the variation in the degree of development of the inner cell mass in blastocysts of the same age. We have been examining rabbit blastocysts 6 days postcoitum, and we have found great variability in (*a*) size of blastocysts, (*b*) degree, and (*c*) pattern of development of inner cell mass. Some blastocysts are four times as large as others. The inner cell mass may develop in diameter or in depth. The asynchronous and synchronous blastocysts that you referred to did not vary more than one day. I am wondering about deriving conclusions from such slight variations in chronological age of the two stages of blastocysts.

A. ENDERS: In recent studies with the electron microscope (Schlafke and A. Enders, 1963, J. Anat.) changes in distribution of organelles in both the trophoblast and the inner-cell-mass cells of the rat blastocyst could be seen on days 5, 6, 7, and later days in delayed implantation. These progressive changes appeared to be the same in grossly different blastocysts. That is, blastocysts from day 5 showed considerable variation in cell number and shape but cytologically were more similar to one another than to later blastocysts.

TYNDALE-BISCOE: I was much interested in Dr. Noyes's results on transplantation. I have attempted to do a few synchronous and asynchronous transfers in the wallaby with the idea of seeing the relationship of the blastocyst and the uterus. Synchronous transfers were successful up to 6 days after resumption of development. With asynchronous transfers, I got results opposite to Dr. Noyes's. The only certain results are those in which the fetus developed to full term. Delayed blastocysts transferred to the uterus either 4 or 6 days after removal of the pouch young resumed development, that is to say, the younger blastocyst developed in the older uterus. Blastocysts that had been developing for 4–6 days failed to develop to full term in the uterus of an animal in which the pouch young had been removed at the time of transfer. The delayed blastocyst is at approximately the stage reached 3 days after ovulation, and it is already lying in the uterus at the time of transfer.

KREHBIEL: Have you tried taking ova from delayed implantation and putting them into the 5-day uterus? Something may happen to the egg in delay.

NOYES: I think we can expect these blastocysts to be very delicate. In the rat our 5–3 were bad, even though we did them in the morning of day 5.

ALDEN: I should like to mention that in limited instances we have obtained a kind of implantation by segmenting ova of mice, which bears on this point. I wonder how you deal with the normal variation in blastocyst appearance in normally mated animals, that is, the normally observed variation in degree of blastocyst development seen within the same cornu?

NOYES: To keep variation to a minimum, the strain is important. You should use F_1 hybrids.

RUNNER: I am somewhat worried about extrapolations from your observations. I wonder whether you do not have a little bit of an uncontrollable factor. You make an incision in the 4- or 5-day uterus and then introduce blastocysts. The interpretation that both egg and endometrium synchronously pass through a narrowly restricted optimal period may be influenced by the operation. That is, the sharp peak of responsiveness described by Dr. De Feo in traumatized uteri is an experimental artifact almost certainly superimposed upon your transplantation experiment. The non-operated progestational uterus may remain optimally receptive for longer than the experiments would indicate. Such latitude would seem necessary to accommodate the variations seen within a single clutch of eggs.

NOYES: There are decidua at the puncture site. Transferring the eggs through the cervix might not obviate this. However, I do not think that handling the uterus does anything. Eggs do not implant on decidua.

G. MAYER

Delayed Nidation in Rats: A Method of Exploring the Mechanisms of Ovo-implantation

In the majority of species during pregnancy, the ovular and maternal phenomena unfold in a continuous way from fertilization to nidation, and, when the ovum has reached the blastocyst stage, it implants in an endometrium ready to receive it. The ovum can implant in territories by no means made to welcome it (eye, duodenum, kidney), as demonstrated by transplantation of ova in mice and rats, male or female, castrated or hypophysectomized (Fawcett *et al.*, 1947; Nicholas, 1950; Runner, 1947).

But, when the ovum is in the uterus, it is very sensitive to the environment in which it is found and whose variations depend on sex hormones. Therefore, it is the uterine environment as well as the determination of its establishment that must be defined in order to understand the mechanism of nidation.

Under normal conditions implantation of the ovum takes place, in most species, in the first days of gravidity. When the egg starts its development and migration down the oviduct, the uterus is preparing the cradle to welcome it. But the succession of phenomena is too fast and their intricacy is too great for man to be able to analyze with confidence. To take only one example, it is difficult to define precisely, in these conditions, the role played by the estrogen secreted by the ovary at the moment of estrus preceding the progestational phase in providing a uterine environment adequate for nidation. In the same way, it is difficult to state precisely whether an event that takes place in the ovum is autonomous and spontaneous or whether it is provoked by the uterine environment (Mayer, 1959*a*, 1959*b*).

DR. GASTON MAYER is professor of histology and embryology in the Faculty of Medicine, Bordeaux, France.

In order to analyze the phenomena, it would be useful to be able to interrupt the development of the ovum experimentally and to produce a resumption, after a certain time, by determining the precise conditions of the uterine environment that favor this resumption.

The rat seems to be a favorable species in this respect for two reasons. On the one hand, the existence of delayed implantation during lactation proves that halting development is possible and that the date of nidation is therefore not determined in this species (Latase, 1887, 1891; Bloch, 1959; Weichert, 1942); on the other hand, the rat is an animal in which we can relatively easily intervene with the different levels of the hormonal regulation of its uterine environment (Mayer, 1960, 1962*b*).

I. Analysis of Hormonal Mechanisms of Nidation by Method of Delayed Ovo-implantation in the Female Rat

During normal gravidity, the ova implant on day 6, if we consider the first day that in which the discovery of the vaginal plug, or intravaginal sperm, is made. The problem to solve is that of the factors responsible for implantation and to analyze how and why, at a precise moment in pregnancy, implantation takes place.

A. Role of the Ovary

The role of the ovary was explored by study of the course of pregnancy after ovariectomy and replacing the ovarian hormones by administration of progesterone alone or in association with estrogen. We should distinguish in this respect the experiments of castration done before the fourth day and those done after. As of day 4 the ova are in the uterus, where they are in the free blastocyst state until they implant. Before day 4 the ova migrate through the oviducts and divide. The needs of the ovum can therefore be different before and after the blastocyst stage, depending on its position in the uterus or in the oviduct.

1. *Ovariectomy on Day 4.* In 1956 we observed (Canivenc, Laffargue, and Mayer, 1956) that female rats castrated on day 4 and injected thereafter daily with progesterone, in general, do not implant, an effect that we could verify by laparotomy after the normal date of implantation. We then observed that the same results were obtained with different daily doses of progesterone (10, 5, 2.5, or 1 mg.).

Yet, to find that the ova implant, it is sufficient to add, at a given moment, a small dose of estradiol to the progesterone administered. In our first experiments we used 1 μg., while we now administer 0.1 μg. When estrogen is given on day 4, nidation takes place at about the normal date. When it is injected later on, at a given moment of progesterone therapy, implantation is delayed, as compared with the normal.

Nevertheless, nidation takes place within forty-eight hours of estradiol administration. Under these conditions, as long as the administration of progesterone lasts, the blastocysts can stay in a lethargic state for several weeks, until a revealing treatment—estrogen—leads them out of it.

Blastocysts of rats castrated on day 1 of gravidity implant normally with progesterone alone. In fact, a daily dose of progesterone of 10 or 5 mg. beginning on day 5 results in a normal implantation demonstrated and verified by laparotomy on day 10.

In conclusion, the needs of the rat for implantation of the ovum are different on day 4 of gravidity from those on day 5.[1] On day 4 progesterone and estrogen are needed; on day 5 progesterone alone suffices. These results raise a double problem: that of the role of progesterone and that of estrogen. The technique of experimentally induced delayed nidation can help us answer these questions.

a) Progesterone Necessary for Ovo-implantation but not for Survival of Blastocyst. Survival: Canivenc and Laffargue (1957) showed that the blastocyst of the rat does not die after castration on the fourth day, even without any administration of progesterone to the animal. The proof that these blastocysts are still living is given by the fact that even after five or six days of privation of ovarian hormones, they can implant and develop when progesterone (10 mg.) and estrogen (1 μg.) are injected into the rat.[2]

One could speculate that the adrenal cortex produces certain substances with progesterone effects and that its activity compensates for the absence of ovaries. It does not seem to be so, for we have seen (Mayer, Thevenot-Duluc, and Meunier, 1958) that the blastocyst of the rat can stay in lethargy in the uterus, in the absence of ovaries and the adrenal cortex, and that it can resume its development some days later if the rat is injected with progesterone and estrogen.

This method of delayed implantation permits the exploration of the sensitivity of the intrauterine blastocyst to different hormonal interventions—a thing difficult to accomplish during normal gravidity that de-

[1] Cochrane and Meyer (1957) obtain an interruption of the development of the ovum in the rat by castration on day 3 and injection of progesterone, yet with a normal implantation, when the ovaries are removed on day 4. Possibly these results are due to variations in different strains of rats employed.

[2] Progesterone alone does not seem to be sufficient to initiate development of blastocysts deprived of sex hormones at the beginning of day 4. In fact, in rats castrated on day 4 (10.00 hr.) the grafting of a pellet of 1 mg. of progesterone in contact with one of the two horns of the uterus does not induce implantation in that horn. But the same animal, subjected to the associated action of progesterone (5 mg.) and estradiol (0.1 μg.) by systemic injection, undergoes implantation in the two horns after such a treatment (Mayer, unpublished).

This result differs from that obtained by operating on whole rats, non-ovariectomized, pregnant, and lactating. In this case, the local injection of a suspension of progesterone induces implantation at the site of the injection and allows the realization of superfetation (Canivenc, Drouvillé, and Mayer, 1953).

velops in a continuous manner, in which the blastocyst stage is very brief. In fact, we can administer during this period of lethargy different hormones and substances to see whether they are detrimental to the blastocyst, the test being the induced implantation of the blastocyst after the treatment. This technique has shown that if progesterone is not essential for the survival or the intrauterine retention of the blastocyst in lethargy, it seems nevertheless to favor that lethargy, while estrogen is noxious in the absence of progesterone.

But a reservation should be made as to the value of the method; the action of the various administered substances on the blastocyst is appreciated by the subsequent possibility or the impossibility of obtaining implantation. Yet the substances being tested may induce the expulsion of ova before the application of the revealing treatment. On the other hand, the administration of various hormones during the period of lethargy can modify the uterine environment as well as the reaction of the

TABLE 1

SPONTANEOUS NIDATIONS IN OVARIECTOMIZED RATS

Ovariectomy		Spontaneous Implantations (Day-8 Laparotomy)		Induced Implantations (Day-15 Laparotomy)	
Day	Hour	N/T	NT/N	N/T	NT/N
5.........	10.00	0/5⁻	0	0/5	0
6.........	10.00	7/10	49/7	0/3	0

N = Number of animals with implantations. T = Total number of experimental animals. NT = Total number of implantation sites.

uterus to the revealing treatment. In both these cases the revealing treatment can be ineffective without proving to be a particular detrimental action on the blastocyst. This technique must then be checked by transplantation of the experimental blastocysts into a new uterine environment, a process that may make allowance for the reservations expressed above.

Implantation: The results of castration at different moments of the preimplantation stage (days 4–6) show that the blastocyst needs progesterone to implant. Laparotomy performed on day 8 shows that ova do not implant in the absence of progesterone if castration is done on day 5 (10.00 hr., 16.00 hr., and 18.00 hr.), but they do implant if castration is done on day 6 (10.00 hr.) (Table 1). Yet there is a very fast involution of the implantation sites in the absence of progesterone (Mayer and Thevenot-Duluc, unpublished).

One might ask what is the threshold of progesterone required to obtain nidation, for instance, after castration on day 5 at 10.00 hours, that is to say, from that moment in which progesterone alone becomes sufficient to induce implantation. This threshold seems to lie between 0.25 and 0.50 mg.—the first dose does not result in nidation, while the second sometimes allows it.[3]

We also wondered whether blastocysts on day 5 of pregnancy could undergo a lethargic state for some time and then resume development. In rats castrated on day 5 of gravidity (10.00 hr.) the administration of the revealing therapy (progesterone and estrogen) beginning on day 10 did not result in ovo-implantation; but these preliminary experiments do not permit us to conclude that the blastocysts were dead as a result of the absence of ovarian hormones after having reached the day-5 stage —for a washing of the uterine horns is necessary to see whether the blastocysts are no longer in the uterus.

b) *Importance of Role of Estrogen in Implantation.* In rats castrated on day 4 and injected with progesterone daily (for example, 5 mg.) the experimenter can induce nidation at will by administering a small dose of estradiol (0.1–0.5 μg.). One fact is that it is possible to bring the blastocyst out of its lethargy at will with estrogen; another fact is that implantation in rats castrated on day 5 requires only progesterone, while both progesterone and estrogen are required in rats ovariectomized on day 4. These two results and other converging facts, especially those obtained by Shelesnyak and Kraicer on decidualization, indicate estrogen release by the ovary between days 4 and 5.

According to this theory, if castration is performed before the release of estrogen, progesterone alone is not sufficient for implantation. If performed after estrogen release, progesterone becomes sufficient.

When does this turning point occur? We can have an approximate idea about it by castrating rats at different moments during day 4 of gravidity. This experiment shows that progesterone alone is insufficient when castration is performed in the first half of day 4; the first positive cases appear during the second half of day 4, the period that would correspond to the action on the uterus of estrogen released by the ovary (Fig. 1).

It is probable that in this respect there are individual variations, and there may be seasonal ones, which can affect the moment of estrogen release on day 4. One should insist on the fact that in this experimental field, possibly more than in other fields, one should operate on animals of a well-standardized colony, as far as weight, food, temperature, and light are concerned, and see that the operations are performed at a definitive hour of the day, the same for the tested animals and for the controls.

[3] These threshold doses correspond somehow to those obtained by Chambon (1949*a*) through another technique in rats spayed on the second day of gravidity.

2. *Ovariectomy before Day 4.* Admitting the theory of estrogen release between days 4 and 5 of gravidity, and supposing that estrogen released during day 4 is responsible for implantation in a rat under the action of progesterone, then castration done before day 4 should result in the absence of nidation in spite of the administration of sufficient doses of progesterone.

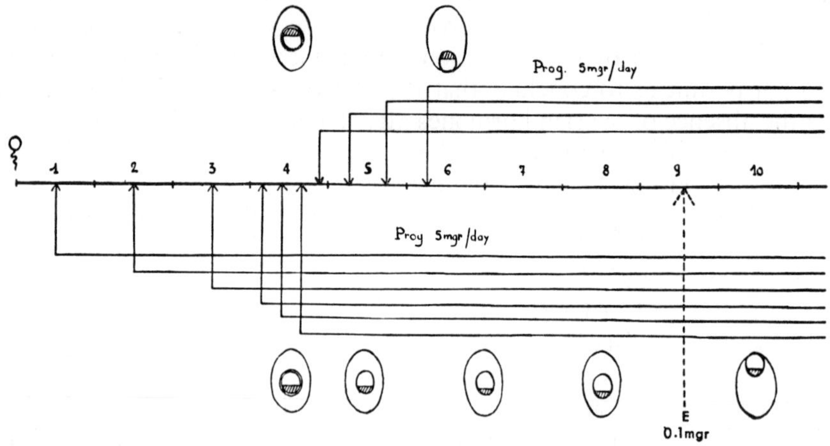

FIG. 1.—Diagram showing the importance of the time of ovariectomy on ovo-implantation and the difference in physiological hormonal requirements before and after day 4 (day 1 is the day of discovery of the vaginal plug). *Lower part:* If the ovariectomy is performed before day 4 or early on day 4, nidation does not take place in animals injected daily with progesterone as of the day of castration; the blastocysts remain free in the uterine lumen, in a dormant state. But injection of estrogen (0.1 μg. estradiol) at any time during the lethargic phase provokes the nidation of the eggs (delayed nidation). *Upper part:* If the animals are ovariectomized after day 4, the ovo-implantation does occur at day 6 in rats receiving progesterone alone (4 mg/day). The reason for these different results seems to be the occurrence of an estrogen surge on day 4, which plays an important role in nidation.

Our first results, in 1956, do not support this conclusion because we obtained implantation in rats castrated on day 2 of gravidity with the sole administration of progesterone. Similar results had already been recorded by Chambon in 1949. We have done these experiments again, using a chemically pure progesterone and taking care to remove the ovaries completely without injuring the oviduct where the ova are (Table 2). Under these conditions progesterone alone (and at the daily dose of 5 mg.) does not result in implantation; yet it is sufficient to inject 0.1 μg. estradiol into rats in the second half of day 4 to obtain nidation on day 6. If estrogen is injected later on, delayed implantation is obtained, the delay depending on the time of estrogen administration.[4]

[4] In this we agree with Psychoyos and Alloiteau (1962), who in their observations come to the conclusion that the results of ovariectomy on day 4 (before noon) do not oppose those obtained by castration on day 2.

To sum up, the experimental study of delayed nidation has allowed us to establish the role of estrogen in launching the phenomena of ovo-implantation and to induce nidation at will within forty-eight hours after the injection of estradiol. These results and those of Shelesnyak and Kraicer led to a working theory, that of the physiological release of estrogen during day 4, which would be responsible under normal conditions for implantation on day 6 (Fig. 2). These results make it necessary to explore the factors responsible for the activity of the ovary during progestation with regard to the mechanism conditioning the secretion of progesterone, as well as that responsible for the release of estrogen.

TABLE 2

DELAYED IMPLANTATION IN RATS OVARIECTOMIZED DAY 2

PROGESTERONE ADMINISTRATION (5 MG/DAY) (DAYS)	ESTRADIOL ADMINISTRATION (1 INJECTION, 0.1 μG.) (DAY)	IMPLANTATION					
		Day 8		Day 10		Day 15	
		N/T	NT/N	N/T	NT/N	N/T	NT/N
2–14	10	....	....	0/11	....	10/11	58/10
2–7	4	8/12	37/8	....	....	....	....

N = Number of animals with implantations. T = Total number of experimental animals. NT = Total number of implantation sites.

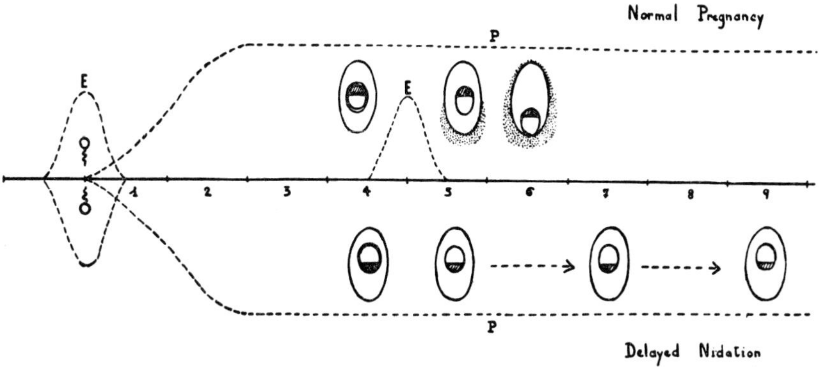

FIG. 2.—Diagram concerning the theory of estrogen surge at day 4. *Upper part:* During normal pregnancy, after estrus (*E*) and fertilization, the corpora lutea secrete progesterone (*P*). At day 4 the eggs are in the uterine lumen (blastocyst stage). At day 4 an estrogen surge begins. The blastocysts implant on day 6. *Lower part:* During delayed nidation (during lactation of numerous young, for example) the extrogen surge at day 4 does not take place. Despite the presence of progesterone, the blastocysts do not implant and remain free in the uterus until the conditions for nidation become favorable (that is, until estrogen secretion occurs).

B. THE ROLE OF THE HYPOPHYSIS

As we have seen, in order to implant, the ovum needs progesterone and estrogen, which are furnished by the ovaries under normal conditions. But the activity of the ovaries is governed by that of the anterior lobe of the hypophysis; the latter must intervene indirectly in the phenomena of implantation by sustaining the secretion of progesterone and by inducing that of estrogen. We know that the first is due to the action of prolactin—which is the luteotrophic hormone (LTH) in the rat—while the second results from the action of FTH (FSH + LH).

The suppression of the two groups of gonadotrophins of the hypophysis can be accomplished by hypophysectomy. When it is complete, it provokes, of course, the suspension of all the ovarian activity, and that in itself is harmful for implantation—for it does not take place—yet we can provoke implantation with progesterone and estradiol (Meunier, 1961).[5]

The selective suppression of FTH (FSH + LH) can be obtained, at least in the rat, by disconnecting the hypophysis from the hypothalamus. We know from the research of Everett (1954, 1956), Desclin (1956), Harris (1955), Meunier (1961), and Alloiteau (1962) that the secretion of LTH seems to be the product of the autonomous activity of the hypophysis and that it is released after elimination of suppression by the hypothalamus. The hypothalamic pituitary disconnection should result in a hormonal picture characterized (*a*) by the secretion of progesterone by the maintained corpora lutea and (*b*) by the absence of the release of ovarian estrogen. Such an endocrine state is that which characterizes the phase of lethargy in delayed implantation (Mayer, 1962*a;* Meunier, 1961).

Autotransplantation of the hypophysis in the kidney is a good means of liberating the pituitary from the action of the hypothalamus. In the virgin rat operated at estrus it permits establishment of a hormonal equilibrium analogous to that provoked by lactation. This system is characterized by the presence of progesterone and by the absence of estrogen; the corpora lutea are large, the vaginal mucosa has a bilaminar epithelium indicating the absence of estrogen, and the mammary glands show signs of secretion in spite of their small development (Everett, 1954, 1956; Desclin, 1956; Nikitowitch-Winner and Everett, 1958).

[5] In a certain number of our experiments, the daily injection of 10 mg. of progesterone has permitted us to obtain normal implantation in rats hypophysectomized on the first day of gravidity. The examination of the sella turcica did not reveal the presence of a fragment of the hypophysis. This observation does not seem to fit in the general framework of our results, that in the rat castrated before day 4 progesterone alone does not permit implantation. These results join the problem of normal or delayed implantation sometimes observed in rats ovariectomized on the beginning of day 4 and submitted only to a progesterone treatment.

Applied to gravidity, autotransplantation of the hypophysis permits the establishment of delayed nidation (Table 3). When the hypophysis is grafted under the kidney during the first day of gravidity, implantation does not take place but the ova stay in lethargy in the uterus. The administration of estradiol (0.1 μg.) induces their implantation, more or less late, depending on the moment of the injection (Table 4), while the needs of progesterone are furnished by the corpora lutea maintained by the hypophyseal graft (Meunier and Mayer, 1961; Meunier, 1961). Similar results have been obtained by Meyer, Prasad, and Cochrane (1958), Cochrane (1961), and Cochrane, Prasad, and Meyer (1962).

TABLE 3

ACTION OF AUTOTRANSPLANTATION OF THE HYPOPHYSIS ON IMPLANTATION IN THE RAT

Day of Operation	Spontaneous Implantation Observed		Histological Structures			
	Day 12	Day 20	Corpora Lutea	Vaginal Epithelium	Mammary Gland D	Mammary Gland L
1	0/15	0/15	+++	LM	(+)	++
2	0/5	0/5	+++	LM	(+)	++
3	0/6	0/6	+++	LM	(+)	++
4	4/15	0/7	+++	LM	(+)	++
5	1/7	0/6	+++	LM	(+)	++

LM = Lactation type of mucification. D = Development. L = Lactation.

TABLE 4

ACTION OF AUTOTRANSPLANTATION OF THE HYPOPHYSIS ON NIDATION IN THE RAT: ACTION OF PROGESTERONE AND ESTRADIOL

Day of Hypophysectomy	Day of Autotransplantation	Treatment: Progesterone		Treatment: Estradiol		Day of Autopsy	Nidations	
		Dose per Day	Duration (Days)	Dose per Day	Duration (Days)		N/T	NT/N
1	1	0	....	....	....	12	0/15	0
1	1	10 mg.	1–12	....	....	13	9/12	51/9
1	....	10 mg.	1–12	....	....	13	6/9	7/6
1	1	0	....	0 μg. 1	1–8	9	4/5	....
1	1	0	....	0 μg. 1	4, 5, 6	12	4/6	....
1	1	0	....	0 μg. 1	19, 20, 21	25	6/8	....

N = Number of animals with implantations. T = Total number of experimental animals. NT = Total number of implantation sites.

When the graft of the hypophysis is made on day 4, a certain number of ovo-implantations is obtained without the aid of estrogen administration. We can suppose that in these cases the ovary had already received the stimulus of the hypophysis to secrete enough estradiol to induce nidation.

On the condition that the treatment be started immediately after estrus, different drugs, such as reserpine (Mayer, Meunier, and Ronault, 1958) or certain tranquilizers (Psychoyos, 1958), provoke in the virgin rat a hormonal picture similar to that produced by hypophyseal transplants: lactogenesis, maintenance of active corpora lutea, and absence of estrogen secretion. The administration of estradiol modifies

TABLE 5

RESERPINE AND OVO-IMPLANTATION

Day of Treatment			Implantation			
Reserpine	Estradiol	Progesterone	Day 10		Day 15	
100 μg/100 gm	0.25 μg.	5 mg.	N/T	NT/N	N/T	NT/N
4	0	0	8/15	67/8	...	...
4	10–14	10–14	0/7	0	2/7	8/2
1–9	0	0	3/24	22/3	...	...
1–9	1–9	0	7/10	48/7	...	...
1–9	0	1–9	2/10	6/2	...	...
1–9	10–14	10–14	...	...	1/7	10/1

N = Number of animals with implantations. T = Total number of experimental animals. NT = Total number of implantation sites.

these histophysiological results; it transforms the bilaminar vaginal epithelium into a mucous multilaminar one and closes the mammary alveoli by developing the tubuloalveolar system of the mammary glands. The daily injection of reserpine (100 μg/100 gm weight) during the first eight days prevents normal implantation in general, while the administration of estradiol as of day 4 allows it (Table 5) under the same conditions (Mayer and Meunier, 1959).

Finally, it should be noted that in a certain number of cases the administration of reserpine during the first eight days of gravidity (Table 6) provokes delayed nidations that, in general, take place spontaneously about eight days after cessation of the treatment (Mayer, Meunier, and Thevenot-Duluc, 1960). It is possible in these cases that ova implant when the ovarian secretion of estrogen is resumed after it has been suspended by the administration of reserpine. In spite of the fact that the action of this substance is complex, we are nevertheless surprised by the histophysiological results that it gives—that of pharmacological disconnection between the hypothalamus and the hypophysis. We are equally surprised by the fact that the rats injected with reserpine present a histophysiological state analogous to that of lactation and that this substance can provoke delayed nidation as the suckling of numerous young. Similar results have been obtained by Chambon (1955) with chlorpromazine.

The analysis of the action of the hypophysis in ovo-implantation through the study of delayed nidation leads to the theory of an autonomous participation of the pituitary in the functional maintenance of the corpora lutea and the secretion of progesterone and to the theory of a

TABLE 6

ACTION OF RESERPINE ON IMPLANTATION

Treatment with Reserpine 100 μg/100 gm of Weight from Day to Day (Inclusive)	Total No. of Treated Animals	No. Animals with Pregnancy	Duration of Pregnancy	
			No. Animals	Day of Parturition
1–2	4	3	0	21
1–4	9	3	2	25
			1	26
1–6	7	2	1	23
			1	29
1–8	28	12	2	23
			1	24
			2	29
			3	30
			3	31
			1	32

hypothalamohypophyseal intervention in the release of estrogen responsible for implantation. If we admit the existence of FTH release on day 4 of a normal gravidity, there remains to be determined under what influence it is brought about and what it represents in relation to the periodic release of estrogen during the course of ovarian cycles.

Finally, the analysis of the hormonal factors of ovo-implantation by delayed nidation has furnished the experimenter with a method that can be used with profit in the study of the tissues and cytological mechanisms of implantation.

II. Analysis of the Cytological Mechanism of Nidation by Delayed Ovo-implantation in the Rat

Little is known concerning the cytological mechanism of nidation, but the technique of delayed nidation can be of great help in its exploration.

Research done on normal nidation pointed out the modifications that the endometrium and the egg undergo before implantation (for this latter point see Alden, 1957; Enders, 1961; Vokaer and Leroy, 1962). On the one hand, the study of the development of blastocysts washed from the uterine horns between days 4 and 6 has shown that the zona pellucida disappears toward day 5, while the blastocyst takes a characteristic elongated aspect on day 6 (Psychoyos, 1961). On the other hand, the endometrium also undergoes definite modifications, which are demonstrated by its tendency toward "decidualization." Shelesnyak and Kraicer (1960) have shown, by the technique of pyrathiazine, that the maximum sensitivity of the endometrium for decidualization lies on day 5 at about 10.00 hours, that is to say, a short time after the supposed intervention of estrogen released before implantation.

The technique of delayed nidation, which permits implantation to be induced at will, can be used to determine the role of estrogen in the development of the modifications of the blastocyst and those of the endometrium.

This work has already shown that estrogen does not seem to be responsible for the disappearance of the zona pellucida. In fact, blastocysts rid themselves of it in rats castrated on the beginning of day 4 and injected with progesterone, that is, before the eventual release of estrogen. The blastocysts in lethargy in the uterus are consequently free of zona pellucida. This means that the disappearance of the zona is not a sufficient condition for implantation. The blastocysts' reactivation allows us to study in a precise way the morphological variations of the blastocysts after injection of estrogen and before implantation. In preliminary research done by our team at Bordeaux, together with Kraicer of the group at Rehovoth, it seems that the first modifications appear nearly eighteen hours after the administration of estradiol. But these investigations should be completed.

In the field of endometrial modifications, the major problem is to know the factor, or the factors, responsible for the appearance and the disappearance of uterine sensitivity toward traumatism or toward the presence of a foreign body in the uterus. We have seen that a blastocyst in lethargy *in utero* can provoke, in the castrated rat injected with progesterone, the decidual reactions of implantation following an injection of a small dose of estrogen (Mayer, 1960; Psychoyos, 1962). Does the uterus react in the same way to mechanical traumatism in analogous conditions?

Recently, we at Bordeaux have approached this problem. Rats castrated at estrus are injected with 5 mg. of progesterone daily. The uterus is injured by a longitudinal thread inserted and left in the uterine horn, either on the fifteenth day or on the twenty-fifth day following the administration of progesterone. Some animals, examined four days after traumatization, respond by weak decidual reactions generally. The administration 24 hours before the trauma, of 0.1 μg. of estradiol (a dose sufficient to induce implantation in rats castrated and injected with progesterone) did not modify in a significant way the reaction to traumatization.

Another experimental series makes use of rats castrated a month previously. A longitudinal thread is inserted into and left in the uterine horns, and a dose of 5 mg. of progesterone is injected daily. The presence of the thread in the uterus does not induce macroscopic decidual reactions, and neither does the administration of 0.1 μg. of estradiol during the course of the progestrone treatment.

Along this line of thought, it should be pointed out that an intrauterine blastocyst is not able to launch a decidual reaction, while this can be obtained by a traumatization inflicted on the endometrium under the same hormonal conditions. This is the case in rats castrated on the beginning of day 4 of gravidity and injected with progesterone, in whose uteri blastocysts do not implant and whose endometria react to the passage of a thread by the appearance of a decidual reaction (Mayer, Thevenot-Duluc, and Meunier, 1958). Here, also, new investigations are necessary to determine precisely the role of the blastocyst in the induction of the decidual reaction and what the release of estrogen does to it from this point of view.

It seems from these data that the endometrium subjected to the action of estrogen becomes sensitive to the presence of the blastocysts and that the modifications that the latter undergo after estrogen administration are not sufficient to confer upon them the quality of inducing decidual reactions in a rat subjected to progesterone alone. It is possible that the release of estrogen confers upon the ovum "aggressive" potentialities and upon the endometrium an increased sensitivity to the presence of blastocysts.

In summary, the method of experimental delayed nidation permits the elucidation of certain problems that arise concerning the physiology of ovo-implantation in the rat. It has demonstrated the important role of estrogen, which, by acting on a uterus primed by progesterone, initiates nidation. It gives the experimenter the possibility of studying by means of convergent methods the modifications of the uterus and of the blastocysts at the preimplantation period. It draws attention, finally, to those qualities of the blastocyst which, in 1891, had allowed M. F. Lataste to compare the fertilized mammalian ovum to the fertilized ovum of birds before incubation, or even to a seed before germination, which can wait a certain time until the realization of all the conditions necessary for their development.

But we should take care not to extend the results obtained in the rat to other species. Thus, in the rabbit (Courrier, 1945; Chambon, 1949*b*; Hafez and Pincus, 1956) and in the hamster (Prasad, Orsini, and Meyer, 1960) the needs of the ovo-implantation are different from those in the rat. These authors found that the administration of exogenous progesterone alone to ovariectomized animals of these species is sufficient to assure implantation, while in the ovariectomized guinea pig nidation takes place in the absence of exogenous progesterone (Deanesly, 1960).

References

ALDEN, R. H. 1947. Implantation of the rat egg. II. Alteration in osmiophilic epithelial lipids of the rat uterus under normal and experimental conditions. Anat. Rec., **97**:1–13.

ALLOITEAU, J. J. 1962. Le contrôle hypothalamique de l'adenohypophyse. III. Régulation de la fonction gonadotrope femelle: Activité LTH. Biol. Med., **51**:250–59.

BLOCH, S. 1959. Weitere Untersuchungen über die hormonalen Grundlagen der Nidation. Gynaecologia, **148**:157–74.

CANIVENC, R., C. DROUVILLÉ, and G. MAYER. 1953. Développement simultané d'embryons d'âges différents chez la ratte: Réalisation expérimentale. C.R. Acad. Sci. Paris, **237**:1036–38.

CANIVENC, R., and M. LAFFARGUE. 1957. Survie des blastocystes du rat en l'absence d'hormones ovariennes. C.R. Acad. Sci. Paris, **245**:1752–54.

CANIVENC, R., M. LAFFARGUE, and G. MAYER. 1956. Nidations retardées chez la ratte castrée et injectée de progestérone: Influence du moment de la castration sur la chronologie de l'ovo-implantation. C.R. Soc. Biol., **150**: 2208–12.

CHAMBON, Y. 1949*a*. Réalisation du retard de l'implantation par de faibles doses de progestérone chez la ratte. C.R. Soc. Biol., **143**:756–58.

———. 1949*b*. Besoins endocriniens qualitatifs et quantitatifs de l'ovoimplantation chez la lapine. *Ibid*., **163**:1172–75.

———. 1955. Action de la chlorpromazine sur l'évolution et l'avenir de la gestation chez la ratte. Ann. Endocrin., **16**:912–22.

COCHRANE, R. L. n.d. Studies on the mechanisms of delayed implantation in the mink and rat. Ph.D. thesis, University of Wisconsin, 1961.

COCHRANE, R. L., and R. K. MEYER. 1957. Delayed nidation in the rat induced by progesterone. Proc. Soc. Exp. Biol. & Med., **96**:155–59.

COCHRANE, R. L., M. R. N. PRASAD, and R. K. MEYER. 1962. Delayed nidation in the rat induced by autografts of the hypophysis, with a case report of "asynchronous implantation." Endocrinology, **70**:228–32.

COURRIER, R. 1945. Endocrinologie de la gestation. Paris: Masson et Cie.

DEANESLY, R. 1960. Implantation and early pregnancy in ovariectomized guinea-pigs. J. Reprod. & Fertil., **1**:242–48.

DESCLIN, L. 1956. Hypothalamus et libération d'hormone lutéotrophique: Expérience de greffes hypophysaires chez le rat hypophysectomisé. Action lutéotrophique de l'ocytocine. Ann. Endocrin., **17**:586–95.

ENDERS, A. C. 1961. Comparative studies on the endometrium of delayed implantation. Anat. Rec., **139**:483–97.

EVERETT, J. W. 1954. Luteotrophic function of autografts of the rat hypophysis. Endocrinology, **54**:685–90.

———. 1956. Functional corpora lutea maintained for months by autografts of rat hypophysis. *Ibid.*, **58**:786–96.

FAWCETT, W. DON, G. B. WISLOCKI, and C. M. WALDO. 1947. The development of mouse ova in the anterior chamber of the eye and in the abdominal cavity. Am. J. Anat., **61**:413–44.

HAFEZ, E. S. E., and G. PINCUS. 1956. Hormonal requirements of implantation in the rabbit. Proc. Soc. Exp. Biol. & Med., **91**:531–34.

HARRIS, G. W. 1955. Neural Control of Pituitary Gland. London: Arnold.

LATASTE, F. 1887. Recherche de zooéthique sur les mammifères de l'ordre des rongeurs. Cadillac sur Garonne: Vital Raoul Lataste.

———. 1891. De la variation de durée de la gestation chez les mammifères et des circonstances qui déterminent ces variations. Mem. Soc. Biol., **43**:21–31.

MAYER, G. 1959*a*. L'ovo-implantation et la vie latente de l'œuf. Bull. Soc. Roy. Belge Gynéc. & Obstét., **29**:1–41.

———. 1959*b*. Recent studies on hormonal control of delayed implantation and superimplantation in the rat. In Implantation of Ova, pp. 76–83. Mem. Soc. Endocrin., No. 6. Cambridge: Cambridge University Press.

———. 1960. Une méthode d'exploration de l'ovo-implantation: L'Interruption du développement de l'œuf. Ann. Endocrin., **21**:501–12.

———. 1962*a*. Fonction gonadotrope des greffes hypophysaires chez la femelle (Étude sur la ratte). Biol. Med., **51**:274–85.

———. 1962*b*. The experimental control of ovoimplantation. In Techniques in Endocrine Research: Nato Advanced Study Institute, Stratford upon Avon, September 2–12. (In press.)

MAYER, G., and J. M. MEUNIER. 1959. Réserpine et progestation chez la ratte: Survie des œufs en phase latente et ovoimplantation normales ou retardées provoquées par l'œstrogène. C.R. Acad. Sci. Paris, **248**:3355–57.

MAYER, G., J. M. MEUNIER, and J. E. ROUAULT. 1958. État hormonal provoqué chez la ratte par l'administration de réserpine: Action de l'œstrogène. C.R. Acad. Sci. Paris, **247**:524–27.

MAYER, G., J. M. MEUNIER, and A. J. THEVENOT-DULUC. 1960. Prolongation de la grossesse par retard de nidation obtenue chez la ratte par l'administration de réserpine. Ann. Endocrin., **21**:1–13.

MAYER, G., A. J. THEVENOT-DULUC, and J. M. MEUNIER. 1958. Action chez la ratte de différents équilibres hormonaux sur l'ovoimplantation et la vie latente de l'œuf. C.R. Acad. Sci. Paris, **246**:1911–14.

MEUNIER, J. M. n.d. Étude expérimentale par la technique des greffes hypophysaires et l'administration de réserpine de la régulation hypothalamique de l'activité gonadotrope chez la ratte. Thèse Doct. Sci., Bordeaux, 1961.

MEUNIER, J. M., and G. MAYER. 1961. Autogreffe d'hypophyse et ovoimplantation chez la ratte injectée de progestérone. C.R. Acad. Sci. Paris, **252**: 4049–51.

Meyer, R. K., M. R. N. Prasad, and R. L. Cochrane. 1958. Delayed implantation in the rat induced by autografts of the hypophysis. Anat. Rec., **130**:339.

Nicholas, J. B. 1950. Experiments on developing rats. VII. Transplantations to intestinal mucosa. J. Exp. Zool., **113**:741–60.

Nikitowitch-Winer, M., and J. W. Everett. 1958. Comparative study of luteotropin secretions by hypophyseal autotransplants on the rat. Effects of site and stages of the estrous cycle. Endocrinology, **62**:522–32.

Prasad, M. R. N., N. W. Orsini, and R. K. Meyer. 1960. Nidation in progesterone treated, estrogen deficient hamsters (*Mesocricetus auratus* Waterhouse). Proc. Soc. Biol. & Med., **104**:48–51.

Psychoyos, A. 1958. Considérations sur les rapports de la chlorpromazine et de la lutéotrophine hypophysaire. C.R. Soc. Biol., **152**:918–20.

———. 1961. Nouvelles recherches sur l'ovoimplantation. C.R. Acad. Sci. Paris, **252**:2306–7.

———. 1962. Le déterminisme de l'ovoimplantation: Recherches complémentaires. *Ibid.*, **255**:775–77.

Psychoyos, A., and J. J. Alloiteau. 1962. Castration précoce et nidations de l'œuf chez la ratte. C.R. Soc. Biol., **156**:46–49.

Runner, M. N. 1947. Development of mouse eggs in the anterior chamber of the eye. Anat. Rec., **98**:1–18.

Shelesnyak, M. C., and P. F. Kraicer. 1960. Décidualization: Une étude expérimentale. In Les fonctions de nidations utérine et leurs troubles, pp. 87–101. Paris: Masson & Cie.

Vokaer, R., and F. Leroy. 1962. Experimental study on local factors in the process of ova implantation in the rat. Am. J. Obstet. & Gynec., **83**:141–48.

Weichert, C. K. 1942. The experimental control of prolonged pregnancy in the lactating rat by means of oestrogen. Anat. Rec., **83**:1–14.

DISCUSSION (*Chairman:* R. K. Meyer)

Buchanan: In rats ovariectomized on day 4 (day 1 is the day sperm are found), blastocysts are recoverable for how long?

Mayer: We did not try to get the maximum of survival of the eggs after ovariectomy day 4, but we observed that in animals spayed and injected with progesterone, eggs are recoverable 15 or 20 days after ovariectomy. In rats spayed at day 4 of the pregnancy and without any hormonal treatment after spaying, eggs are recoverable 11 days after the operation. But maybe these delays are not maximal.

Buchanan: In rats ovariectomized and adrenalectomized?

Mayer: We observed the presence of intrauterine eggs 6 or 7 days after the operation performed on day 4.

De Feo: Do tranquilizers, such as chlorpromazine, which also activate corpora lutea but do not produce a body weight loss as does reserpine, also cause a delayed implantation?

Mayer: Yes, it seems to do so. Chambon (1958, Bull. Acad. N. Med.,

142:243) has found some shortening of delay with chlorpromazine. In our experiments we used very high doses of reserpine, and it is possible that the drug produces stress. But we must emphasize that the histo-physiological picture of the ovary and the vagina is the same in reserpine animals as in animals bearing a hypophyseal autograft.

YOCHIM: Can you speculate on the possible source of estrogen just before and after implantation?

MAYER: Before the implantation, and particularly at day 4, the source of estrogen seems to be the ovary. After the implantation, there is an intervention of a new organ in the endocrinological balance: the placenta. It is probable that the trophoblastic cells intervene very soon to induce the secretion of estrogen by the ovary. The problem is to know whether or not an interruption of estrogen secretion takes place between day 4 of pregnancy and the period of the onset of estrogen secretion that is due to the intervention of the placenta.

MEYER: What is the source of estrogen on day 4?

MAYER: From the cytological point of view, it seems to be the interstitial tissue of the ovary (theca). In Alloiteau and Acker's (1960, C..R Acad. Sci. Paris, **250**:1566–68) view, the corpus luteum can, in certain circumstances, elaborate estrogen by transformation of an ovarian androgen. In our problem the point is to know whether the estrogen jet at day 4 is evidence of a persistence of the ovarian cycle during progestation.

YOCHIM: We have performed experiments on rats ovariectomized the day after estrus. Estrogen is necessary in both the pre- and the postimplantation period. Daily injections of estrone with progesterone will limit the period of uterine sensitivity to day 4 of treatment. After the period of uterine sensitivity, injection of estrogen with progesterone is necessary for maximal decidual growth.

MAYER: I do not know what happens in the physiological process. What I can say is that implantation can occur at a normal time in rats ovariectomized on day 2, injected daily with progesterone (5 mg/day), and receiving only a single estrogen injection (0.1 μg.) on day 4. These animals have implantation sites of normal size at day 10.

SHARMAN: Dr. Mayer, is it likely that the estrogen surge observed on day 4, and to a lesser extent on day 8, is due to some cyclical phenomenon that is going on even after ovariectomy? Is it possible that the "estrous" cycle continues, perhaps because of cyclical hormone production by some other organ, for example, the adrenal?

MAYER: Yes, it is possible that the implantations that sometimes occur spontaneously in rats ovariectomized on day 4 and injected with progesterone alone are due to an eventual production of estrogen by the adrenals. But the intervention of the adrenal is very complex, and there are now some contradictory facts concerning this point. For instance, we observed in certain cases that implantation can occur in adrenalectomized ovariectomized rats (complete castration in the first half of day 4) injected with progesterone alone.

NOYES: If you ovariectomized rats and let them go for 3 weeks, then gave 5 mg. of progesterone every day, put eggs in from a donor, that is, 5-day blastocysts, then gave 0.1 microgram of estradiol, would they implant in 48 hours?

MAYER: Psychoyos (1961, C.R. Acad. Sci., **252**:2306–7) got implantation of eggs coming from donor rats ovariectomized on day 4 and injected with progesterone, then transferred into host rats ovariectomized 15 days before and injected with progesterone. The eggs do not implant, but they do after injection of estrogen (0.5 μg.) during the progesterone treatment.

NOYES: Is there no need for priming with estrogen for the endometrium to function? Will an atrophic uterus plus 0.1 microgram of estradiol be enough to cause implantation?

MAYER: The problem is different in rats ovariectomized and injected with progesterone and in rats receiving no hormones after castration day 4. In the latter case, the delay in obtaining nidation after the beginning of the hormonal treatment (progesterone plus estrogen at day 10, for example) is longer than in the case of rats injected daily with progesterone alone after day 4 and receiving estrogen on the same day.

The eggs, after a stay in an atrophic uterus, can implant if one injects progesterone and estrogen into the mother. But I do not know whether these eggs can develop in a normal way.

NOYES: Four days is not long enough. Estrogen is still in the system. If you wait 2 weeks, you will get an atrophic uterus, and then I would be surprised if 0.1 microgram would be enough estrogen to give implantation.

MAYER: It may be that, in experimental conditions where the uterus is atrophic, the amount of estrogen necessary to obtain nidation must be higher compared to the amount used for the implantation in a conditioned uterus.

YOCHIM: In castrated rats we gave progesterone for 8 days and tried to produce maximum sensitivity with the addition of estrogen. We could observe maximum sensitivity only if the animals was first "recycled" through an estrogenic phase.

DICKMANN: I think that the estrogen/progesterone story, in relation to implantation in the mouse, has been worked out very beautifully by Smithberg and Runner.

RUNNER: The experiments that Dr. Noyes speaks of have been done with the mouse, if I understand his point correctly. Mated prepuberal animals fail to develop corpora lutea of pregnancy and fail to recycle promptly. These mice offer unusually convenient and ample experimental material because their blastocysts are delivered to the uterus but implantation does not ensue, although the blastocysts are capable of promptly attaching in the anterior chamber of the eye or promptly implanting in prepared host uteri. Initiating daily injections of progesterone to these prepuberal mice at successively later days after mating results in implantation when progesterone, and progesterone alone, is instituted as late as 18 days postcoitum. Our interpretation is that an estrogen peak, that is, estrogen priming, occurred at the time of mating and that, as the estrogen effect tailed off, the ability of progesterone by itself to initiate implantation became progressively reduced to zero by 18 days.

When animals comparable to those used above were castrated by the day after mating, blastocysts were recovered up to 45 days postcoitum and the blastocysts were capable of implantation up to about 40 days. After 18 days postcoitum, however, success was obtained only when estrogen accompanied the administration of progesterone. Both the experiments included estrogen priming, but the time relations of when estrogen was required for nidation seem to be different from that reported in the experiments with rats.

EHARD F. NUTTING AND ROLAND K. MEYER

Implantation Delay, Nidation, and Embryonal Survival in Rats Treated with Ovarian Hormones

DELAYED NIDATION was described in several species of rodents as early as 1887 by Lataste (1891). This French investigator associated the prolongation of pregnancy following postpartum mating in mice with nursing of at least three young. The prolonged pregnancy occurring in these circumstances was attributed to a retardation in the development of the ova after reaching the uterus. The delay of implantation in mice caused by nursing has been reported in many studies, and the same phenomenon has been observed in rats and in several other species. Artificially delayed nidation in non-lactating rats was demonstrated by Chambon (1949*b*) to occur as a consequence of ovariectomy and treatment with progesterone. Modifications of this procedure were subsequently used by Cochrane and Meyer (1957), Canivenc and Laffargue (1956), and Mayer, Thevenot-Duluc, and Meunier (1957) to investigate the regulation of delayed implantation.

Neither anterior pituitary secretions nor adrenal secretions appear to be directly involved in producing delay of implantation of blastocysts in rats (Cochrane and Meyer, 1956; Meyer and Cochrane, 1962). Most of the data in the literature on delayed implantation supports either the theory of Pincus (1936), Whitten (1955, 1957, 1958), and Snyder (1938) that it is the result of an excess of progesterone or the theory of Bloch (1948, 1958), Krehbiel (1941*a*, 1941*b*), and Weichert (1940, 1941, 1942, 1943) that it is the result of estrogen deficiency. The hypothesis of Greenwald (1958), however, that progesterone associated with negligible amounts of estrogen postpones nidation, may be a more accurate description of the actual hormonal conditions.

DR. EHARD F. NUTTING is in the Division of Biological Research, G. D. Searle and Company, Chicago, Illinois.

Hoping to define these hormonal requirements more precisely, we began a program of experimentation to explore the relationship between progesterone and estrone for delayed nidation and implantation of blastocysts. Non-nursing ovariectomized pregnant rats were used exclusively in these studies. This report deals mainly with the results from a series of investigations designed to determine the requirements of progesterone in these processes. Some data from additional studies now in progress will also be presented in the discussion to provide a more complete picture of the role of steroids in delayed implantation.

Material and Methods

GENERAL

Mature virgin female rats weighing 190–230 grams (Holtzman Company and Badger Research, Inc.; Madison, Wisconsin) were caged with adult males in the evening. Insemination was confirmed the next

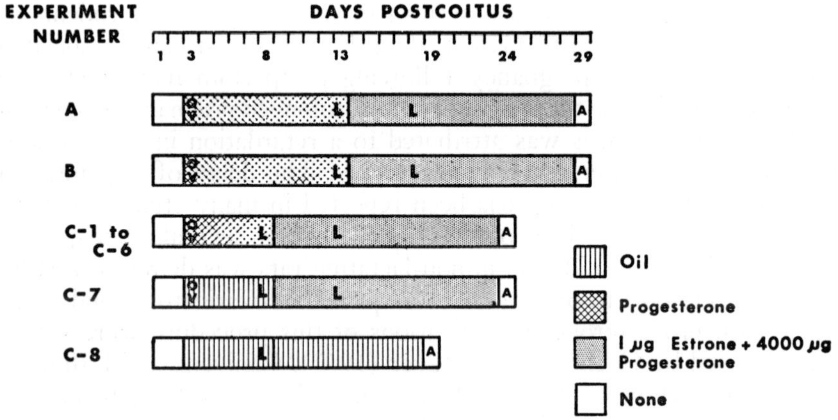

Fig. 1.—Graphic outline of various experimental procedures used in studying the effect of progesterone on delayed implantation. (*OV* = time of ovariectomy; *L* = time of laparotomy; *A* = time of autopsy.)

morning before 10:00 A.M. by the presence of spermatozoa in vaginal smears. The day sperm were found was designated as day 1 of pregnancy and hereafter referred to as day 1 postcoitus. Ovariectomies and first laparotomies were performed through dorsal lateral incisions. Second laparotomies were done through mid-ventral incisions. All ovariectomies were done on day 3 of pregnancy, while the times of the first and second laparotomies varied with the different experiments. The technique used for ovariectomy was as follows: the mesovarium was ligated; the bursa was slit open, exposing the ovary; the hilus was grasped with fine watchmakers' forceps; and the ovary was carefully excised with a small iris scissors. During the entire procedure 3× binocular loupe magnifiers were employed in order to minimize trauma to the oviduct and assure completeness of the ovariectomies. Ether was used as an anesthetic, and clean, but not sterile, conditions were maintained during all surgical procedures. Progesterone or combinations of progesterone with estrone were administered throughout as subcutaneous injections in 0.25 ml. of corn oil daily.

This study was divided into three separate experiments. The procedures and methods used in each are discussed below in detail and are illustrated graphically in outline form by Figure 1.

EXPERIMENT A

This experiment was performed to study the effect of various quantities of progesterone on delayed nidation in ovariectomized animals. The effect of treatment was measured by the ability of the blastocyst to undergo subsequent nidation and successfully maintain itself throughout pregnancy. The experimental design consisted of 11 groups, each composed of 5–6 females. Assignment to treatment groups was not done on a random basis. Sufficient numbers of bred females to form suitable groups in a short space of time were not available because of the relatively small size of the breeding colony at this time. Also the preliminary nature of this study precluded the selection in advance of all the doses eventually used. Animals were ovariectomized as described above, and daily doses of progesterone, ranging from 3.9 to 4,000 μg. at equally spaced logarithmic intervals, were administered to individuals in each treatment group from day 3 through day 13 postcoitus. Animals were laparotomized on day 13, and uteri were examined for the presence or absence of implantation sites. Any animals having implantation sites at this time were noted and eliminated from further experimental consideration. Beginning on the following day, day 14, and continuing through day 28, all animals were injected with 1 μg. estrone and 4,000 μg. progesterone in an attempt to induce nidation of blastocysts and maintain their subsequent development. Animals were laparotomized a second time on day 18, and the uteri were again observed for the presence of implantation sites. All animals were continued on the experiment regardless of whether or not they showed positive signs of pregnancy on day 18. Autopsies were done on day 29 postcoitus, at which time the number of live fetuses, dead fetuses, and placentomas or placental scars were recorded.

EXPERIMENT B

The purpose of this experiment was to determine the reproducibility of some of the results obtained in Experiment A, using an improved experimental design to insure randomness. Except for the number of groups, the treatment and operation schedules were identical with that in Experiment A and will be described here only briefly. Progesterone was administered to two groups, each composed of 17 inseminated and ovariectomized females, which were assigned at random to their respective groups. The two groups were given daily doses of 4,000 μg. and 125 μg. progesterone per female, respectively, from day 3 through day 13, and 1 μg. estrone plus 4,000 μg. progesterone per day from day 14 through day 28. The first and second laparotomies were done on days 13 and 18, respectively, and autopsies were done on day 29. A chi-square analysis (Snedecor, 1957) was used to compare treatment groups for the number of barren females per animals treated in each group and number of live fetuses per number of implantation sites in each group. An analysis of variance (Snedecor, 1957) was used for comparing groups for the average number of placentation sites on day 18 per animal treated.

EXPERIMENT C

This experiment was designed to produce a shorter period of delay in implantation, which was deemed more desirable for future work. In addition, we wanted to establish with this new procedure the nature of the dose-response relationship between quantities of progesterone administered during the time preceding implantation and the subsequent nidation and development of the blastocyst. Inseminated animals were distributed at random between 8 treatment groups, each composed of 10 females. Groups were numbered from 1 to 8. Animals in groups 1–6 were injected daily from day 3 through day 8 with graded doses of progesterone ranging from 125 to 4,000 μg. Animals were laparotomized late in the afternoon or evening of day 8, and their uteri were examined for the presence of implantation sites. Animals having implantation sites at this stage of the experiment were noted and checked for completeness of the ovariectomy. The results were not used for further analysis. Beginning on the following day, day 9 postcoitus, and continuing through day 23, all animals were injected with a combination of 1 μg. estrone and 4,000 μg. progesterone contained in a single volume of oil. This treatment was used to induce nidation of blastocysts and maintain their continued development through the remainder of pregnancy. A second laparotomy was done on day 13 to examine again the uteri for implantation sites. Autopsies were done on day 24, at which time the number of live fetuses, dead fetuses, and placentomas or placental scars were recorded.

Group 7 was treated the same as groups 1–6 except that corn oil alone was injected from day 3 through day 8. Thus this group functioned as a control for the several progesterone treatments.

Group 8 was also injected daily with corn oil alone from day 3 to day 8 and continued through day 18. However, unlike group 7, ovariectomies were not performed and a single laparotomy was done on day 8 to inspect the uteri and record the number of sites. Autopsies were done on day 19 postcoitus, at which time it was hypothesized that fetal development would have reached a stage in development corresponding to that observed in the other groups on day 24 postcoitus.

A chi-square analysis (Maxwell, 1961) was used to compare treatment groups for number of barren females per animals treated in each group and number of live fetuses relative to number of implantation sites in each group. The observed number of implantation sites (S) in each female was transformed to values of $Y = \sqrt{S + 0.375}$. This transformation was used to stabilize the variance of the number of implantation sites that varied directly with the mean number of sites per group. The transformed values were used in comparing the groups for number of implantation sites per treated female by the method of analysis of variance.

Results

Experiment A. A résumé of the results of this experiment is presented in Table 1. The data were interpreted without the aid of statistical methods because of the non-random manner employed in the selection and assignment of experimental animals to the various treatment groups. The reasons for not employing a more elegant experimental design have been stated in the previous section.

Implantation usually did not occur until after the initiation of treatment with estrone in combination with progesterone. There were only three instances in which nidation occurred before this time in the 66 ovariectomized animals treated with progesterone. Ovarian remnants were subsequently found in 2 of these animals at autopsy. As the quantity of progesterone was decreased from 4,000 μg. to 15.6 μg., the mean number of implantation sites, both per rat treated and per rat with sites, was reduced. The response appeared to be linear for at least the upper portion of the dose range. Nidation was not observed in rats receiving less than 15.6 μg. progesterone. Examination of uteri at autopsy on day 29 revealed no evidence of the occurrence of implantation after day 18 (Table 1).

Postimplantation embryonic survival did not occur in any of the 5 pregnant animals that had been treated with 15.6–125 μg. progesterone before implantation. In contrast, pregnancy was at least partially maintained in 12 of 13 animals receiving 250 μg. progesterone or more. There was no evident correlation between the mean number of live fetuses and the preimplantation dose of progesterone in this group. Since the number of viable fetuses resulting from any one treatment was small, no definite conclusions can be drawn regarding the effect of progesterone on embryonic mortality.

Experiment B. In contrast to the procedure in Experiment A, the placement of animals into treatment groups of this experiment was done on a random basis and the data were analyzed with the aid of appropriate statistical methods, as described in the previous section. Implantation

TABLE 1

EFFECT OF PROGESTERONE TREATMENT FROM DAY 3 TO DAY 13 ON DELAY OF IMPLANTATION, SUBSEQUENT NIDATION, AND EMBRYONAL SURVIVAL IN OVARIECTOMIZED RATS

EXPERIMENT No.	DAILY DOSE PROGESTERONE (μG.)	NO. ANIMALS			TOTAL NO. SITES*	TOTAL NO. LIVE FETUSES†
		Treated	With Sites (Day 13)	With Sites (Day 18)		
A........	4,000	6	1‡	4	26 (5.2)§	7 (1.8)‖
	2,000	6	1‡	5	34 (6.8)§	13 (2.6)
	1,000	6	0	2	9 (1.5)	7 (1.2)
	500	6	1	1	4 (0.8)	2 (0.4)
	250	5	0	2	12 (2.4)	6 (1.2)
	125	5	0	1	3 (0.6)	0
	62.5	6	0	1	3 (0.5)	0
	31.2	6	0	2	6 (1.0)	0
	15.6	6	0	1	1 (0.2)	0
	7.8	6	0	0	0	0
	3.9	6	0	0	0	0
B........	4,000	17	0	14	72 (4.2)	56 (3.3)
	125	17	0	8	32 (1.9)	15 (0.9)

* Numbers in parentheses are the mean number of sites.

† Numbers in parentheses are the mean number of live fetuses.

‡ Remnant of ovarian tissue present.

§ Based on 5 rats in which nidation did not occur.

‖ Calculated on 4 rats owing to death of one pregnant animal before autopsy.

did not occur in any of the 34 treated animals prior to the addition of estrone to the treatment (Table 1). The difference in the numbers of barren females following treatment with 125 or 4,000 μg. progesterone was not significant ($\chi^2 = 3.22$, 1 d.f., $P > 0.05$). The number of implantation sites per treated female was significantly larger ($P < 0.05$) in the group treated with 4,000 μg. progesterone (Table 2). This confirms the dose response relationship suggested by the data in Experiment A. Re-examination of uteri at autopsy on day 29 postcoitus confirmed the number of nidation sites observed at the laparotomy on day 18 and revealed no evidence of the occurrence of implantation after that time. Postnidation embryonic survival represented by the total number of live fetuses relative to the number of implantation sites was significantly higher ($\chi^2 = 9.23$, 1 d.f., $P < 0.01$) with 4,000 μg. progesterone than with 125 μg.

Experiment C. Implantation did not occur in any of the 70 ovariectomized animals (groups 1–7) during the preimplantation treatment period (Table 3). Eight of 10 intact control rats (group 8), however, were

TABLE 2

ANALYSIS OF VARIANCE OF NUMBER OF SITES (S) FROM DATA IN TABLE 1, EXPERIMENT B, USING INDEX OF RESPONSE (Y), WHERE $Y = \sqrt{S + 0.375}$

Term	D.F.	Sum of Squares	Mean Square	F
1. Between doses.......	1	3.7728	3.7728	4.74*
2. Within doses.........	32	23.6169	0.78302	....

* $P < 0.05$.

TABLE 3

EFFECT OF PROGESTERONE TREATMENT FROM DAY 3 TO DAY 8 ON DELAY OF IMPLANTATION, SUBSEQUENT NIDATION, AND EMBRYO SURVIVAL IN OVARIECTOMIZED RATS AND INTACT ANIMALS

GROUP No.	DAILY DOSE PROGESTERONE (μG.)	NO. ANIMALS			TOTAL NO. SITES*	TOTAL NO. LIVE FETUSES†
		Treated	With Sites (Day 8)	With Sites (Day 13)		
1......	4,000	10	0	9	74 (7.4)	64 (6.4)
2......	2,000	10	0	8	49 (4.9)	42 (4.2)
3......	1,000	10	0	5	25 (2.5)	20 (2.0)
4......	500	10	0	9	33 (3.3)	21 (2.1)
5......	250	10	0	5	24 (2.4)	13 (1.3)
6......	125	10	0	5	19 (1.9)	5 (0.5)
7......	....	10	0	0	0	....
8‡.....	....	10	8	....	78 (7.8)	62 (6.2)

* Numbers in parentheses are the mean number of sites.
† Numbers in parentheses are the mean number of live fetuses.
‡ Ovaries were not removed from this group.

pregnant on day 8. Forty-one of the 60 females treated with progesterone (groups 1–6) had sites within 5 days after injections with estrone and progesterone were commenced. In contrast, none of the 10 rats in the ovariectomized control group (group 7) became pregnant. Clearly, progesterone is an essential component in the hormonal environment of the blastocyst during the preimplantation period.

Data from only those groups treated with progesterone (groups 1–6) were subjected to a statistical analysis, since implantation did not occur in ovariectomized control animals (group 7) and data from intact control animals (group 8) were not strictly comparable to those obtained from animals that had a delay of nidation. The differences in the number of barren females between treatments were not significant ($\chi^2 = 2.06$, 5 d.f., $P > 0.05$). Treatment with progesterone, however, did result in a significant difference in the number of implantation sites per treated female ($P < 0.05$, Table 4). A regression analysis of the number of sites per treated female indicated that the response slope was highly significant ($P < 0.01$) and linearly related to the dose (Table 4). The slope, b, of the dose response line was 0.791. The regression line was fitted to the transformed values (Fig. 2). The dose response relationship between progesterone and number of implantation sites suggests that this technique could be used as a method for the bioassay of progesterone.

TABLE 4

ANALYSIS OF VARIANCE OF NUMBER OF SITES (S) FROM DATA IN TABLE 3, GROUPS 1–6, USING INDEX OF RESPONSE (Y), WHERE $Y = \sqrt{S + 0.375}$

Term	D.F.	Sum of Squares	Mean Square	F
Slope*..................	1	9.9134	9.9134	10.3827†
Non-linearity..........	4	3.0669	0.7667	0.8030
Between doses.........	5	12.9803	2.5961	2.7190‡
Within doses..........	54	51.5592	0.9548	....

* Slope of dose response line was $b = 0.791$.
† $P < 0.01$.
‡ $P < 0.05$.

The total number of live fetuses, dead fetuses, and placental scars observed in each rat at autopsy on day 24 corresponded to the number of sites observed at the second laparotomy (day 13). Thus, in all three experiments, nidation occurred within 5 days after initiation of treatment with a combination of estrone and progesterone. Females found to be barren at this time remained barren in spite of a continuation of the treatment.

A summary of the chi-square analyses of the number of live fetuses relative to the number of implantation sites is given in Table 5. There was a highly significant difference in the distribution of number of live fetuses relative to the number of implantation sites between treatments ($P < 0.01$). The variation between these values due to linear regression was also highly significant; while the deviation from linearity was not significant ($P > 0.05$). This suggests that fetal survival is related to the dose of progesterone. To illustrate this relationship, the relative number of live fetuses was calculated, expressed as a percentage, and plotted for each dose of progesterone (Fig. 3). Postimplantation embryonic survival was found to vary directly with the amount of progesterone administered during the preimplantation period.

Discussion

These results indicate that a delay in nidation of blastocysts occurs when rats are ovariectomized and treated with progesterone. Adequate quantities of progesterone appear to be necessary to maintain the viabili-

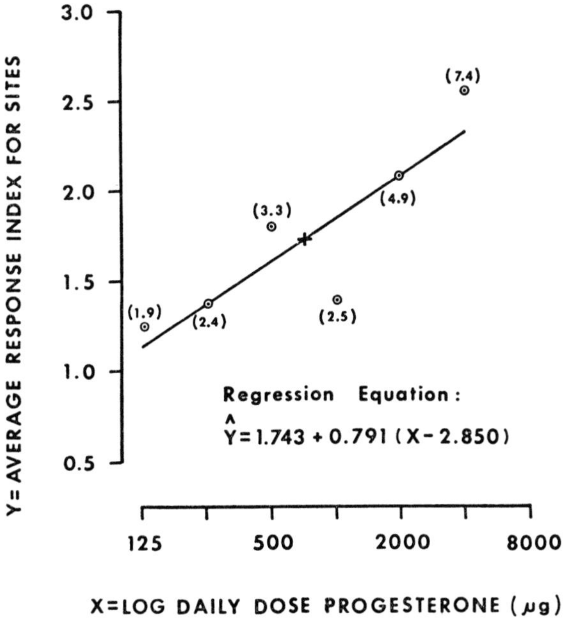

Fig. 2.—Dose response relationship in ovariectomized rats between the index of number of sites (Y) and log-dose progesterone (X) from data in Tables 3 and 4. $Y = \sqrt{S} + 0.375$, where S is the observed number of implantation sites for each animal. Each point represents the mean index (Y) of 10 rats. Numbers in parentheses are the means of the observed number of implantation sites for the same 10 animals. The solid line is the line of regression representing the regression equation.

TABLE 5

Chi-Square Analysis of Number of Live Fetuses Relative to Number of Implantation Sites from Data in Table 3

Variation	D.F.	χ^2
Linear regression.....	1	34.130*
Deviation...........	4	4.693
Between doses.......	5	38.823*

* $P < 0.01$.

ty of blastocysts during the period development is arrested. Nidation usually does not occur until a small amount of estrone is added to the progesterone. Only 3 of 178 ovariectomized animals used in this study had implantation sites before treatment with estrone was commenced, as compared to 8 of 10 rats when the ovaries were not removed. These results are in complete agreement with Cochrane and Meyer (1957) and Cochrane (1961). They likewise reported occasional instances in which implantation occurred without estrogen treatment and associated these

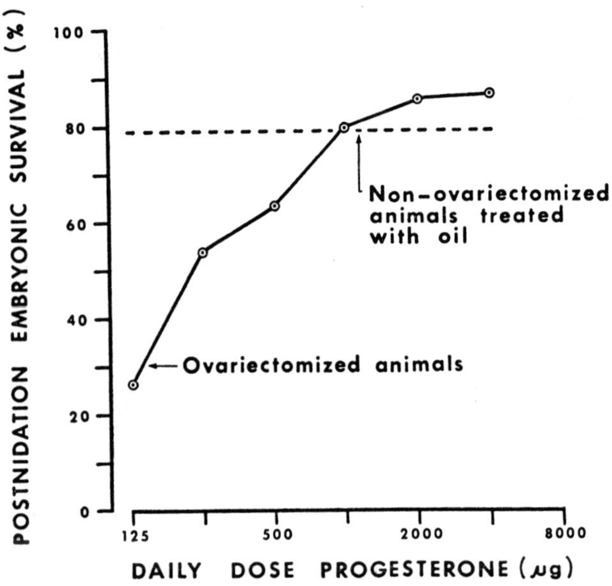

FIG. 3.—Relationship between postnidation embryonic survival and prenidation treatment with progesterone from data in Table 3. Each point represents the ratio of the total number of live fetuses to the total number of implantation sites.

cases with the stressful influence of temperature fluctuations in animal quarters at certain times. Changes in temperature cannot account for implantation in our studies, since the temperature in animal quarters was regulated and maintained at a uniform level. The occurrence of natural estrogenicity in corn oil, as reported by Booth, Bickoff, and Kohler (1960), offers another possible explanation. An alternate and perhaps more plausible explanation is the possibility of the occurrence of incomplete ovariectomies, resulting in the retention of small ovarian remnants large enough to secrete estrogen. Indeed, 2 of the 3 rats that underwent implantation without estrogen treatment were found to have small identifiable remnants of ovarian tissue. The fact that these three animals were ovariectomized relatively early in this study, when the operation may have been done with less skill, also tends to favor the idea of incomplete ovariectomies. Additional support for this explanation was given by Psychoyos and Alloiteau (1962), who obtained no spontaneous nidation when operations were done with the aid of a binocular microscope; a high incidence was found when magnification was not used, as well as when small fragments of ovarian tissue were purposely left intact. Thus, it is mandatory that extreme care be exercised to insure complete ovariectomy in order to assure a delay in nidation.

Investigators have generally agreed that the administration of small quantities of estrogen can induce nidation in ovariectomized rats being treated with progesterone. However, studies attempting to determine the effectiveness of various amounts of estrogen for producing implantation under these conditions have not been reported. Some information on this subject was required before studies of the interaction between progesterone and estrone could be undertaken. Consequently, an experiment was done to determine the optimal and maximal doses compatible with a delay of implantation. The experimental procedure employed was similar to that described earlier in this paper. Briefly, rats ovariectomized on day 3 postcoitus were treated daily from day 3 through day 8 with 4,000 μg. progesterone in combination with various quantities of estrone ranging from 0.01 to 10 μg. Eleven animals were assigned to each group at the beginning of the experiment. Animals were laparotomized on day 8 and examined for the presence of implantation sites. If none were present on day 8, a combination of 4,000 μg. progesterone plus 1 μg. estrone was given daily, beginning on day 9, and uteri were again examined 5 days later.

Implantation occurred before day 8 in only two of 43 ovariectomized animals receiving treatments containing 0.01, 0.03, 0.1 μg. estrone or no estrone (Table 6). Both animals were inspected grossly at time of autopsy for the presence of ovarian remnants. None were found. Implantation sites were found in 25 of the remaining 41 rats on day 13 postcoitus and within five days after initiating the standard implantation treatment. Sixteen of these 41 animals remained barren even though treatment with estrone and progesterone was continued until day 24 postcoitus.

In contrast to this situation, the remaining treatment groups were characterized by an absence of delayed nidation. Implantation occurred by day 8 in 25 of 43 animals receiving 0.3, 1, 3, and 10 μg. estrone in combination with progesterone and in 10 of 10 non-ovariectomized control rats treated with oil. Only one of the remaining 28 animals, treated with 0.3 μg. estrone, subsequently underwent nidation. Practically complete sterility resulted when animals were treated with 10 μg. estrone, as evidenced by only 1 of 10 rats undergoing implantation in the course of the experiment.

These results show that the effect of estrone on pregnancy in the ovariectomized rat treated with progesterone depends upon the daily amount administered. A relatively large dose of 10 μg. estrone interferes to such an extent that practically no implantation occurs. The antifertility property displayed by the 10 μg. dose of estrone was not unexpected, since the effect of large doses of estrogens administered before implantation is well known (Smith, 1926; Burdick and Pincus, 1935; Burdick, Whitney, and Pincus, 1937; and Dreisbach, 1959). The maximal daily quantity of estrone compatible with a delay of implantation is approximately 0.1 μg., and the minimal dose to cause nidation consistently at the normal time is between 0.3 and 1 μg.

TABLE 6

EFFECT OF ESTRONE ON NIDATION IN OVARIECTOMIZED RATS TREATED WITH STANDARD DOSE OF PROGESTERONE

Treatment Days 3–8		No. Animals Treated	No. Animals with Sites	
Dose P (μg.)	Dose E (μg.)		Day 8	Day 13
4,000	10	11	1	0
4,000	3	11	7	0
4,000	1	11	10	0
4,000	0.3	10	7	1
4,000	0.1	11	1	6
4,000	0.03	11	1	8
4,000	0.01	10	0	5
4,000	....	11	0	6
....	....	10	10	....

The studies with estrone were extended to determine the effect of small amounts of estrone, using less than the minimal effective dose for nidation, on the dose-response relationship between progesterone and the number of implantation sites. The procedure was identical to that used in Experiment C groups 1–6 (Fig. 1) of this paper and also in the estrone studies just discussed. All possible combinations of 0, 250, 1,000, and 4,000 μg. progesterone were made with 0, 0.01, and 0.1 μg. estrone, using a factorial experimental design. Ten animals were assigned to each of the 12 resulting treatment groups. These treatments were administered from day 3 to day 8. All animals were then injected daily with 1 μg. estrone in combination with 4,000 μg. progesterone from day 9 to day 24 postcoitus. Implantation did not occur in the absence of exogenous hormones and occurred in only 1 of 20 rats receiving estrone in the absence of progesterone (Fig. 4). These results confirm those obtained in Experiment C and are essentially in agreement with those reported by Cochrane and Meyer (1957). However, they are contrary to those of Canivenc and Laffargue (1957). This discrepancy will be discussed later in the paper. The number of implantation sites was related to the dose of progesterone in the absence of estrone. This

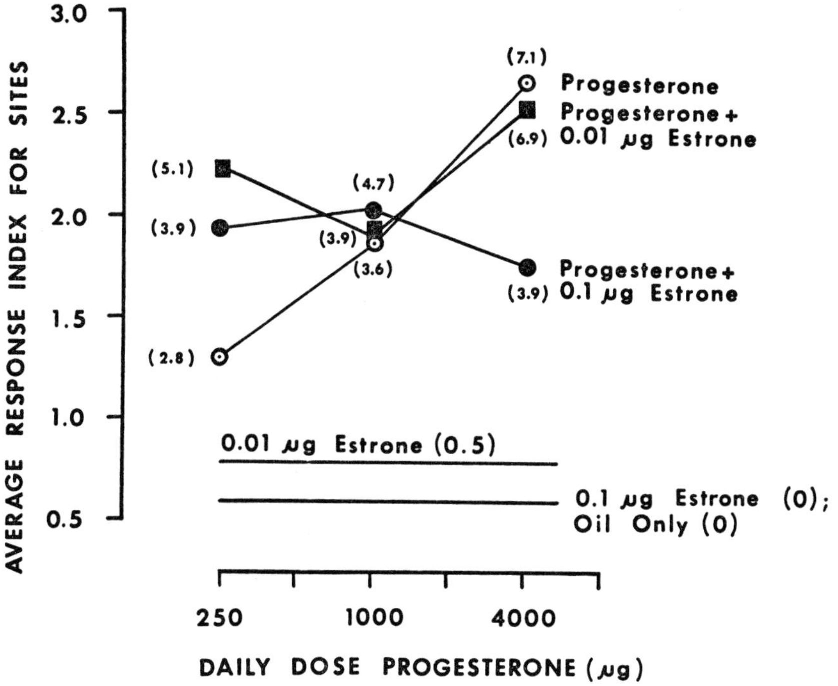

FIG. 4.—Dose response relationship in ovariectomized rats between the average response index for number of implantation sites described in the text and the daily dose of progesterone alone and in combination with estrone. Horizontal lines in the lower portion of the graph represent the response levels in the absence of progesterone for the treatments indicated. Each point represents the mean index of response for 9 or 10 animals. Numbers in parentheses are the means of the observed number of implantation sites for the same animals.

confirms the results reported in the preceding section. When a specified quantity of estrone is administered concomitantly with progesterone, the magnitude of the response appears to vary depending upon the quantity of progesterone. However, this apparent trend in the responses, suggesting an interaction between the two hormones, was not considered to be significant (Nutting and Meyer, 1963).

The time at which ovariectomy is performed has been considered to be another important factor affecting delayed nidation. Although no attempt was made to measure the effect of this variable in the present studies, a discussion of this factor is considered pertinent to understanding the general requirements for delay of implantation and induction of nidation. Except for the rare event of spontaneous nidation, a delay in nidation occurred in our studies when ovariectomy was done on day 3. Cochrane and Meyer (1957) had similar results when females were ovariectomized on day 3 but variable results when spaying was done on day 4. Canivenc and Laffargue (1956) obtained delayed nidation in rats castrated on day 4 and treated with progesterone. Later Canivenc, Laffargue, and Mayer (1956) confirmed this and in addition reported variable results when ovariectomies were done on day 3 and no delay when they were done on day 2, 5, or 6. The contradictory results obtained when ovariectomy was done on day 4 appears to have been resolved by Psychoyos (1960). He found that nidation regularly occurred when the operation was performed before noon of day 4 but that it was variable if it was postponed until later in the day. The failure of Canivenc *et al.* (1956) to obtain delayed nidation when animals were spayed on day 2 was essentially in agreement with the earlier studies of Chambon (1949*b*). However, Psychoyos and Alloiteau (1962) consistently obtained delayed nidation when ovariectomy was done on day 2. Extensive studies done in our laboratory confirm those of Cochrane and Meyer (1957), Psychoyos (1960), and Psychoyos and Alloiteau (1962). In addition, we have found that a delay of nidation is consistently obtained when ovariectomy is done on day 1 postcoitus.

Thus, opposing viewpoints on the effect of time of ovariectomy are evident. The results of Canivenc suggest that delayed nidation can be established in the ovariectomized rat only during the short period corresponding approximately to the time that the fertilized ovum is entering the uterus. The combined results from the present investigation and those of other investigators indicate that delayed nidation can be instituted following ovariectomy any time between the afternoon of day 1 and the morning of day 4 postcoitus. Failure to obtain delayed nidation when animals are spayed later than this might well be due to the endogenous release of estrogen prior to the operation. Clarification of this issue requires further study using techniques that insure complete removal of ovaries and minimal injury to the oviducts.

The data presented in the preceding section demonstrated that progesterone did not induce nidation. This does not agree with the studies of Chambon (1949*a*, 1949*b*), which suggest that progesterone is capable of inducing nidation. According to his data, daily quantities of 0.25 mg. progesterone resulted in delayed nidation, doses of 0.5, 2, 4, and 8 mg. did not interfere with the occurrence of nidation at the normal time, and 0.1 mg. failed to maintain the viability of the blastocysts. In addition to being contrary to our results, Chambon's view is not in accordance with the data presented by Canivenc and Laffargue (1956), Canivenc, Laffargue, and Mayer (1956), and Psychoyos and Alloiteau (1962), in which delayed nidation was obtained using 10 mg. progesterone daily; or with those of Canivenc, Laffargue, and Mayer (1956) and Psychoyos (1962), in which daily treatment with 5 mg. progesterone resulted in delayed implantation. Additional evidence showing that large amounts of progesterone are compatible with delayed nidation has been given by Johnson and Shelesnyak (1958), who used 6 mg. progesterone; Psychoyos and Alloiteau (1962), Cochrane and Meyer (1957), and Nutting and Meyer (1962), with 4 mg.; and Mayer, Thevonot-Duluc, and Meunier (1959), with 1 mg. progesterone. The preponderance of evidence disavows the concept that relatively large doses of progesterone alone can cause implantation.

As mentioned previously, Canivenc and Laffargue (1957), contrary to our data, found that they could obtain delayed nidation by withholding hormonal treatment from spayed rats until day 14 or 15. Nidation was then induced with estrone and progesterone. In contrast, Cochrane and Meyer (1957) withheld hormonal treatment until day 9 and subsequently obtained nidation in only 2 of 20 rats after attempting to induce it with estrone and progesterone. These last results are essentially in agreement with those we have presented.

There are several possible explanations for the lack of agreement regarding the effect of absence of ovarian hormones on delay of nidation and subsequent implantation. Animals were not ovariectomized at comparable times in these various studies. Ovariectomy was done on day 3 postcoitus in our studies and in those of Cochrane and Meyer. Canivenc and Laffargue, on the other hand, ovariectomized their animals on day 4. The latter procedure would have given the uterus a longer time to prepare for the accommodation of the unimplanted blastocyst prior to the removal of the ovaries. Another important factor that might lead to the disparities shown in the response could be the hormonal treatment used to induce nidation. The treatment used by Canivenc and Laffargue may have been nearer the optimum for blastocyst implantation. The possibility of the adrenal glands' being involved in these differences must also be considered. Lyons, Li, and Johnson (1953) found that they could get formation of deciduomata in ovariectomized-hypophysectomized immature rats after treatment with a preparation of highly purified adrenocorticotrophin. Balfour, Comline, and Short (1957) have presented evidence for progesterone secretion from adrenals of cattle, sheep, and swine. Canivenc and Mayer (1955) and Canivenc, Radenac, and Mayer (1955) have, by burning small areas of the pregnant female's skin, caused delayed nidation in the nursing rat suckling a small litter. These findings suggest that the adrenal may be capable of maintaining unimplanted blastocysts during conditions of stress. Thus, the control of environmental conditions and improvement in technique to remove stressful influences, the time of ovariectomy, and the hormonal treatment used for the induction of nidation must all be considered when attempting to explain the differences.

The data presented in this study indicate that embryonic survival after implantation is affected by the dose of progesterone administered before nidation, suggesting that postimplantation survival decreases as the preimplantation dose of progesterone is decreased. Other information obtained by Meyer and Nutting (1963), however, introduces some doubt concerning this conclusion. Therefore, additional study is required to clarify this point. This aspect of fertility should be pursued, since it may be of significant importance in the understanding of abortion and fetal mortality in humans and farm animals.

The controversial character of the literature concerned with delayed nidation and the induction of nidation certainly prohibits all but a few definite conclusions on the subject. However, we wish to present our view of these conditions, based largely on our studies, even though some of the reasoning may be speculative in nature.

It appears that neither an excess of progesterone nor a deficiency of estrogen can be considered the cause of delayed nidation. Once the blastocyst reaches the lower portion of the oviduct or the lumen of the uterus, its continuing survival is dependent mainly on the quantity of progesterone available to the animal. In the absence of this steroid, or when quantities are negligible, nidation occurs only infrequently or not at all. This is true even if small amounts of estrogen are administered. Under some experimental conditions survival of blastocysts has been reported to occur even in the absence of ovarian hormones (Canivenc and Laffargue, 1957). According to our studies, however, the role of progesterone appears to be vitally concerned with maintaining the viability of the blastocyst during the extended preimplantation period. In contrast, estrogen plays an active part in determining whether or not implantation will occur, but only if relatively large quantities of progesterone are available to insure the presence of viable blastocysts. If a sufficient quantity of progesterone is present, delay of nidation will occur while the amount of estrogen is below the threshold level. Conversely, implantation occurs when the amount of estrogen exceeds the threshold level.

Our studies were not designed to determine mechanisms of action beyond that of the hormonal requirements for obtaining a delay of implantation when subsequent nidation was induced with a standard treatment of estrogen and progesterone. A different combination of steroid hormones may be more effective in inducing nidation of blastocysts following a period of delay. Thus, the prenidation reduction in the number of embryos is merely an assumption based on indirect evidence. Until it is demonstrated otherwise, improper synchronization between development of the blastocyst and uterus must also be considered as a possible cause of differential nidation. The necessity for such synchronization has been shown by Noyes and Dickmann (1960, 1961). In any event, it is still not known whether progesterone exerts its effect on prenidation viability by acting directly on the blastocyst or indirectly through its influence on the uterus or by a combination of the two routes.

References

Balfour, W. E., R. S. Comline, and R. V. Short. 1957. Secretion of progesterone by the adrenal gland. Nature, **180**:1480–81.

Bloch, S. 1948. 8. Zum Problem der Nidationsverzögerung bei der säugeden Maus. Bull. Schweiz. Akad. med. Wiss., **4**:309–32.

———. 1958. Experimentelle Untersuchungen über die hormonalen Grundlagen der Implantation des Säugerkeimes. Experientia, **14**:447–49.

Booth, A. N., E. M. Bickoff, and G. O. Kohler. 1960. Estrogen-like activity in vegetable oils and mill by-products. Science, **131**:1807–8.

Burdick, H. O., and G. Pincus. 1935. The effect of oestrin injections upon the developing ova of mice and rabbits. Am. J. Physiol., **11**:201–7.

Burdick, H. O., R. Whitney, and G. Pincus. 1937. The fate of mouse ova tube-locked by injections of oestrogenic substances. Endocrinology, **21**:568.

Canívenc, R., and M. Laffargue. 1956. Survie prolongée d'œufs fécondés non implantés, dans l'utérus de rattes castrées et injectées de progestérone. Compt. rend. Acad. Sci., **242**:2857–60.

———. 1957. Survie des blastocystes de rat en l'absence d'hormones ovariennes. Compt. rend. Acad. Sci., **245**:1752–54.

Canivenc, R., M. Laffargue, and G. Mayer. 1956. Nidations retardées chez la ratte castrée et injectée de progestérone: Influence du moment de la castration sur la chronologie de l'ovoimplantation. Compt. rend. Soc. Biol., **150**:2208–12.

Canivenc, R., and G. Mayer. 1955. Nidation retardée par brûlure chez la ratte. Compt. rend. Acad. Sci., **240**:1273–75.

Canivenc, R., J. Radenac, and G. Mayer. 1955. Étude de mechanisme de la nidation retardée par brûlure chez la ratte: Action de la progestérone. Compt. rend. Soc. Biol., **149**:1258–60.

Chambon, Y. 1949*a*. Absence d'influence sur l'implantation de fortes doses de progestérone chez la ratte. Compt. rend. Soc. Biol., **143**:753–56.

———. 1949*b*. Realisation du retard de l'implantation par les faibles doses de progestérone chez la ratte. *Ibid.*, pp. 756–58.

Cochrane, R. L. n.d. Studies on the mechanisms of delayed implantation in the mink and rat. Ph.D. thesis, University of Wisconsin, 1961.

Cochrane, R. L., and R. K. Meyer. 1957. Delayed nidation in the rat induced by progesterone. Endocrinology, **96**:155–59.

DREISBACH, R. H. 1959. The effects of steroid sex hormones on pregnant rats. J. Endocrin, **18**:271–77.

GREENWALD, G. S. 1958. Formation of deciduomata in the lactating mouse. J. Endocrin., **17**:24–28.

JOHNSON, T. H., and M. C. SHELESNYAK. 1948. Histamine-oestrogen-progesterone complex associated with the decidual cell reaction and with ovum implantation. J. Endocrin., **17**:xxi–xxii.

KREHBIEL, R. H. 1941*a*. The effects of lactation on the implantation of ova of a concurrent pregnancy in the rat. Anat. Rec., **81**:43–61.

———. 1941*b*. The effects of theelin on delayed implantation in the pregnant lactating rat. *Ibid*., pp. 381–92.

LATASTE, M. F. 1891. Des variations de durée de la gestation chez les mammifères et des circonstances qui déterminent ces variations: Théorie de la gestation retardée. Compt. rend. Soc. Biol., **151**:565–66.

LYONS, W. R., C. H. LI, R. E. JOHNSON, and R. D. COLE. 1953. Evidence for progesterone secretion by ACTH-stimulated adrenals. Proc. Soc. Exp. Biol. & Med., **84**:356–58.

MAXWELL, A. E. 1961. Analysing Quantitative Data. London: Methuen & Co. Ltd.

MAYER, G., A. J. THEVENOT-DULUC, and J. M. MEUNIER. 1957. Progestation et surrenalectomie: Action de la surrénalectomie chez la ratte gravide castrée et injectée de progesterone. Compt. rend. Soc. Biol., **151**:95–99.

———. 1959. Évolution de la grossesse chez des rattes traitées par des stéroids sexueles ou corticossurrénaux durant la phase de vie latente des œufs fécondés. *Ibid*., **153**:605–9.

MEYER, R. K., and R. L. COCHRANE. 1962. Induction of implantation in the ovariectomized progesterone-treated rat after adrenalectomy. J. Endocrin., **24**:77–82.

MEYER, R. K., and E. F. NUTTING. n.d. (In preparation.)

NOYES, R. W., and Z. DICKMANN. 1960. Relationship of ovular age to endometrial development. J. Reprod. & Fertil., **1**:186–96.

———. 1961. Survival of ova tansferred into the oviduct of the rat. Fertil. & Steril., **45**:67–80.

NUTTING, E. F. n.d. (In preparation.)

NUTTING, E. F., and R. K. MEYER. 1962. Failure of transient progesterone deprivation to induce ova implantation in ovariectomized rats. Proc. Soc. Exp. Biol. & Med., **111**:372–75.

———. n.d. (In preparation.)

PINCUS, G. 1936. The Eggs of Mammals. New York: Macmillan Co.

PSYCHOYOS, A. 1960. Nouvelle contribution à l'étude de la nidation de l'œuf chez la ratte. Compt. rend. Acad. Sci., **251**:3073–76.

PSYCHOYES, A., and J. J. ALLOITEAU. 1962. Castration précoce et nidation de l'œuf chez la ratte. Soc. Biol., **156**:46–49.

SMITH, M. G. 1926. On the interruption of pregnancy in the rat by the injection of ovarian follicular extracts. Bull. Johns Hopkins Hosp., **39**:203.

SNEDECOR, G. W. 1957. Statistical Methods Applied to Experiments in Agriculture and Biology. 5th ed. Ames, Iowa: Iowa College Press.

SNYDER, F. F. 1938. Factors concerned in the duration of pregnancy. Physiol. Rev., **18**:578–96.

WEICHERT, C. K. 1940. The experimental shortening of delayed pregnancy in the albino rat. Anat. Rec., **77**:31–48.

———. 1941. The effectiveness of estrogen in shortening delayed pregnancy in the rat. *Ibid.*, **81**:106 (supplement).

———. 1942. The experimental control of prolonged pregnancy in the lactating rat by means of estrogen. *Ibid.*, **83**:1–17.

———. 1943. Effect of environmental stilbestrol in shortening prolonged gestation in the lactating rat. Proc. Soc. Exp. Biol. & Med., **53**:203–4.

WHITTEN, W. K. 1955. Endocrine studies on delayed implantation in lactating mice. J. Endocrin., **13**:1–6.

———. 1957. The effect of progesterone on the development of mouse eggs *in vitro*. *Ibid.*, **16**:80–85.

———. 1958. Endocrine studies on delayed implantation in lactating mice. II. Role of the pituitary in implantation. *Ibid.*, pp. 435–40.

DISCUSSION (*Chairman:* M. N. RUNNER)

YOCHIM: How did you determine the hormonal combination for the postimplantation period? What method was used to determine it?

NUTTING: Studies of delayed implantation by Cochrane and Meyer (Proc. Soc. Biol. & Med., 1957, **96**:115) had previously demonstrated that treatment with 4,000 μgm. progesterone and 1 μg. estrone would induce implantation and promote embryonal survival in ovariectomized rats treated with progesterone. This particular combination was also used by Lyons (1943, Proc. Soc. Biol. & Med., **54**:65) to obtain maintenance of pregnancy in hypophysectomized ovariectomized rats.

YOCHIM: This is the same combination of hormones that will maintain growth of deciduomata.

HAFEZ: Dr. Nutting, I think that your regression line is a classical contribution to quantitative studies on implantation. I wonder how you calculated your response index. What is the significance of the value 3; does this represent the maximum number of implanted blastocysts, or didn't you count the number of corpora lutea in both ovaries?

NUTTING: The response index of 3 was chosen arbitrarily for use in the graphs and would correspond to an observed mean of approximately 8.6 implantation sites. A mean of this magnitude was not obtained in any of the treated groups of animals. The index value of 3 does not represent the maximum number of blastocysts, since the average number of implantation sites in untreated control animals in our laboratory is usually 10.5–11.5, corresponding to an estimated response index of 3.2–3.5.

HAFEZ: Would the number of viable blastocysts increase with the increase of doses of progesterone?

Nutting: We have treated animals with 8,000 μg. progesterone daily in one of our studies and subsequently obtained fewer implantation sites than resulted after administration of 4,000 μg. progesterone daily. Thus, the dose-response relationship does not appear to be valid when more than 4,000 μg. progesterone is administered daily during the preimplantation period.

Hafez: Are the massive doses of progesterone harmful to the survival of blastocysts?

Nutting: The smaller number of implantation sites following treatment with 8,000 μg. progesterone daily suggests a possible harmful effect. However, I have not tried larger quantities of progesterone.

Noyes: In what state is the ovariectomized animal on day 3? If all the estrogen molecules were isotopically tagged, where would they be?

Nutting: I do not really know the exact hormonal conditions existing at the time of ovariectomy. Any estrogen that may have been present at the time of ovariectomy or secreted from an extra-ovarian source after the ovaries were removed was either rapidly eliminated from the animals or was not present in large enough quantities to induce implantation. Regarding the location of tagged molecules, studies by Jensen and Jacobson (1962, Rec. Prog. Hormone Res., **18**:387) on the fate of tritiated estradiol in immature rats have shown that the radioactive estrogen was rapidly incorporated by the uterus and vagina. However, it was retained by these tissues for only a few hours.

Deanesly: Chambon (1949, C.R. Soc. Biol., **143**:756) obtained delayed implantation in rats with low doses of progesterone and further development with 1 mg. daily. In a further paper (1955, C.R. Soc. Biol., **149**:518) Chambon and Lefrein stated that in view of later work the dose with which some rats went to term was probably slightly larger than that.

The research reported in the preceding chapter was supported by USPH A-804 (C) 15, and by funds from the Wisconsin Alumni Research Foundation.

RUTH DEANESLY

The Corpus Luteum Hormone during and after Ovo-implantation: An Experimental Study of Its Mode of Action in the Guinea Pig

ANY DETAILED consideration of delayed implantation is bound to focus attention on the interaction of the fertilized ovum and the endometrium, on the part played by each as the process begins, and on the nature of the stimuli causing a return to or acceleration of functional activity after the resting period. It is not the theory so much as the details of the process that need elucidation.

Extensive experimental studies of delayed implantation both in lactating and in ovariectomized rats and mice have provided much information on the hormone background of ovo-implantation in these species. Nevertheless, the conclusions drawn from these experiments should not be applied without reserve to totally different species. Ovo-implantation after delay may entail a renewed vitality or aggressiveness by the fertilized egg and not merely its passive response to an actively developing glandular endometrium, stimulated by an increase in sex hormones. This resumed activity by the egg may itself depend, it is true, on uterine secretions stimulated by sex hormones, but the study of uterine secretions is still biologically in its infancy. From the experiments of Corner (1928) and others on the rabbit, it was deduced that fertilized eggs died in the uterus after ovariectomy, before the time of implantation, because they could not be nourished in the absence of the progestational endometrium. More recent experiments have shown that rat and mouse eggs, unlike those of the rabbit, can remain viable for long periods in the uteri of ovariectomized females with inactive uterine

DR. RUTH DEANESLY is in the School of Agriculture of the University of Cambridge, England.

endometria, while the fertilized eggs of armadillos can actually be stimulated to become implanted if the ovaries are removed (Buchanan, Enders, and Talmage, 1956), possibly reacting to an increase in adrenal secretions.

Species differences in the endocrinology of ovo-implantation are well seen if the guinea pig is compared with the rat. Some twenty years ago, Krehbiel (1941), during experiments in accelerating implantation in lactating rats with exogenous estrogens, observed that a traumatic deciduoma could be stimulated in a lactating female, while the fertilized eggs of postpartum mating remained unimplanted. Here was a reactive endometrium, in the luteal phase, but unresponsive blastocysts.

TABLE 1

STIMULATION OF DECIDUOMATA IN GUINEA PIGS OVARIECTOMIZED 6 DAYS AFTER MATING

Day of Ovariectomy	Guinea Pigs Not Injected (Animals with Deciduomata/ Animals Traumatized)	Guinea Pigs Injected, 1 Mg. Progesterone (Animals with Deciduomata/ Animals Traumatized)
3	0/6	4/4
4	2/6	1/1
5	1/5	
6	1/1	

In the guinea pig the reverse condition can be found. If mated females are ovariectomized before the eggs have implanted (days 3–5 post-coitum [p.c.]), nidation takes place normally (day 6–6½ p.c.) (Deanesly, 1960*a*). This is not because a progestagen is unnecessary but because so little is required that the uterus is adequately sensitized by the developing corpora lutea in 2½–3 days from ovulation. Attempts to stimulate traumatic deciduomata (Loeb, 1908) in such uteri, however, were unsuccessful unless additional progesterone (1 mg.) was given. Some of these guinea pigs were mated to vasectomized males, and others were mated to normal males but had ligatures placed round the Fallopian tubes; they were ovariectomized 3–6 days after mating (Table 1). In these experiments the blastocyst showed itself a more efficient agent for inducing decidualization than a needle and thread—an indication perhaps that it carried some locally effective hormone or enzyme.

The guinea pig differs from the rabbit in hormone requirements; no exogenous estrogen is necessary for deciduoma formation after either recent or long-standing ovariectomy, whereas in the ovariectomized rabbit the traumatic deciduoma requires both estrogen and progesterone (Kehl and Chambon, 1950), although ovo-implantation requires only progesterone—a further indication of a contribution from the blastocyst.

The differences between common laboratory animals in the hormone requirements for ovo-implantation, as well as in the actual modes of implantation, make it clear that further work on different species will be required before implantation mechanisms can be clarified.

Ovo-implantation and placenta formation in the guinea pig have been studied by Duval (1892), and many morphological embryologists, including, recently, Davies, Dempsey, and Amoroso (1961). Blandau (1949), in an experimental study, noted that the blastocysts of guinea pigs had a greater capacity for proteolysis in culture than had rat blastocysts. The uterus of the guinea pig, on the other hand, was less ready to form experimental deciduomata than the rat uterus, which responds in this way to a great variety of stimuli.

TABLE 2

GUINEA PIGS OVARIECTOMIZED ON DAY 2 POST-COITUM AND GIVEN PROGESTERONE INJECTIONS ON DIFFERENT DAYS

Days Injected P.c.	No. Females	No. with Implantations	Day Killed P.c.
2	8	7	10–11
3–11	4	3	12
4, 5	3	3	10
7–14	2	0	15
11–16	6	1	17
11–20	2	0	21

It was an attempt to delay implantation in the guinea pig by ovariectomy, 3–5 days after mating, that led directly to confirmation of Loeb's original findings (on 4 females) that removal of the ovaries at that time did not inhibit normal implantation (Loeb and Hesselberg, 1917). Further experiments (Deanesly, 1960*a*) showed that ovariectomy one day earlier, on day 2 p.c., effectively prevented implantation unless progesterone was given not later than day 4. The transport of eggs through the tube was normal, but apparently the uterus had not by that time become progestationally sensitized (Table 2).

The normality of the implantations in ovariectomized guinea pigs was established by giving exogenous progesterone from day 11 and killing on or about day 21 (Table 3). Differentiation had proceeded, and some embryos were equal to the best controls, though others were smaller and some had died. Early work had confirmed Loeb and Hesselberg's statement that the embryos in ovariectomized females were tending to regress after about day 14 p.c. This is a time of very rapid embryonic growth and differentiation (Plate I), when the embryo develops from a primitive streak to a fetus with head, heart, somites, and allantoic placenta (Harman and Prickett, 1932; Scott, 1936). Obviously, the progestagen requirements increase, as they do in the ovariectomized pregnant rabbit after implantation (Courrier, 1945). In the normal guinea pig there is an increased concentration of progesterone in the corpus luteum from about day 11 (Rowlands and Short, 1959), probably indicating greater activity.

The period of pregnancy for which an ovarian or exogenous progestagen is required is extremely short in the guinea pig, presumably because of the early production of placental sex hormones (Deanesly, 1960*b*). Experimental work (Herrick, 1928; Courrier, Kehl, and Raynaud, 1929; Nelson, 1934) had shown that the ovaries ceased to be necessary for the maintenance of pregnancy after about 40 days p.c. Courrier *et al.* found that in one case pregnancy continued after ovariectomy on day 20 p.c. without exogenous hormones, and this observation has been confirmed in the course of present work.

TABLE 3

EMBRYONIC DEVELOPMENT IN 25 GUINEA PIGS OVARIECTOMIZED DAYS 3–5 POSTCOITUM AND KILLED DAY 21; PROGESTERONE INJECTED FROM DAY 11 POSTCOITUM

Injections, Day 11–Day 20	No. Females	No. with Implantations	No. with Live Embryos
10 mg. progesterone. .	15	13	11
5 mg. progesterone+ 1 μg. estradiol.	10	9	3

Taken together, the various experiments indicated that the crucial period during which ovarian progestagen was necessary to the developing embryo was from day 14 to day 19 or 20 p.c. It was decided to study this postimplantation period in the embryos of normal and ovariectomized females to see whether light was thrown on the mode of action of progesterone, or the ovarian progestagen, on the early embryo and its placenta. It seemed possible that there would be a critical stage in time or development beyond which the progestagen-deficient embryo would not be able to go.

Two series of embryos from normal and ovariectomized guinea pigs 13–18 days p.c. were examined. The first series comprised embryos from 20 normal and 31 ovariectomized guinea pigs, together with 11 others ovariectomized and given progesterone. The embryonic swellings were measured, weighed, and sectioned. Ovariectomies were carried out 3–5 days after mating unless otherwise stated. The females, with the exception of a few in the second series, had not previously been pregnant.

In the second series of 18 normal and 17 ovariectomized guinea pigs the entire uteri were cleared in benzyl benzoate by the method of Orsini (1962), and the embryonic swellings were examined in situ under the binocular microscope.

From the weights, after fixation, of the uterine swellings (Table 4), it was clear that the average size was below normal in ovariectomized

TABLE 4

GROWTH OF EMBRYONIC SWELLINGS IN NORMAL AND OVARIECTOMIZED PREGNANT GUINEA PIGS (SERIES I)

Day P.C.	Normal			Ovariectomized		
	No. Females	Swellings		No. Females	Swellings	
		Range (Mg.)	Largest (Mg.)		Range (Mg.)	Largest (Mg.)
13	3	482– 651	617	4	177–518	439
14	4	402– 730	650	4	365–557	522
15	3	653– 951	904	8	451–736	694
16	4	771–1182	1042	9	522–847	831
17	4	804–1233	1138	2	735–834	722*

The weights are of fixed swellings in 70 per cent alcohol, excluding those obviously shrunken and regressed. Figures for the largest are the average of 4.

* Average of 3.

females, although a good many of the swellings were within the normal range. This growth retardation appeared as early as day 12 p.c., but there was no general arrest of growth until day 16 p.c. (Fig. 1). From day 17 p.c. no living embryos were found in the untreated ovariectomized series.

Sections through what appeared to be healthy swellings on each successive day showed normal development of the placental membranes and normal differentiation of the embryos. At all stages, however, there were both dead and retarded young and on day 16 only 5 of 18 ovariectomized females contained living embryos, though embryos had developed up to about the 15-day stage with head, heart, somites, and allantoic placenta. The amount of variation and the extent of development in some embryos of the experimental series made it impossible to pick out any crucial stage of progestagen deficiency before the end of day 16, although many embryos were obviously affected and the amniotic cavities were not fully developed. By day 16 in the normal embryo, the body wall closes, except for the umbilical vessels, and this change may temporarily reduce the progestagen available from the developing placenta. Certainly it is a stage beyond which untreated embryos, with one exception, seemed unable to survive (Deanesly, 1963).

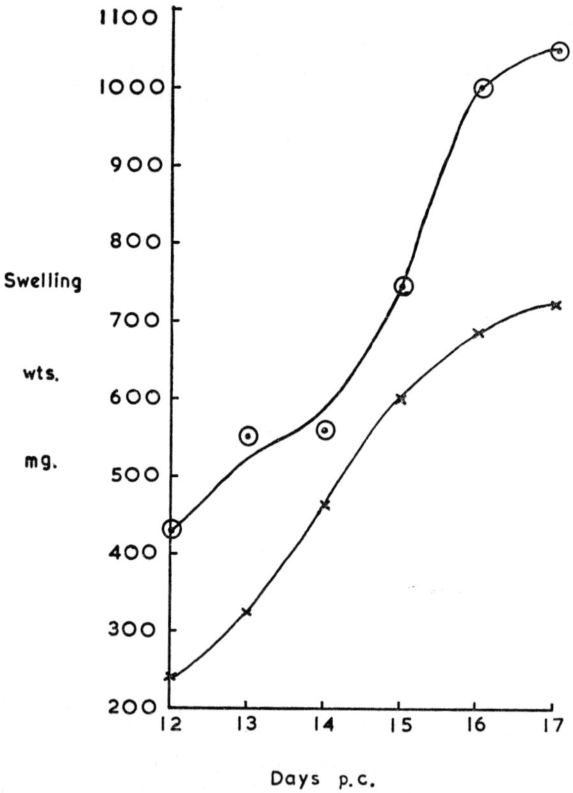

FIG. 1.—Average weights of swellings in normal (⊙) and ovariectomized (×) pregnant guinea pigs.

In a group of ovariectomized guinea pigs receiving 5 mg. progesterone daily from day 9 or 10 p.c. supplemented by a daily absorption of about 1 mg. from subcutaneous progesterone tablets, the largest embryonic swellings were of full normal size and development (1 gm.) on day 16 p.c. No estrogen was given.

The survival of embryos in ovariectomized females was tested by beginning progesterone treatment in groups of guinea pigs at 13, 14, 15, and 16 days p.c. and continuing it until one day before autopsy (days

PLATE I

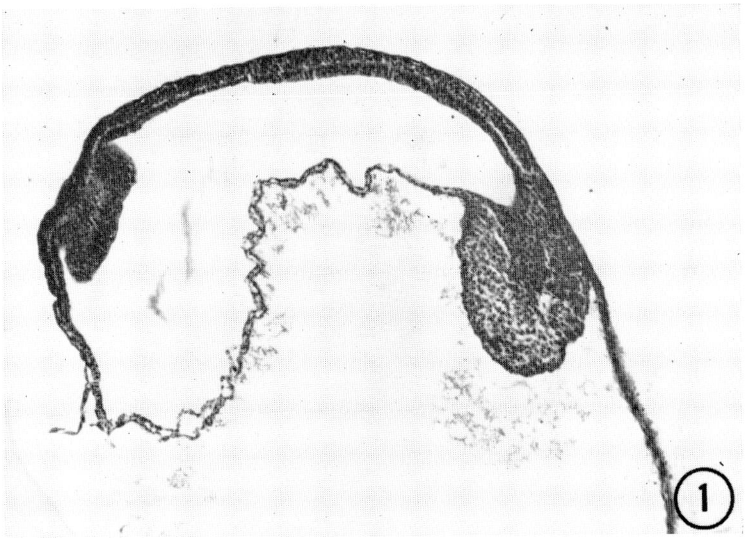

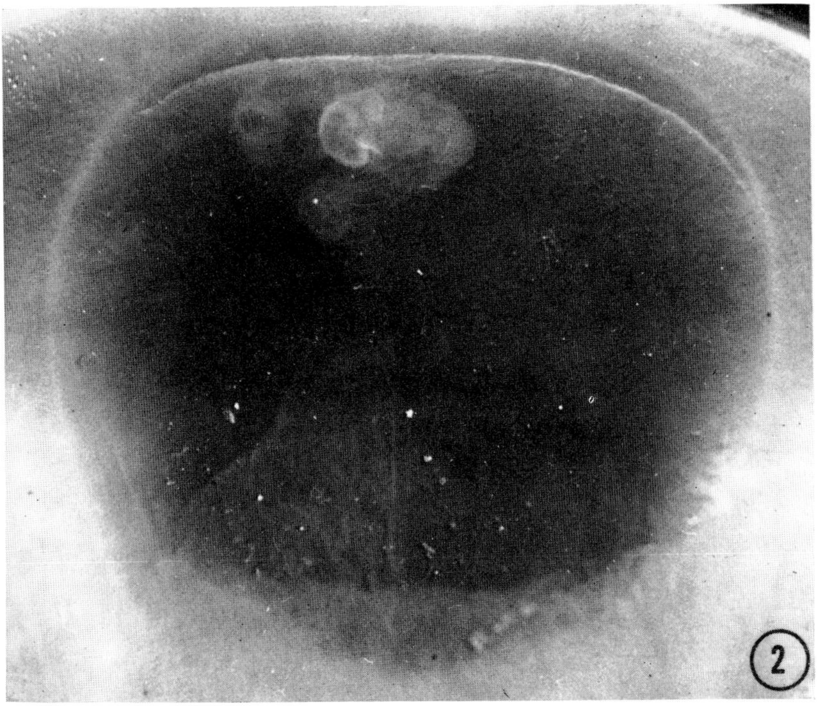

1, Normal guinea-pig embryo in section at 14 days postcoitum. ×54.

2, Normal guinea-pig embryo in situ at 16 days postcoitum, showing head, heart, and allantoic placenta.

20–28 p.c.). Table 5 shows the results of this experiment and the marked reduction in the viability of the embryos by day 16. Actually only 2 out of 13 embryos were alive at autopsy as compared with 7 out of 9 in the 15-day group.

The experiments, as a whole, illustrate the effectiveness of ovarian and perhaps of placental progestagens in the guinea pig and their close connection with the rapidly forming 14–20-day embryo. The small quantities required for ovo-implantation and the persistence of the progestational condition of the uterus between ovariectomy on day 3 and implantation 3–3½ days later suggest that the progestagen is less rapidly excreted and metabolized than progesterone in the rabbit and human.

TABLE 5

EMBRYONIC SURVIVAL IN GROUPS OF PREIMPLANTATION, OVARIECTOMIZED GUINEA PIGS; PROGESTERONE GIVEN FROM DAY 13, 14, 15, OR 16 POSTCOITUM

Progesterone Treatment Begun (Day P.c.)	Proportion of Females with Living Embryos	Proportion of Living Embryos	Killed (Days P.c.)
13	7/7	19/22	21, 24, 28
14	4/11	14/30	17, 20, 21
15	3/3	7/9	21
16	2/6	2/13	21, 28

As to how the progestagen acts in the postimplantation period, the exact effect that it has on the uterus, whether and in what state it is taken up, we still know very little, though in work on the rabbit it has been shown to be locally active. From the present experiments it can be stated definitely that the full normal growth of the embryonic swellings does not occur in progestagen-deficient females. The early stages of organ differentiation and placenta formation can take place normally without ovarian or exogenous progestagens in ovariectomized females, although there is an increase in fetal mortality. The largest swellings usually contain the largest and most advanced embryos, but this is not always the case; lack of expansion does not seem to inhibit embryonic differentiation or to cause death (Deanesly, 1963). As Courrier (1945) found in the rabbit and cat, the embryos appear more vulnerable than the placentae when progesterone is deficient, which suggests that some factor essential to growth is lacking. It is difficult to explain the death of well-formed embryos that have continued to develop up to day 16 on any other explanation. Dewar (1957) finds that the extra-uterine weight gain of pregnant mice is under progesterone control, and it is reasonable to suppose that the uterus and embryos are also affected.

Ovo-implantation in any species depends on two different factors—the presence of the appropriate sex hormones to condition the uterus and the capacity of the blastocysts for what has been termed "aggressive" action or, alternatively, for survival. The sex-hormone requirements will be related to the cyclically varying hormones characteristic of the species.

Work on the guinea pig emphasizes the clear differences that separate it from rats and rabbits and the need to extend detailed studies as widely as possible among mammals. It would be especially valuable to study closely related species, in which one shows delayed implantation but the other does not. Examples of this are the European stoat and weasel (*Mustela mustela* and *Mustela nivalis*); the former shows delayed implantation, but the latter does not. For delayed implantation, fertilized eggs must reach the uterus while it is under the influence of seasonal anestrous conditions, and they must be able to survive though unable to implant. How far implantation, when it comes, is induced by the increased ovarian estrogens stimulated by increased pituitary gonadotrophins is difficult to say, but it may be noted that, in the stoat, unimplanted blastocysts can still be found when uterus and mammary glands in the spring already show marked estrogenic effects (Deanesly, 1943). Apparently they do not respond to as little estrogen as the rat blastocyst.

Only by extending detailed study to as many species as are available can the mechanisms of ovo-implantation yield their secrets.

References

Blandau, R. J. 1949. Embryo-endometrial inter-relationship in the rat and guinea-pig. Anat. Rec., **104**:331.

Buchanan, G. D., A. C. Enders, and R. V. Talmage. 1956. Implantation in armadillos ovariectomized during the period of delayed implantation. J. Endocrin., **14**:121.

Corner, G. W. 1928. Physiology of the corpus luteum. I. The effect of very early ablation of the corpus luteum upon embryos and uterus. Am. J. Physiol., **86**:74.

Courrier, R. 1945. Endocrinologie de la gestation. Paris: Masson & Cie.

Courrier, R., R. Kehl, and R. Raynaud. 1929. Neutralisation de l'hormone folliculaire chez la femelle gestante castrée. C.R. Soc. Biol. **100**:1103.

Davies, J., E. W. Dempsey, and E. C. Amoroso. 1961. The sub-placenta of the guinea-pig: Development, histology and histochemistry. J. Anat. **95**:457.

Deanesly, R. 1943. Delayed implantation in the stoat (*Mustela mustela*). Nature,., **151**:365.

———.1960*a*. Implantation and early pregnancy in ovariectomized guinea-pigs. J. Reprod. & Fertil., **1**:242.

———. 1960*b*. Endocrine activity of the early placenta of the guinea-pig. J. Endocrin., **21**:235.

———. 1963. Early embryonic growth and progestagen function in ovariectomized guinea-pigs. J. Reprod. & Fertil., **6.**
Dewar, A. D. 1957. Body weight changes in the mouse during the oestrous cycle and pseudopregnancy. J. Endocrin., **15**:230.
Duval, M. 1892. Le placenta des rongeurs. III. Le placenta du cochon d'Inde. J. Anat. & Phys., **28**:57.
Harman, M. T., and M. Prickett. 1932. The development of the external form of the guinea-pig (*Cavia cobaya*) between the ages of 11 days and 20 days of gestation. Am. J. Anat., **49**:351.
Herrick, E. H. 1928. Duration of pregnancy in guinea-pigs after removal and also after transplantation of ovaries. Anat. Rec., **39**:193.
Kehl, R., and Y. Chambon. 1950. Nouvelles précisions sur le conditionnement du déciduome par traumatisme chez la lapine. C.R. Soc. Biol., **144**:254.
Krehbiel, R. H. 1941. The production of deciduomata in the pregnant lactating rat. Anat. Rec., **81**:67.
Loeb, L. 1908. The production of deciduomata and the relation between the ovaries and the formation of the decidua. J. Am. Med. Assoc., **50**:1897.
Loeb, L., and C. Hesselberg. 1917. The cyclic changes in the mammary gland under normal and pathological conditions. Part III. J. Exp. Med., **25**:305.
Nelson, W. O. 1934. Studies in the physiology of lactation. III. The reciprocal hypophysial-ovarian relationship as a factor in the control of lactation. Endocrinology, **18**:33.
Orsini, M. W. 1962. Technique of preparation, study and photography of benzyl-benzoate cleared material for embryological studies. J. Reprod. & Fertil., **3**:283.
Rowlands, I. W., and R. V. Short. 1959. The progesterone content of the guinea-pig corpus luteum during the reproductive cycle and after hysterectomy. J. Endocrin., **19**:81.
Scott, J. P. 1936. The embryology of the guinea-pig. I. A table of normal development. Am. J. Anat., **60**:397.

DISCUSSION (*Chairman:* M. N. Runner)

Greenwald: The fact that the animal needed only 1 mg. of progesterone on day 2 after ovariectomy to implant ova suggests that the guinea pig is very thrifty in utilizing progesterone. Have you tested this in any other way, such as ovariectomy followed by progesterone and estrogen, then testing for length of time before vaginal mucification occurs?

Deanesly: In pregnant, ovariectomized guinea pigs receiving only progesterone, there is absence of vaginal mucification, indicating absence of estrogens, until day 18 or day 20 postcoitum. If progesterone is absorbed from subcutaneous tablets, 1.6 mg. daily may suffice for maintenance of pregnancy in ovariectomized females.

Lutwak-Mann: Have you looked at the guinea-pig endometrium?

It is just conceivable that the endometrium may possess luteotrophic activity (as well as, perhaps, luteolytic activity).

DEANESLY: The guinea-pig uterus does not regress conspicuously after ovariectomy. The prolonged maintenance of corpora lutea in hysterectomized guinea pigs has no direct bearing on the present experiments.

LUTWAK-MANN: Could it not be a source of hormone production?

DEANESLY: I rather suspect the placenta.

NOYES: Frazer has shown that, if the embryo is released from the uterus following ovariectomy in the pregnant rat, the embryo will survive. When the ovaries are taken out and the embryo is left, the uterus contracts, ischemia kills the embryo, and the placenta is resorbed.

DEANESLY: These experiments related to a much later stage of pregnancy.

HARTMAN: Both the pregnant and the pseudopregnant opossum uteri are characterized by so high a degree of turgidity that, when a 6- or 7-mm. slit is cut through the myometrium, the whole contents herniate out. In the pregnant uterus the embryos near term are "popped out" one at a time with some force. In the pseudopregnant animal the turgidity of the uterus lasts about 10–11 days; in the pregnant animal up to term ($12\frac{3}{4}$ days). After ovariectomy the uterus collapses dramatically within a period of 12 hours.

ORSINI: Dr. Deanesly's paper points again to what I tried to say yesterday: that there are critical periods in the course of gestation that are probably associated with major morphological changes, such as the vascularization of the chorionic plate by the allantois. At such periods the conceptus is extremely vulnerable to stress and may need higher levels of hormones.

GLASSER: I am interested in the function of progesterone in the post-implantation period. If a pregnant rat is irradiated (250 roentgens delivered to the whole body at day $\frac{1}{2}$ postconception), a corpus luteum forms. However, there is evidence of deficient secretory function. There is no interference, by the radiation, with implantation. There is, in fact, good agreement between the number of ova shed and the number that implant.

On day $14\frac{1}{2}$ postconception extensive fetal wastage may be noted. It is marked by massive hemorrhage. In concurrent experiments animals handled in this fashion were treated with progesterone. Injections (0.5–5 mg/rat/day) were started on the day of exposure. Progesterone obviates all hemorrhage and allowed for an increase in survival from 15 to 60 per cent. A single injection of progesterone was without effect. The effective dose was 5 mg. of progesterone. Smaller doses were not effective; larger doses increased the number of dead embryos.

Analysis of the data implicates placental dysfunction as a major factor in pregnancy wastage in the irradiated rat. Not only is the role of the placenta as a transfer organ impaired, but the endocrine secretory capacity of the placenta is influenced by ionizing radiation. Thus the relationships between the corpus luteum and the placenta in the secretion of progesterone during the postimplantation period seem to be of primary importance and demanding of further definition.

DEANESLY: These experiments appear to illustrate the increased progesterone requirements of embryos in mid-pregnancy.

RUNNER: You are separating implantation from maintenance. How much radiation do you give to the rat?

GLASSER: These results have been obtained with 125 and 250 roentgens of whole-body radiation.

HAFEZ: If chicken eggs are incubated, there are 2 peaks of embryonic mortality: one on day 4 and one on day 18 of incubation. The first peak may be similar to what Dr. Orsini may be referring to. Dr. Deanesly, if ovariectomy on day 2 has no effect, will you conclude that progesterone is not necessary for the transport of embryos in the uterine tube?

DEANESLY: Yes.

HAFEZ: Does the period of rapid embryonic growth coincide with the period of necessary progesterone?

DEANESLY: Yes. It coincides with the period of growth and organ differentiation.

HARTMAN: Marker and I (1940, Anat. Rec., **76**:29; 1940, J. Biol. Chem., **133**:529–37) once had two monkey females pregnant about 90 days (gestation period averages 168 days). One of these received by injection 1.1 gm. of Marker's theelin (estrone) over a 20-day period. On day 115 of pregnancy she aborted. Estrogenic activity was manifested for some months. Monkey No. 2 received 1.035 gm. progesterone over a 20-day period. She carried the fetus to term and nursed the baby. No pregnediol or estrone was recoverable from the urines at any time.

SHARMAN: In marsupials there is evidence that the adrenals may be producing something that maintains pregnancy after ablation of the corpus luteum. Bourne (1949, The Mammalian Adrenal Gland [Oxford]) described an extra, cortical zone present in the female but absent in the male brush possum (*Trichosurus*). The zone showed fluctuations during pregnancy and lactation. The estrous cycle lasts 26 days, pregnancy 17 days, and there is a single corpus luteum, which may be completely removed by taking out the ovary in which it lies. Pregnancy proceeds to term after removal of the corpus on day 11 of pregnancy. In nonmated females the luteal phase is maintained following removal of the corpus at day 11 of the cycle, and the estrous cycle is not shortened as it is following removal of the corpus at day 8. If progesterone is injected following removal of the corpus at day 8, the luteal phase is induced but return to estrus is delayed only by the number of days progesterone is injected. Since the luteal phase is maintained in both pregnant and non-mated animals following removal of the corpus luteum, it seems that the placenta is not implicated.

DEANESLY: In the guinea pig the vaginal epithelium is a sensitive index of circulating estrogens; absence of vaginal mucification shows that they are absent after ovariectomy until about day 20 postcoitum, when the placenta becomes estrogenic (Deanesly, 1960, J. Endocrin., **21**:35). Experiments in which relaxin was given to 10–16 day ovariectomized, pregnant guinea pigs (Zarrow, unpublished) confirmed the absence of estrogens in these animals. Neither the traumatic decidua nor implantation requires estrogen in the guinea pig.

M. C. SHELESNYAK AND P. F. KRAICER

The Role of Estrogen in Nidation

THE OBJECT of this presentation will be to define the role of estrogen in the sequence of events during the onset of gestation that is called "nidation." Much of this report will consist of presenting and interpreting information that signalizes the intrusion of a surge of estrogen secretion during progestation, that interval between fertilization and the fixation of the fertilized ovum in the endometrium either by invasion of the nidus or by engulfment by the nidus. Attention will be directed chiefly to the effects of estrogen on the uterus, particularly to the role of estrogen in the transformation of endometrial cells into the decidua. This transformation of endometrial cells, by growth and differentiation, into decidua is defined as "decidualization."

The general plan of this discussion will consist of a descriptive definition of the process of nidation. Functional and temporal aspects of the estrogen role on the uterus will be correlated with data on histamine and progesterone actions. This interrelationship was explored by using experimentally induced decidualization and natural ovum-associated *déciduome* formation and also by seeking manifestations of estrogen activity during progestation. To search for these manifestations of estrogenic activity, morphological, physiological, and biochemical parameters were examined. The specific problem was approached by investigating natural circumstances or by designed experiment, as the situation dictated.

The late Vilhjalmur Stefansson, thinker and man of deeds, said in his own favorite of his many books that "the accepted facts of a few years ago become the error and folklore of today. You standardize knowledge and while you are on the job, the knowledge changes" (1936). Since our information of many of the episodes and conditions of early gestation is incomplete, permit us to present the following definition of "nidation" as a working definition—for convenience, perhaps even for clarity. We

DR. M. C. SHELESNYAK is professor of endocrine and reproduction physiology; head, Biology of Reproduction (Biodynamics), Weizmann Institute of Science, Rehovoth, Israel.

propose to define "nidation" as *the sequence of biological events that occur in the female of the species ending with the imbedding of the fertilized ovum in the uterus, the major episodes of nidation being, first,* nidus formation, *or preparing the uterine zone into which the blastocyst imbeds, and, second,* nidus invasion, *the active penetration of the ovum into the nidus or passive engulfment of the ovum by the nidus.*

Nidus formation is the primary subject of this discussion, with, of course, the role of estrogen in this process. Nidus formation is a prerequisite for ovum implantation in natural pregnancy; it can be provoked under artificial conditions by experimental means. When the nidus is produced under experimental conditions, it is called a "deciduoma," as distinct from the natural ovum-associated nidus, the "decidua." Extensive use of experimental induction of decidualization was made in exploring the mechanism of nidation, and it is pertinent to stress certain points of technique.

A fundamental element of the work to be reported is the induction of decidualization of the endometrium by systemic administration of a histamine releaser. This technique is based on the results of our early work, which established a role for histamine in the induction of decidualization and the formation of deciduoma (Shelesnyak 1957*a*, 1957*b*, 1960). Much evidence has been adduced by our group implicating histamine as an essential stimulatory metabolite, which acts upon the properly prepared or sensitized endometrial stromal cells to induce decidualization. Our method for inducing decidualization of the progestational endometrium is to inject, via systemic route, a large amount of a histamine liberator. The most efficient material tested to date is pyrathiazine hydrochloride (Pyrrolazote, Upjohn). The most effective time to inject the pyrathiazine is on the morning of the fourth day of the luteal phase of pseudopregnancy (or pregnancy) (Shelesnyak *et al.*, 1961). The systemic administration of pyrathiazine results in the release of histamine from various sources in the body (Marcus *et al.*, 1963). The liberated histamine passes into the blood stream and can reach the endometrium via the vascular network.

This technique for the induction of decidualization is potent and reliable; it is the method of choice in our laboratory. It can be exercised with ease and with precision for studies involving time as a parameter. It requires no surgery or the concomitant physiological stress of surgery. But the greatest advantage derived from the use of the systemic method is that there are none of the complications inherent in the classical method of traumatizing the uterus. Trauma invariably and inevitably produces debris and uterine-tissue reactions to injury, including tissue wounding and regeneration, which are unrelated to decidualization but confound the decidual picture. Freedom from the primary and secondary effects of tissue injury means that the systemic methods permit unambiguous examination of histogenic and biochemical processes that occur in the very earliest stages of decidualization (Shelesnyak, 1962).

It is convenient at this point to introduce some definitions and some standard terminology that will be used. *Induction* of decidualization, as used here, means *the stimulation of a sensitized or sensitive endometrium to begin to transform certain stromal cells to decidual cells*. When conditions are favorable, decidualization begins and the transformation carries on to production of decidual mass or deciduoma. Thus, a "*sensitized*" *endometrium has the potential to decidualize when stimulated by a decidualization inducer*.

A standard terminology for designating the days of pseudopregnancy and pregnancy will be used. Since both conditions are characterized by a persistence of the luteal phase and of leucocytic configuration of the vaginal smear, we refer to these days as L_1, L_2, . . . L_n, L_1 being the first day of appearance of leucocytic vaginal smear after the preceding Co, or cornified cell smear of estrus. According to this convention, the day of discovery of sperm in the vagina is day 0 of pregnancy (which is a metestrous day of vaginal cornification). This terminology has the advantage of making the days of pregnancy and of pseudopregnancy strictly comparable. It also overcomes the difficulty presented by certain animals that show a persistence of the cornified vaginal smear for two consecutive days at the beginning of pseudopregnancy. It has been shown that, in animals with an additional day of cornified cell smear, L_4 is identical, with respect to decidual reactions and biochemical parameters that were measured, to L_4 of an animal with only one day of cornified cells (Shelesnyak *et al.*, 1961).

Let us focus our attention on the estrogen secretion during nidation. The estrogen of estrus, which is considered to be a primer of the endometrium for progesterone action, will not be subjected to examination. We are concerned with that estrogen secretion which takes place during progestation when the uterus is under progesterone dominance. The first hints that the estrogen secretion during progestation was a surge of relatively short duration were provided by correlating certain morphological observations with physiological and biochemical ones.

The usual pattern of cells from the vaginal smears of impregnated rats is a persistent leucocytic configuration. However, Nelson (1929) and, later, Mirskaia and Crewe (1930) noted some cases in which estrous-type vaginal smears of cornified cells appeared during L_4 or L_5 of pregnancies otherwise normal and uneventful. Swezy and Evans (1930), studying the pregnant rat (and, later, Bloch [1958] the pregnant lactating mouse), reported that histological examinations of the ovaries revealed a surge of follicular development four days after the estrus in which the animals had been mated and impregnated. Vokaer's (1952) analysis of athrocytosis in the rat uterus revealed evidence suggestive of estrogenic activity on L_4 of pregnancy. These morphological findings suggested an estrogen surge, but no functional significance in nidation could be assigned to an estrogen surge on the basis of these data.

Westin (1955) reported that mast cells of the uterus were dissipated by estrogen, and Shelesnyak (1959*c*) observed that during the twenty-four hours prior to the time of expected implantation (nidus invasion) the population of mast cells in the uterus of the pregnant rat fell to almost zero. Since a reduction in mast cells can be correlated with the release of histamine (Riley, 1959), these observations suggested a role of estrogen via histamine release in the uterus. However, the case for a histamine-related functional role of estrogen surge in nidation needed a great deal more evidence; some of the necessary data will be presented later in this discussion.

Turning from structural to biochemical aspects, we find that of many enzyme systems, which vary in activity with the amount of available estrogen, two have been studied in the progestational uterus. These are betaglucuronidase (Prahlad, 1962) and glycylglycine dipeptidase (Albers *et al.*, 1961). Changes in uterine concentration of these enzymes resembling those characteristic of estrogen activity have been noted between L_3 and L_5 of pseudopregnancy and pregnancy. But here again the functional significance of estrogen surge in nidation cannot be inferred from the information.

It was evident that the elucidation of the role of estrogen in nidation required rigid experimental approaches. The first step we considered was the elucidation of the role of estrogen in the induction of decidualization. Accepting estrogen as a requirement for decidualization, we reasoned that it was important to delineate the period in the course of progestation during which the decidual reaction could be induced in the non-traumatized uterus. The systemic method for inducing decidualization permitted this investigation. By administering the systemic inducer at different but closely spaced times, we found that the period of uterine sensitivity to decidual induction was very brief (Shelesnyak *et al.*, 1961). The brevity and transience of the uterine sensitivity suggested that there was an earlier event that was also transient and that it sensitized the uterus to respond to the decidual-inducing stimulus.

It was now necessary to identify this event with the estrogen surge. Experiments were performed to study the role of the ovaries in the sensitization of the endometrium. By removing the ovaries of pseudopregnant (and pregnant) rats at different times during progestation, we showed that there is indeed a critical period of estrogen secretion from the ovary that is indispensable for the sensitization of the uterus (Shelesnyak *et al.*, 1963).

Ovaries were removed from rats, and daily injections of progesterone were begun on L_4, which is the day when the uterus is in a state of maximal sensitivity to decidual induction. Administration of pyrathiazine to the animals (on L_4) to induce deciduoma resulted in decidual reactions. The same response occurred if the ovaries were removed at midnight on L_3. Removal of ovaries during the afternoon or evening of L_3 resulted in partial or complete block of decidual response to pyrathiazine given on L_4. If the ovaries were removed at noon on L_3, no deciduoma could be induced by pyrathiazine, despite adequate quantities of exogenous progesterone.

The role of estrogen was then examined. Exogenous estradiol, given during the afternoon of L_3 to rats ovariectomized before noon on L_3, restored the capability of the endometrium to respond to systemic induction of decidualization. From these results it was clear that an ovarian estrogen surge occurred during the afternoon of L_3 that was essential for the sensitization of the progestational uterus.

The accumulated physiological evidence established (*a*) that there is an ovary-derived estrogen surge and (*b*) that this estrogen secretion sensitizes the uterus to decidual induction. What the nature of the estrogen action was, especially at the tissue and cellular level, remained to be explored.

The disappearance of mast cells from the uterus of the rat prior to ovum implantation invited attention to several other relevant data correlating with the estrogen surge. The relationships of estrogen to mast cells (Westin) and of mast cells to histamine (Riley) have been noted. Spaziani and Szego (1958) and Shelesnyak (1959*b*) then demonstrated that estrogens (Spaziani and Szego, estradiol; Shelesnyak, estradiol, estrone, and estriol) have a histamine-releasing action on the rat uterus. That this phenomenon occurs in the uterus of the impregnated rat, in synchrony with the estrogen surge prior to ovum implantation, was established by estimating histamine content of the uterus during progestation (Shelesnyak, 1959*a*). The estimations were made by bioassay of the histamine extracted from L_2, L_3, and L_4 uteri of pregnant rats. We (Marcus and Shelesnyak) have extended our early findings, using chromatographic separation of the histamine and fluorometric determinations, to the uteri of normal estrous cycle, of pregnancy through day L_6, and of pseudopregnancy. Fluctuation of histamine content and concentration followed the estrogen fluctuation of the normal estrus, and the estrogen surge of pregnancy. The picture of uterine histamine during pseudopregnancy is being analyzed.

The information available at this stage of our experiments clearly establishes an ovarian-derived estrogen surge during progestation, and the biochemical data presented so far relate the estrogen to histamine and the induction phase of decidualization. However, we have yet to demonstrate a role of the estrogen as activating the progestational uterus to become sensitive to the histamine stimulus.

Psychoyos (1960) showed that one of the very first reactions to stimuli that provoke decidualization, provided that estrogen is available, is a marked increase in capillary permeability of the uterus. Attempting to link the increased capillary permeability that Psychoyos reported at this stage of progestation and the established permeability activity of estrogen (Hechter *et al.*, 1941) with the massive leucocytic infiltration of the uterus prior to decidualization, and the estrogen surge, suggested a search for an estrogen-dependent leucotaxic substance similar to that reported by Spector and Storey (1958). A plasma kinin would fit their characterization of their unknown substance; plasma kinins are responsible not only for leucotaxis but also for vasodilation. Preliminary results of experiments carried out in our laboratory (by Shelesnyak and Lappé) suggest estrogen-associated changes of kinin-like activity in the uterus. No precise role has been assigned to this substance at this early stage of our investigations, but the existence of a consistent and conforming pattern is real.

One can predict with a degree of confidence that, of the vast array of reputed estrogen-dependent and estrogen-related phenomena that have been observed, many could be detected in association with the estrogen surge. However, again, when we sought to fix a role for estrogen in decidualization, we found it necessary to focus our attention on specific activities. We therefore turned to the relation of estrogen to tissue growth.

We have analyzed the composition of uteri at serial stages of pseudopregnancy, of decidualization, and of the normal estrous cycle (Shelesnyak and Tic, 1963*b*). Estimations were made of the weight, protein, RNA, and DNA.

Cyclic variations in the weight and in the content of RNA, DNA, and protein occurred during the estrous cycle. All four components achieved maxima during the proestrous phase, and minima at diestrus. Since this pattern of biochemical changes parallels the cyclic appearance of cornification, it is reasonable to suspect that both are manifestations of the same hormonal influences.

During pseudopregnancy, the composition of the uterus undergoes revealing changes. On L_1, L_2, and L_3 the values are like those obtained from the diestrous uterus. On L_4 and L_5 the uterus undergoes a change closely resembling the growth seen in proestrus. This transient surge of growth passes, and the uterus returns to a diestrous composition. It will be seen presently that this surge represents synthesis of uterine components essential for decidualization. Both the time of these syntheses and the changes in composition observed support the contention that estrogen secretion is the stimulus. The enhancement of protein and nucleic acid synthesis in the uterus by estrogen has been demonstrated by a number of workers (Jeener, 1948; Mueller, 1957; Mueller *et al.*, 1958; Brody *et al.*, 1961).

When decidualization is induced by the systemic technique on L_4, the uterus grows exponentially for at least four days. However, not all the

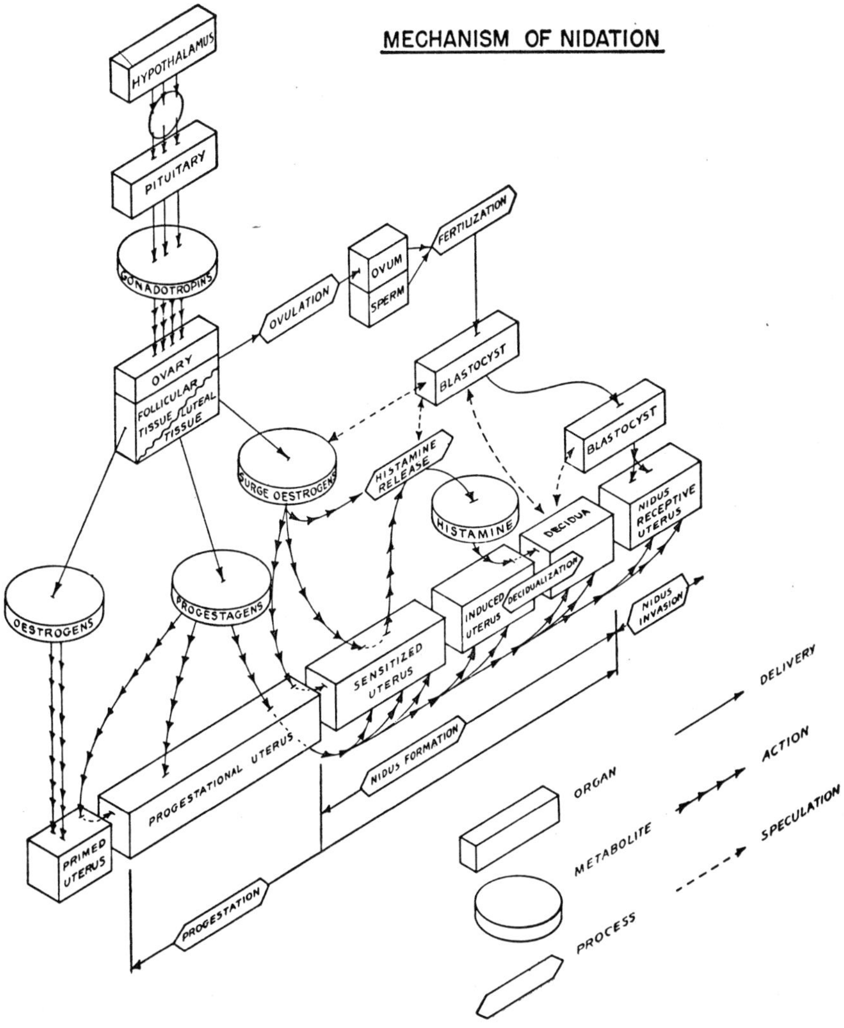

Figure 1

components estimated begin to increase from the time of decidual induction. Mathematical analysis indicates that growth begins on L_3, one day before induction, in terms of weight and RNA increment, and 12–24 hours after induction in terms of protein and DNA. This is, of course, the expected sequence. The growth on L_3–L_4 is the response to estrogen already noted and is not growth of decidual tissue. It is, however, considered to be a predecidual growth of the uterus.

It was shown, by using an anti-estrogen, that, if this predecidual growth is suppressed, then decidualization cannot be evoked. We have injected MER-25 into rats on L_3 of pseudopregnancy or pregnancy (Shelesnyak *et al.*, 1963). Induction of decidualization or nidation was prevented. Determination of the uterine composition and weight showed that the response to the estrogen surge was suppressed and that diestrous values were obtained (Shelesnyak and Tic, 1963*a*). Administration of the anti-estrogen on L_4, after the estrogen surge, did not affect decidualization or nidation. The specificity in time of the action of MER-25 serves to emphasize the brevity of the period of essential estrogenic stimulation.

There is ample evidence from observations during normal progestation and from our experiments that an estrogen surge exists during the postovulatory progestational phase of the cycle, essentially a period of progesterone predominance. This estrogen sensitizes the uterus and makes it capable of responding to decidual-inducing stimuli. In the absence of the estrogen surge, or in the event that it is suppressed, decidual-inducing stimuli are ineffective. These findings fit into the theory of the mechanism of nidation and permit a further elaboration of the theory that was first postulated by one of us (M. C. S.) in 1956 and extended in 1960 (Shelesnyak).

This discussion can thus be summarized by presenting the current and expanded presentation of our theory as shown in Figure 1. There are still many opaque areas, but, to us, this is the challenge.

Acknowledgments

We are greatly indebted to the Population Council, Inc., for their support in this work. I also wish to thank Mr. Joseph Shalom and Mr. Yehoshua Shamash for their loyal and conscientious technical help. Generous supplies of material used are gratefully acknowledged, as follows: Estradiol, Organon N.V., Holland; MER-25, Merrill, U.S.A.; Progesterone, Syntex S.A., Mexico; Pyrathiazine, Upjohn, U.S.A.

References

Albers, H. J., J. M. Bedford, and M. C. Chang. 1961. Uterine peptidase activity in the rat and rabbit during pseudopregnancy. Am. J. Physiol., **201**:554–56.

BLOCH, S. 1958. Experimentelle Untersuchungen über die hormonalen Grundlagen der Implantation des Säugerkeimes. Experientia, **14**:447–50.
BRODY, S., and N. WIQVIST. 1961. Ovarian hormones and uterine growth: Effects of estradiol, progesterone and relaxin on cell growth and cell division in the rat uterus. Endocrinology, **68**:971–77.
CREWE, F. A. E., and L. MIRSKAIA. 1930. Mating during pregnancy in the mouse. Nature, **125**:569.
HECHTER, O., L. KROHN, and J. HARRIS. 1941. The effect of estrogen on the permeability of the uterine capillaries. Endocrinology, **29**:386–92.
JEENER, R. 1948. Acides nucléiques et phosphatases au cours des phénomènes de croissance provoqués par l'œstradiol et la prolactine. Biochim. Biophys. Acta, **2**:439–53.
MARCUS, G. J., P. F. KRAICER, and M. C. SHELESNYAK. 1963. Studies of the mechanism of decidualization. II. The histamine-releasing action of pyrathiazine. J. Reprod. & Fertil. (In press.)
MUELLER, G. C. 1957. A discussion of the mechanism of action of steroid hormones. Cancer Res., **17**:490–506.
MUELLER, G. C., A. M. HERRANEN, and K. F. JERVELL. 1958. Studies on the mechanism of action of estrogens. Recent Prog. Hormone Res., **14**:95–129.
NELSON, W. O. 1929. Oestrus during pregnancy. Science, **70**:453–54.
PRAHLAD, K. V. 1962. A study of the rat uterine β-glucuronidase prior to the implantation of the ovum. Acta Endocrin., **39**:407–10.
PSYCHOYOS, A. 1960. La réaction déciduale est précédé de modifications précoces de la perméabilité capillaire de l'utérus. C.R. Soc. Biol., **154**:1384–87.
RILEY, J. F. 1959. The Mast Cells. Edinburgh and London: Livingstone.
SHELESNYAK, M. C. 1957*a*. Some experimental studies on the mechanism of ova-implantation in the rat. Recent Prog. Hormone Res., **13**:269–317.
———. 1957*b*. Experimental studies on the role of histamine in implantation of the fertilized ovum. Bull. Soc. Roy. Belg. Gynéc. & Obstét., **27**:521–37.
———. 1959*a*. Fall in uterine histamine associated with ovum implantation in the pregnant rat. Proc. Soc. Exp. Biol. & Med., **100**:380–81.
———. 1959*b*. Histamine releasing activity of natural estrogens. *Ibid.*, pp. 713–23.
———. 1959*c*. Histamine and the nidation of the ovum. Mem. Soc. Endocrin., **6**:84–88.
———. 1960. Nidation of the fertilized ovum. Endeavour, **19**:81–86.
———. 1962. Decidualization: The decidua and the deciduoma. Perspect. Biol. & Med., **5**:503–18.
SHELESNYAK, M. C., and P. F. KRAICER. 1961. A physiological method for inducing experimental decidualization of the rat uterus: Standardization and evaluation. J. Reprod. & Fertil., **2**:438–46.
SHELESNYAK, M. C., P. F. KRAICER, and G. H. ZEILMAKER. 1963. Studies on the mechanism of decidualization. I. The oestrogen surge of pseudopregnancy and progravidity and its role in the process of decidualization. Acta Endocrin., **42**:225–32.

SHELESNYAK, M. C., and L. TIC. 1963*a*. Studies of the mechanism of decidualization. IV. Synthetic processes in the decidualizing uterus. Acta Endocrin., **42**:465.

———. 1963*b*. Studies on the mechanism of decidualization. V. Suppression of synthetic processes of the uterus (DNA, RNA and protein) following inhibition of decidualization by an anti-oestrogen, ethanoxytriphetol (MER-25). *Ibid.* (In press.)

SPAZIANI, E., and C. M. SZEGO. 1958. The influence of estradiol and cortisol on uterine histamine of the ovariectomized rat. Endocrinology, **64**:713–23.

SPECTOR, W. G., and E. STOREY. 1958. A factor in the oestrogen-treated uterus responsible for leucocyte emigration. J. Path. & Bact., **75**:387–98.

STEFANSSON, V. 1936. Adventures in Error. New York: Robert M. McBride & Co.

SWEZY, O., and H. M. EVANS. 1930. Ovarian changes during pregnancy in the rat. Science, **71**:46.

VOKAER, R. 1952. Recherches histophysiologiques sur l'endométre du rat en particulier sur le conditionnement de ses propriétés athrocytaires. Arch. Biol. **63**:1–84.

WESTIN, B. 1955. The influence of some ovarian hormones on the occurrence of mast cells in the mouse uterus. Acta Path. Microb. Scand., **36**:337–42.

DISCUSSION (*Chairman:* M. N. RUNNER)

SHELESNYAK: Before beginning the discussion I should like to add some information from our current work. Our basic theory of nidation involves at least three physiological phases required for decidualization, induction, and maintenance. There is an interplay of estrogen and progesterone and histamine. By blocking surge estrogen or blocking histamine, we prevent decidual induction. If progesterone is blocked, decidual tissue does not develop, even though the process of decidualization may be induced. We have accumulated much evidence in the rat that ergocornine prevents the development of decidual tissue by interference with progesterone. We have just completed a study in women to determine whether ergocornine is effective in women (Shelesnyak, Lunenfeld, and Hönig, 1963, Life Sciences, p. 73). The study can be summarized as follows: When a single tablet of 2 mg. of ergocornine methanesulphonate is administered to women who are in the postovulatory phase of their menstrual cycle, there is a sharp drop in the levels of urinary pregnanediol and estrogens. These results, indicating a depression of progesterone in women after ingestion of a single dose of ergocornine, are consistent with observations on the rat.

NOYES: Do you really want to interfere with progesterone metabolism in women?

SHELESNYAK: The indications at the moment are that it is a very transient interference. In the study so far, based on estimation of the urinary steroids, there is recovery in 24–48 hours. If interference is necessary, I prefer 24–48 hours to 20 days.

NOYES: What is the stage of the investigation? Do you want to lower estrogen and elevate 17-ketosteroids in a population that may be hypoestrogenic and hirsute enough already?

SHELESNYAK: Give us about three years; if we are lucky, then, with diligence, industry, and support, we should have a picture of where it works, how it works, and when it works. When we have this picture in a controlled sample, I shall be prepared to discuss the problem of population control.

GREENWALD: If an estrogen surge exists in rats and if you block it, you should be able to delay implantation. Have you tried using nembutal or other blocking agents that might impair the release of LH?

SHELESNYAK: Implantation is delayed in rats after the removal of the ovary prior to the estrogen surge. We have not attempted to block estrogen surge with nembutal. In our studies (unpublished) nembutal administered after the estrogen surge did not prevent decidualization.

GREENWALD: Is there any variation in the time of implantation depending on the length of previous estrous cycles, that is, a difference between animals having a 4- or 5-day cycle?

SHELESNYAK: If our theory is correct, there should be none. In fact, the estrogen surge is independent of estrus. The estrogen surge occurs during progestation and before the phase of sensitivity in the animals in our colony. These include females with 4-day and with 5-day estrous cycles.

DE FEO: We have tried to block the "surge" in pseudopregnant rats by administering nembutal in a dose known to be effective in proestrous rats. This was done not only at the critical 2:00 P.M. period but also at 11:00 A.M., daily from day 1 through day 4. Maximal uterine sensitivity still appeared on day 4 and was lost by day 5 as in normal animals (1963, Endocrinology, **72**:305). We concluded that there is no estrogen surge or else that it cannot be blocked by this method.

YOCHIM: By manipulating the amount of estrogen priming in ovariectomized rats, we have been able to vary the timing of uterine sensitivity after treatment with estrone and progesterone. In one group of animals we observed maximal sensitivity on both the third and the fourth day of treatment. Sensitivity was completely lost by the fifth day.

SHELESNYAK: To animals from which the ovaries had been removed weeks earlier, we administered a single dose of estradiol, a dose that was adequate to induce vaginal estrus. We then gave daily progesterone. Sensitivity as on day L_4 of normal pseudopregnancy was not evident on L_4 of this design. It was necessary to give surge estrogen, and then after 14–18 hours the uterus responded to pyrathiazine induction.

DAVIS: You mentioned mast cell histamine. The work of Schayer in this country and of Kahlson in Sweden indicates that important amounts of non–mast cell histamine are present in most tissues of the body, and the release of this material is an important physiological regulatory mechanism. Does your work support this idea, and would non–mast cell histamine be released in the uterus in response to estrogen?

SHELESNYAK: Mast cell histamine does exist in the rat uterus. In attempting to correlate the physiological picture with the histological one, we noted a depletion of mast cells prior to the beginning of decidualization. We assume that the histamine released from the mast cells played the inducing role.

DAVIS: Does this make a difference in our thinking about the site of action of estrogen in the uterus?

SHELESNYAK: It might.

WIMSATT: Do you have any information on recovery time of mast cells after degranulation is induced by injection?

SHELESNYAK: No, but after the deciduoma runs its course and a second pseudopregnancy is provoked, histamine-releaser will again induce decidualization.

WIMSATT: Did you imply that this mast-cell releasing substance is effective on mast cells only at this time, or any time?

SHELESNYAK: The effectiveness of the inducer (histamine-releaser) is very time-specific. Ordinarily, there are very few mast cells in the rat endometrium. When the time is reached and histamine is needed for induction of decidua, the mast-cell population drops. Recovery of this mast-cell population may be by regeneration or infiltration.

WIMSATT: If you could eliminate histamine before you give estrogen, and then give estrogen, would you get deciduoma?

SHELESNYAK: In experimental procedures by which the histamine has been depleted but the estrogen not manipulated, we failed to get decidualization by histamine-releasers. The experiment about which you ask, namely, giving added estrogen (that is, additional to the animal's surge estrogen) has not been carried out.

GLASSER: I was interested in your graph depicting a progesterone-directed increase in nucleic acid, weight, and protein from L_3 onward. Were these determinations done on the whole rat uterus or prospective and actual deciduoma?

Generally, although we have described biochemical changes within a short period of time after trauma, I have not been pleased with the information derived from such studies. How much of the increase in protein that we describe is myometrial? If the increase in protein is non-parallel with respect to the increase in DNA, as you describe, where is the increased protein coming from? Have you corrected your data for the significant alterations in tissue water that are to be noted? Are your data expressed on a wet weight, dry weight, or milligram nitrogen basis?

SHELESNYAK: Myometrium and decidua tissue are separable only after day L_7. Earlier stages can be studied only together with the myometrium. Any study of early changes that does not employ "systemic" induction of decidualization is, in my mind, open to serious criticism.

BIGGERS: You showed a picture of a uterus from a rat that had been treated with pyrathiazine, in which swellings occurred in different parts of the uterine horns. How do you account for the fact that the drug, which was administered systemically, acted only in certain parts of the uterus?

SHELESNYAK: Alexandre Psychoyos of Paris (Collège de France) and Dr. Orsini should be complimented here on their work. They have shown quite clearly that the first response to stimulus was localized, according to vascular distribution. This is also true following pyrathiazine.

MEYER: What are we to assume about levels of progesterone in the first days?

SHELESNYAK: Do you mean levels on days L_1, L_2, L_3, and L_4?

MEYER: If estrogen is at a given level and sensitization is on day 4, could not this represent an increased output of progesterone for your test? You could study this possibility by giving a constant amount of estrogen with varying doses of progesterone. We do not say anything about where progesterone is before ovulation on day 4.

SHELESNYAK: If we assume that it maintains a constant status, we can be satisfied. A drop in progesterone does not induce pregnancy in delayed nidation, and, although Johnson and I were successful with this once, we cannot reproduce this result at will.

MEYER: I am very much concerned with the hypothesis that sensitivity on day 4 may be due to increased amounts of progesterone without necessarily increasing the amount of estrogen. Suzuki studied pseudopregnant and pregnant rats. He found that progesterone is increasing and reaching higher levels around day 4 in blood from the ovarian vein. We have not tested the question whether sensitivity may be due to increased progesterone level in pseudopregnancies as compared to a normal cycle.

SHELESNYAK: How do you fit the role of increased progesterone in inducing nidation and delaying nidation with the fact that injection of doses of estrogen in an already pregnant endometrium is necessary to get pyrathiazine-induced deciduoma?

MEYER: I must say that we have not tested this hypothesis, but we have not said much about progesterone levels. We assume that it goes to a level after ovulation and stops.

SHELESNYAK: There are so many things that favor estrogen. It seems more direct. In order to be certain, we must try to prove that we are wrong.

DE FEO: While we wholeheartedly agree that pyrathiazine—which, incidentally, has not worked well enough for us as yet—may be a good inducer of spontaneous deciduomata by non-traumatic means, we disagree with its being referred to as "physiological" when (*a*) it is a pharmacologic agent whose entire spectrum of actions is not clearly known and, (*b*) unlike the rat blastocyst, operates from the peritoneal cavity rather than the uterine lumen.

SHELESNYAK: We believe that it is more "physiological" than any other method. We are convinced that histamine plays a role as inducer; we have proof that pyrathiazine releases histamine, and that leads us to suggest that the histamine reaches the uterus via systemic means and approximates a physiological induction. We do not claim that pyrathiazine is a body metabolite.

Success in inducing decidualization by pyrathiazine has been achieved in thousands of rats in our laboratory and also in the laboratories at Birmingham (Anatomy Department), Bordeaux, Rome, and Paris.

Failure may be due to strain differences (although the strains in the various laboratories mentioned differ). Response to antihistamines can vary greatly in different strains (see Ambrus *et al*., 1961, Proc. Soc. Exp. Biol. & Med., **108**:360).

MAYER: The important point is that pyrathiazine acts as decidual inducer only when estrogen acts in synergy with progesterone. Pyrathiazine does not induce deciduoma in ovariectomized rats injected only with progesterone, but it does in a normal pseudopregnancy at day 5, that is to say, after the estrogen release taking place at day 4.

A similar result is observed with the physiological decidual reaction induced by the implantation of the egg. If there is no estrogen (in rats ovariectomized at day 4 and injected with progesterone), the eggs do not implant and do not induce decidual reaction. But they do in rats ovariectomized at day 4 and injected with progesterone and estrogen.

DE FEO: We have studied mast cells in relation to deciduoma formation. The rat uterus, particularly in the region of the mesometrial triangle, has a potent source of stored histamine in the mast cells. However, even if these cells are markedly depleted by 48/80 pretreatment, the uterus still responds to intraluminal inducers on day 4 by formation of deciduomata. In addition, complete elimination of stainable mast cells still enables the uterus to develop the characteristic hydration associated with estrogen administration. We wonder whether we are still dealing with histamine release from the non-stainable mast cells, that is, in a non-storage phase, or else the histamine source may be from cells other than the mast cells.

SHELESNYAK: Have you measured histamine release in mast cell-depletion studies? It is pertinent. If you have removed the mast cells from the uterus and measured histamine release following estrogen, you will be able to correlate whether there is an additional source other than the mast cells.

DE FEO: Do you still believe that the blastocyst induces the decidua via histamine release?

SHELESNYAK: Some speculation exists, but we have yet to rule out the possibility that the estrogen factor is contained in the "stuff" with the blastocyst. That is, the stuff that the blastocyst brings down from the ovary, particularly in the larger blastocysts. We cannot rule out the presence of a certain amount of estrogen in this mass. Very little is necessary to trigger this response.

DICKMANN: In your opinion, what role does the blastocyst play in implantation?

SHELESNYAK: I am greatly interested in the role of the blastocyst in nidation, but I do not know enough about the blastocyst at this time to say. This is, of course, one object of all our studies, in fact of every one who works in this field.

NOYES: Why will not the mature blastocyst stick to decidua?

SHELESNYAK: I really do not know, and you know that I do not know.

ALLEN C. ENDERS

Fine Structural Studies of Implantation in the Armadillo

MOST OF THE studies of placentation made with the electron microscope have been concerned primarily with the nature of the cellular layers interposed between the fetal and maternal blood streams in the well-developed chorioallantoic placenta, as were the original studies of Wislocki and Dempsey (1955*a*, 1955*b*). Studies of the villi or labyrinths of the mature chorioallantoic placenta of the rat, guinea pig, rabbit, cat, sow, mare, armadillo, and human have accumulated substantial information concerning the elaborations of the surface of the trophoblast and the organelles of the cells of the placental membranes (see Wislocki and Padykula, 1961, for a summary of the early literature). The yolk sac also has been studied with the electron microscope, including studies concerning uptake of particulate matter by pinocytotic activity (Dempsey, 1953; Luse, 1957; Luse, Davies, and Smith, 1959). However, early implantation stages have received relatively little attention. Larsen (1961) has studied the fusion of the trophoblast with the maternal epithelium in the first establishment of association at the mesometrial pole in implantation in the rabbit. He reported that the maternal epithelium forms a true syncytium and fuses directly with the trophoblast. He also described the invasion of the lumina of the glands and the eventual penetration of the basement membrane of these glands by the trophoblast. In previous work some aspects of the fine structure of the villi of the armadillo placenta (Enders, 1960*b*) and the fine structure of the armadillo blastocyst (Enders, 1962) have been studied. It was the purpose of this study to discern in detail the intercellular relationships established in the process of implantation in the armadillo.

Patterson (1913), in an excellent monograph, reported the results of his histological investigations of implantation in the armadillo. He de-

DR. ALLEN C. ENDERS was an associate professor of biology in the Department of Biology, Rice University, Houston, Texas, at the time of the symposium. At present he is associate professor of anatomy at Washington University School of Medicine, St. Louis, Missouri.

termined that the single blastocyst formed after fertilization enters the uterus simplex in the horizontal groove at the fundic end of this organ and that implantation occurs in this position after a period of delay. He further established that Rauber's layer is involved in the early implantation, that mesoderm is formed precociously from the trophoblast, and that there is an early inversion of the yolk sac. He described in detail the formation of the four identical quadruplets, starting with the division of the embryonic shield. In describing early implantation, he brought to completion a description of placentation and polyembryony in the armadillo that he had initiated with Newman (Newman and Patterson, 1910) several years earlier.

In studying the later stages of development, Newman and Patterson (1910) stripped the embryonic vesicle from the uterus and consequently were not aware of the relationship of the endometrium to the villi of the developing and mature hemochorial placenta. Patterson (1913) pointed out, however, that the endometrium of the fundic tip constituted a placental attachment region. Enders and Buchanan (1958) noted that in this region the endometrial sinuses are particularly close to the surface and that the villi of the armadillo placenta invade the anastomotic network of these venous sinuses at an early stage. The subsequent growth of the placenta is by enlargement of these maternal blood spaces and is accomplished without destruction of the maternal endothelium and, consequently, leaves the vascular pathways relatively undisturbed in the body of the uterus. For purposes of description, Enders (1960*a*) divided placental growth into three stages: that of placental establishment, including initial attachment, yolk sac inversion, and formation of the closing plate; that of placental enlargement, including formation of the cell columns and vascular villi; and the period of the mature placenta, which exists from the disappearance of the cell columns until parturition. It is the stage of placental establishment that constitutes the subject of the present study.

Preparation of Implantation Sites

Twenty-three implantation sites of less than 2 mm. in diameter were used for the study with the electron microscope. An additional eight implantation sites of this level of development were studied with the light microscope. Several times as many later stages have been studied previously, with both the light and the electron microscope. Of the early implantation sites, roughly half came from normal animals killed in November and December. The remaining implantation sites were produced experimentally by bilateral ovariectomy during the delay period. This method merits a somewhat fuller explanation.

Buchanan, Enders, and Talmage (1956) first determined that bilateral ovariectomy of armadillos in delayed implantation was followed by implantation, provided that the ovariectomy was performed more than a month before the normal time of implantation. In further studies it was found that implantation did not occur if only the ovary containing the corpus luteum was removed and that exogenous hormones did not appear to alter the time sequence of implantation following ovariectomy (Enders and Buchanan, 1959). No implantation stages have been found prior to day 16 postovariectomy, nor have any free blastocysts been found later than day 25. On days 18, 19, and 20 more implantation sites than free blastocysts have been found. Consequently, implantation can be said to occur approximately 18 days after bilateral ovariectomy, and early implantation stages can be obtained routinely by this method.

In our hands, fixation with potassium permanganate, followed by rapid dehydration in cold ethyl alcohol and imbedding in epoxy resin, provides the best preservation of implantation sites for studies with the electron microscope. This procedure, however, introduces some limitations. To locate the blastocyst or implantation site, the uterus has to be inverted, risking the possibility of stretching the site or producing desiccation if the search is prolonged. Therefore, the fundic tip of the uterus is usually dipped in 0.9 per cent sodium chloride to determine whether a free blastocyst or an implantation site is present. Permanganate penetrates poorly and renders the fixed tissue opaque. Consequently, a small block containing the implantation site must be cut from the uterus prior to fixation in such a fashion that it can be subsequently oriented. This trimming-down is usually done under saline solution.

Eight of the early implantation sites were fixed in osmium-containing fixatives, despite the inferior quality of such preparations, in order to check the distribution of ribosomes and to act as a check on our standard fixation procedure.

Observations

In the initial stages of implantation the size of the site is of little value in estimating the age or stage. Blastocysts suspended in fluid range in diameter from 0.3 to 0.5 mm. However, when flattened on the surface of the uterus, they may measure as much as 0.7 or 0.8 mm. in width. (It should be noted that more collapsed blastocysts are found at implantation than at any other time.) Early implantation sites showing various degrees of development range from 0.4 to 1 mm. in width. From the 1-mm. stage on, expansion is rapid and there is better correlation between the size of the implantation site and the stage of development.

Our earliest implantation site was an attached blastocyst that adhered to the endometrium throughout the imbedding procedures and gave indications of possible destruction of several uterine epithelial cells but showed no structural modifications. The next two sites both became detached in preparation. The earlier of these two stages had a symplasmic mass and evidence of differentiation of endoderm but was otherwise unaltered. The other detached site had, in addition to well-developed symplasmic masses, two adhering uterine epithelial cells and the beginnings of inversion of the germ layers (entypy). All subsequent sites remained firmly attached. The extent of development of these sites could be followed roughly by the following events, which occur in this approximate sequence: formation of the exocelom, inversion of the yolk sac, and formation of the separate embryonic shields.

Shortly after the formation of the exocelom, this structure begins to expand rapidly, concomitant with an expansion of the closing plate. The expansion of the exocelom and placental membranes fills the uterine lumen and then rapidly distends the fundic portion of the uterus, leaving the body of the uterus relatively unaffected until the villi form at the beginning of the period of placental expansion.

It is convenient to start our description with the stage just prior to inversion of the yolk sac, by which time the majority of structures present in the early implantation site have been formed.

The implantation site projects into the uterine lumen only somewhat more than a hemisphere, the outer covering of which is the abembryonic trophoblast (Pl. I, *1*). The embryonic shield and amnion constitute a separate vesicle situated beneath the apex of the projection (Pl. I, *2*). Between the embryonic shield and the abembryonic trophoblast is the yolk sac epithelium, which is difficult to distinguish where it is in contact with the embryonic shield but which otherwise forms a definite layer of cuboidal cells lying beneath the abembryonic trophoblast and somewhat separated from it. In the earlier stages there are only a few scattered mesenchyme cells in the embryonic cavity between the amnion and the trophoblastic plate. These rapidly form into two or more vesicles, which unite, forming the extraembryonic celom, which then obliterates the extraembryonic cavity. Peripherally, both the abembryonic trophoblast and the yolk sac epithelium are fused to a ring of cytotrophoblast (Pl. I, *3*). Mitotic figures are numerous in this cytotrophoblast, and it appears to be the principal region of proliferation of trophoblast tissue during this stage. Toward the center of the implantation site, the cytotrophoblast forms a single layer of cells, which constitutes the conversion of the trophoblastic plate into a closing plate in this region. Just lateral to the cytotrophoblast, irregular masses of symplasma ring or partially ring the implantation site. Beneath the implantation site in the central region deep to the trophoblastic plate are irregular cells that are in close association with the maternal tissue and constitute the invasive trophoblast.

ABEMBRYONIC TROPHOBLAST

At the time of implantation the cells of the abembryonic trophoblast are similar in structure to the previous stage (Pl. II, *4* and *5*). Indeed, more differences are found between the trophoblast cells of the blastocyst with zona pellucida and the delay blastocyst than between the latter and the early implantation stage. After implantation, however, the trophoblast cells persist for a period of time, but, as the exocelom increases in size and the yolk sac cells become enlarged, the entire abembryonic trophoblast disintegrates and is lost. At no time does the yolk sac epithelium form a vesicle beneath the abembryonic trophoblast. Rather, it fuses with it at the margin of the implantation site. It is from the margin of this region outward that the trophoblast is lost.

YOLK SAC

In the unimplanted blastocyst some of the cells at the margin of the embryonic cell mass are elongated and in a position in which it can be assumed that they will form endoderm, but cytologically there is little difference between these cells and other embryonic cell mass cells. With the commencement of implantation the endodermal cells become clearly demarked by an increase in density of cytoplasm and a marked extension in length (Pl. III, *6*). At first these cells are squamous, but they shortly become more cuboidal, starting with the region between the point of fusion of the trophoblast and the margin of the developing embryonic shield. As development continues, the mesenchyme cells come to underlie the portion of the endoderm that will form the yolk sac epithelium, after which disintegration of the abembryonic trophoblast occurs, leaving the yolk sac epithelium exposed to the uterine lumen. The inverted yolk sac thus formed persists as a columnar epithelium throughout the period of placental establishment and also the period of placental expansion. It is eventually pressed against the endometrium sometime during the period of the mature placenta.

The cells of the early yolk sac have relatively unmodified surfaces, uniformly distributed strands of endoplasmic reticulum, and Golgi membranes of moderate proportions (Pl. III, *7*). After the mesenchyme becomes associated with these cells, they become more columnar in shape, develop regular microvilli, terminal bars, and a more extensive juxtanuclear Golgi zone (Pl. IV, *8*). Large amorphous granules are common inclusions in the yolk sac epithelium, and, occasionally, cellular debris is found adhering to the surface, but lipid droplets are not commonly present, and only a few vesicles are found in these early stages.

By the end of implantation, the yolk sac constitutes a membrane of differentiated cells situated in an excellent position to absorb the products elaborated by the uterine glands.

SYMPLASMIC MASS

The symplasmic mass is one of the first structures to appear and is in many respects the most enigmatic. This tissue probably arises from the trophoblast. In the early implantation sites it is located at the margin of the site and may extend as a tab some distance from it. Well before the end of the period of placental establishment the symplasmic mass or masses disappear.

The numerous nuclei in the symplasmic mass are clumped together near the center and are surrounded by cisternal elements of the endoplasmic reticulum. Golgi membranes are present in groups between the nuclei and the marginal cytoplasm. In the marginal cytoplasm there is a distinct zonation, with mitochondria present in the inner aspect but largely absent more peripherally. Characteristically, highly branched tubules of the endoplasmic reticulum ramify throughout the marginal cytoplasm (Pl. IV, *9*). Small lipid droplets and larger amorphous granules are the most common cytoplasmic inclusions. The surface of the symplasma is studded with numerous short microvilli.

The functional significance of this tissue is not known. The symplasma appears to be sticky when touched by a glass rod in manipulating implantation sites. The peripheral position of this tissue might serve to stabilize the orientation of an implanting blastocyst or to prevent uterine overgrowth.

PERIPHERAL TROPHOBLAST

The cytotrophoblast forms a continuous mass of cells in the early implantation site, which constitutes the trophoblastic plate (Pl. V, *10*). As development continues, the invasive trophoblast gradually separates from the cytotrophoblast centrally. As the width of the site increases, a thick peripheral ring of cytotrophoblast, in which mitotic figures are numerous, develops, as does a thin central closing plate. The cytotrophoblast persists in its peripheral position until the end of the period of placental establishment, at which time it gives rise to some of the cell columns, and may contribute to the marginal attachment of the closing plate to the endometrium.

The cells of the cytotrophoblast are small, which large nuclei, scant cytoplasm, and few surface elaborations (Pl. V, *11*). The endoplasmic reticulum is in the form of flattened cisternae. The membranes and vesicles of the Golgi complex are compact but surprisingly abundant. Mitochondria are rounded and not very numerous. The cytoplasm is uniform in structure, of little density, and contains very few inclusions.

The cytological features of these cells are consistent with the interpretation that the peripheral cytotrophoblast is the major site of cellular

PLATE I

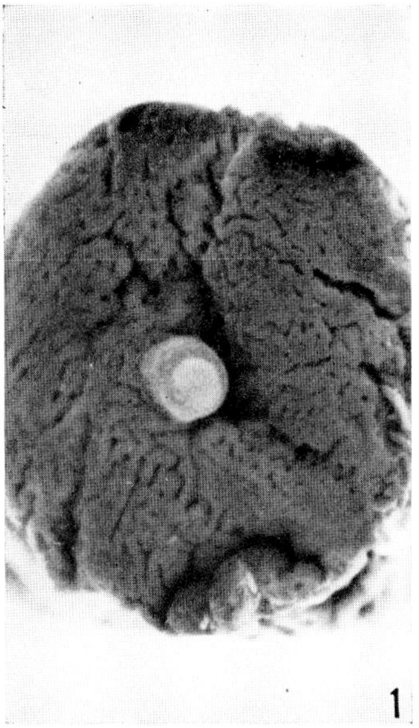

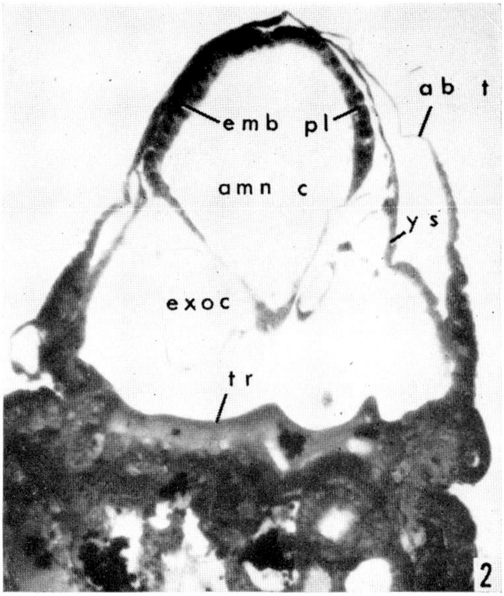

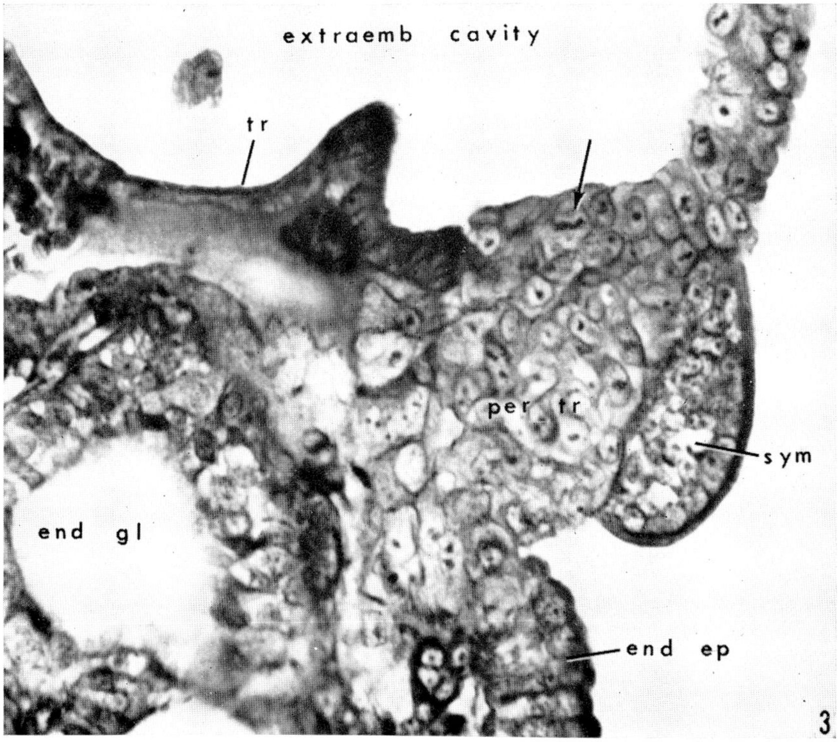

1, Surface view of an implanting blastocyst. The lighter sphere within the implanting blastocyst is the embryonic cell mass and amnion. Note the openings of the glands on the surface of the uterus. ×12.

2, A section through the implantation site seen in *1*. The maternal tissues lie at the base of the picture. Note the presence of the abembryonic trophoblast (*ab t*), yolk sac (*y s*), embryonic plate (*emb pl*), amnionic cavity (*amn c*), beginning exocelom (*exoc*), and trophoblast (*tr*) overlying the eroded maternal tissue. ×135.

3, A higher magnification of the section shown in *2*, taken from the area of the lower right corner of that figure. Note the presence of a mitotic figure (*arrow*) in the peripheral trophoblast (*per tr*); a symplasmic mass (*sym*) and central trophoblast (*tr*) can be seen in addition to an endometrial gland (*end gl*) and endometrial epithelium (*end ep*). ×550.

PLATE II

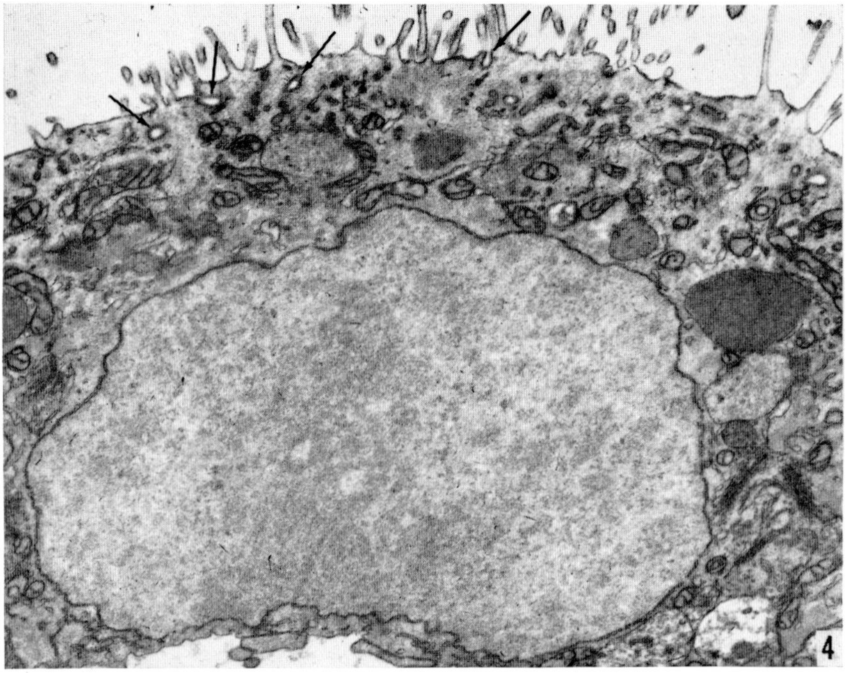

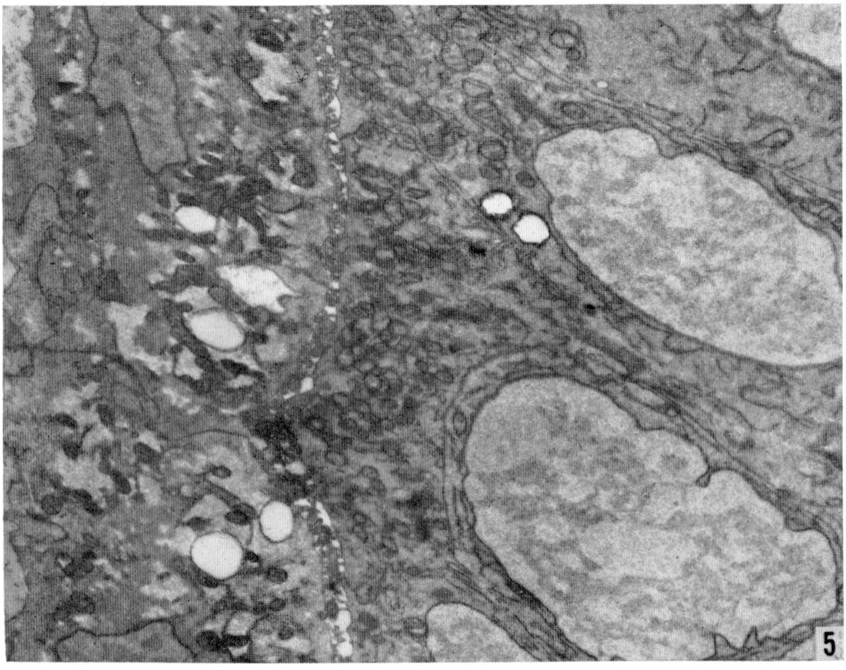

4, Abembryonic trophoblast from a blastocyst just commencing implantation. Note evidence for pinocytosis at arrows. ×12,400.

5, Trophoblast (*right*) adhering to uterine epithelium (*left*). Note intermingling of microvilli and coincidence of contour at border between the epithelia. ×8,200.

PLATE III

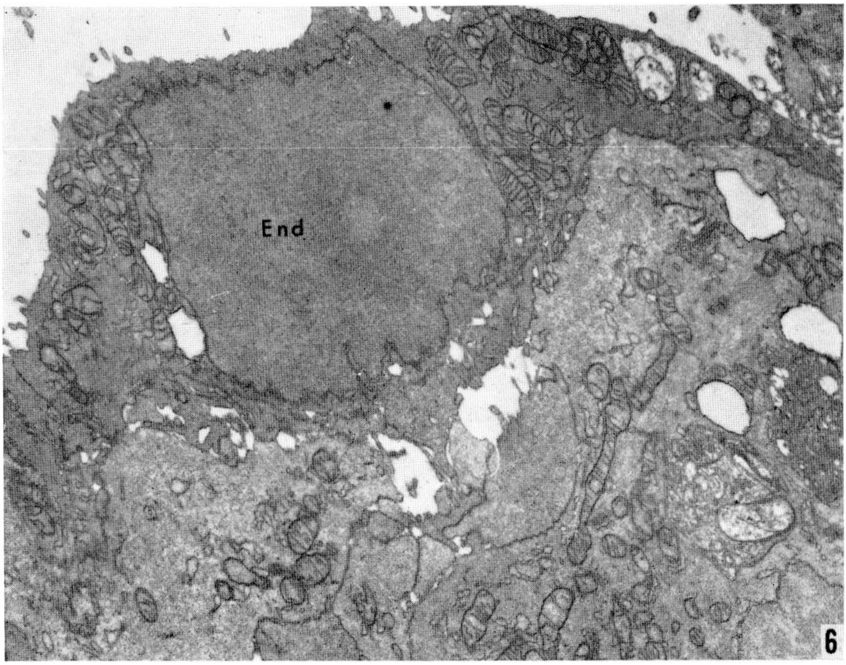

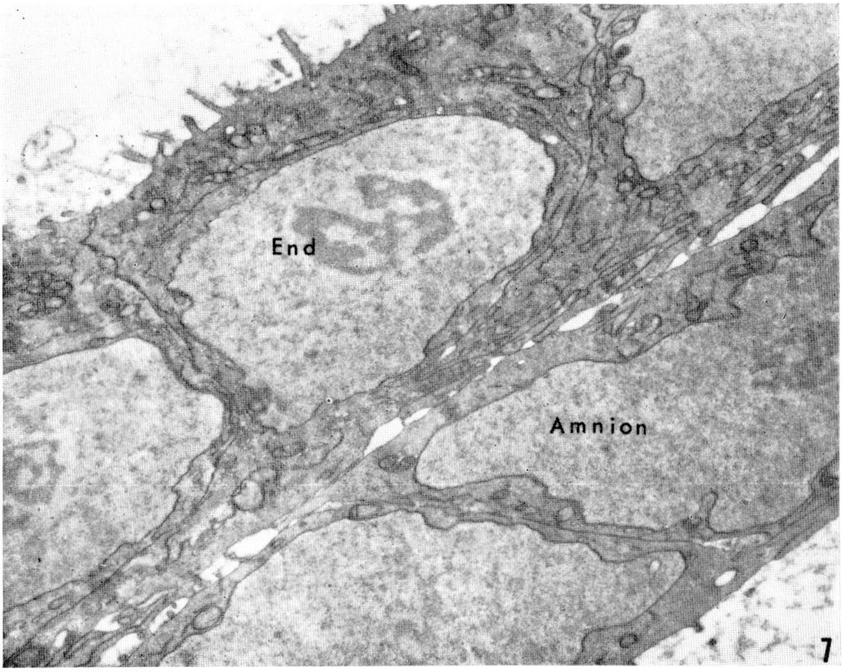

6, Differentiation of endoderm (*End*) from other cells of the embryonic cell mass (*bottom*) in a blastocyst at the onset of implantation. ×10,000.

7, The endoderm (*End*) of the yolk sac is shown where it overlies the amnion prior to the stage of formation of the exocelom. ×8,000.

PLATE IV

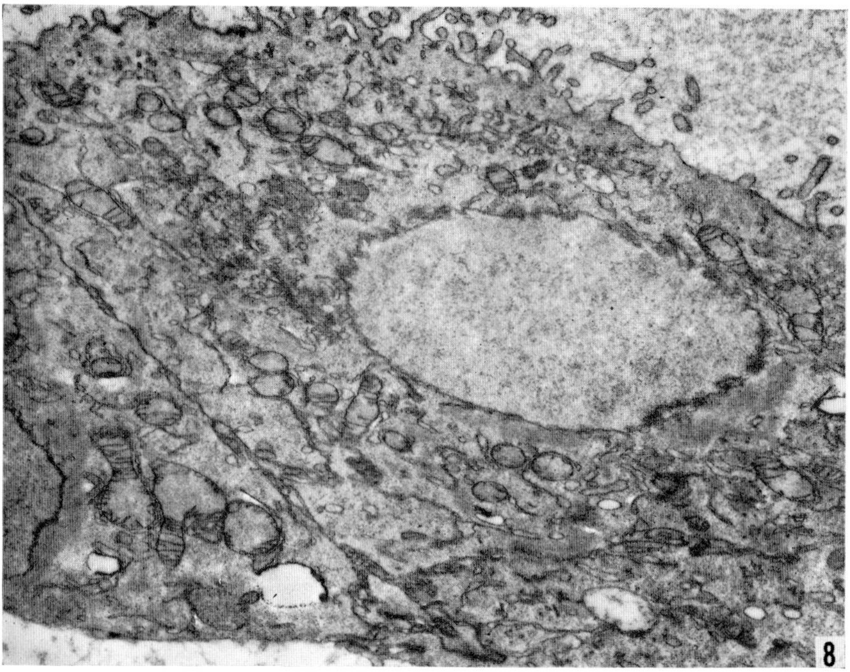

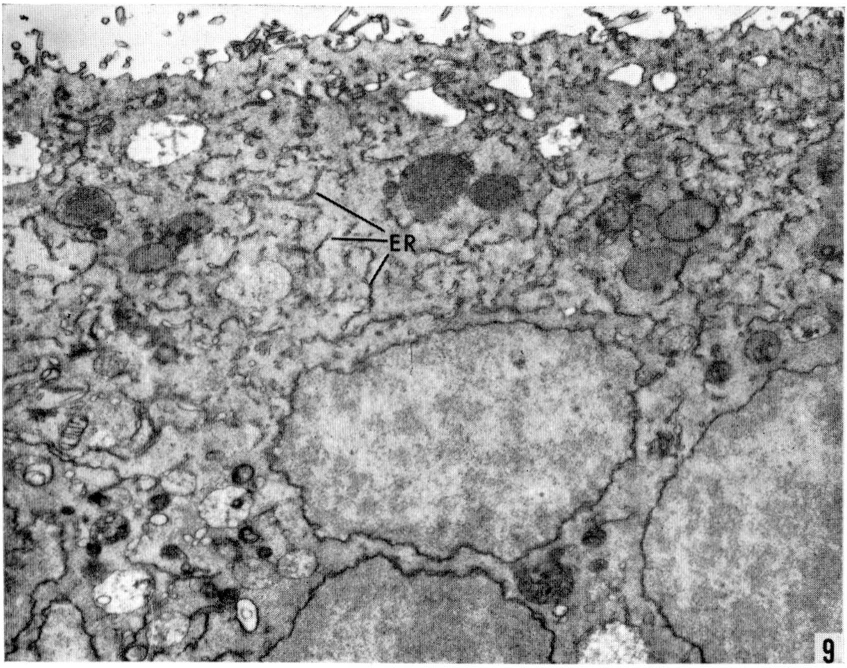

8, The endoderm of the yolk sac after inversion. Note the Golgi complex to the left of the nucleus in this slightly tangential section. ×9,300.

9, Margin of a symplasmic mass. Note the absence of cell membranes between the nuclei at the bottom of the picture and the abundant tortuous endoplasmic reticulum (*ER*). ×7,500.

PLATE V

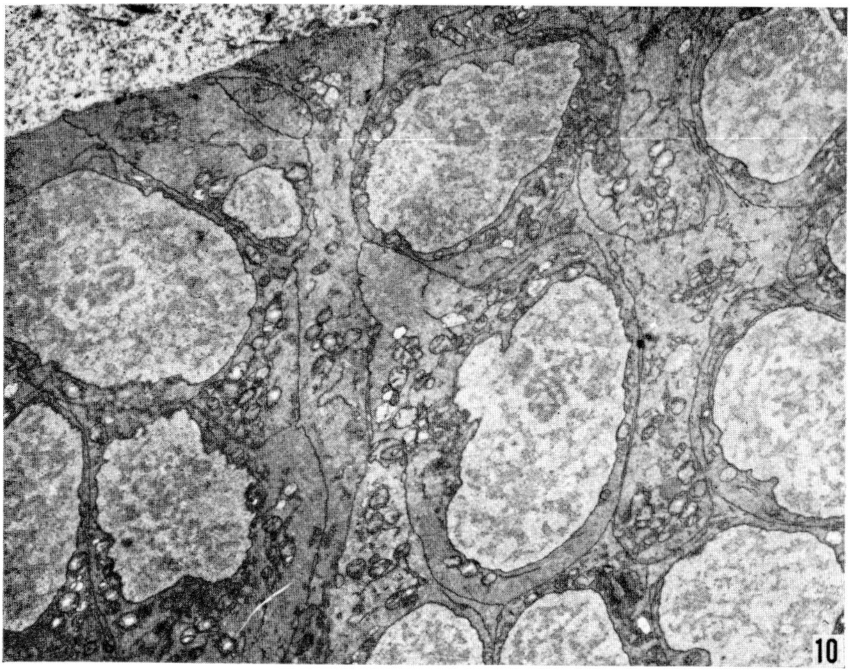

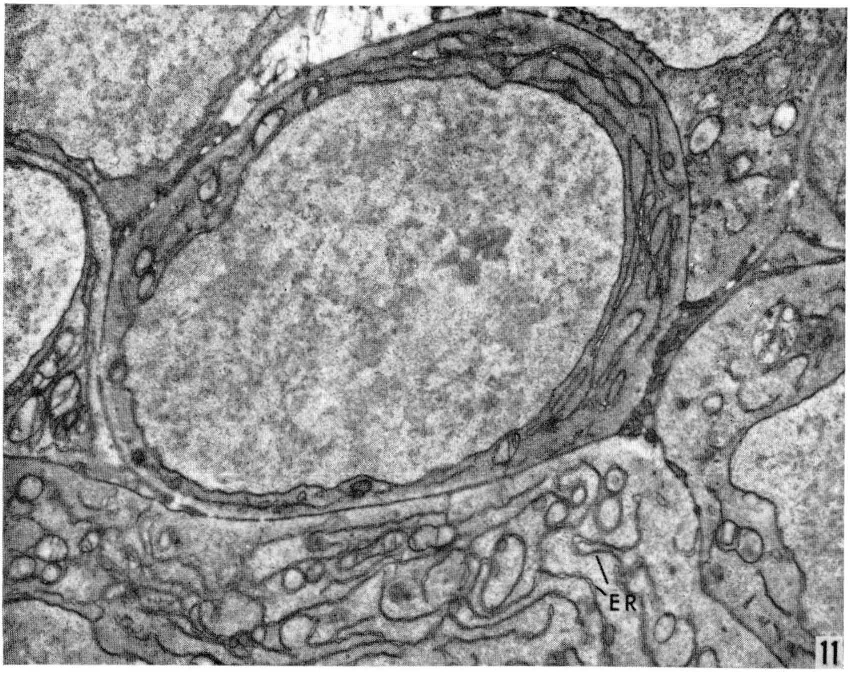

10, The cytotrophoblast forming the trophoblastic plate. In the upper left is the extraembryonic cavity. Note the relatively uniform, uncomplicated nature of these cells. ×4,500.

11, Cytotrophoblast cells from the peripheral ring of cytotrophoblast. Note the relatively simple borders and the profiles of cisternal elements of the endoplasmic reticulum (*ER*). ×7,800.

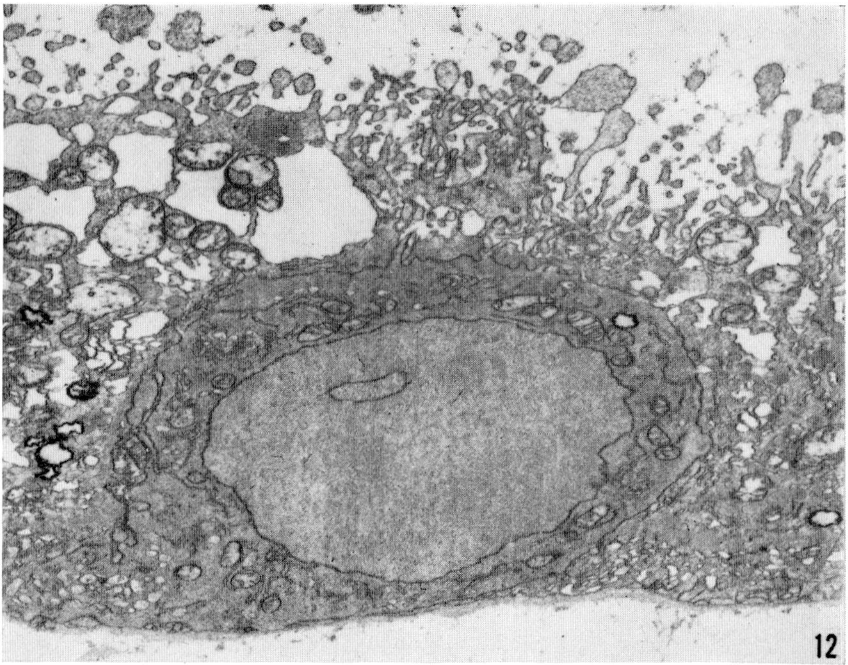

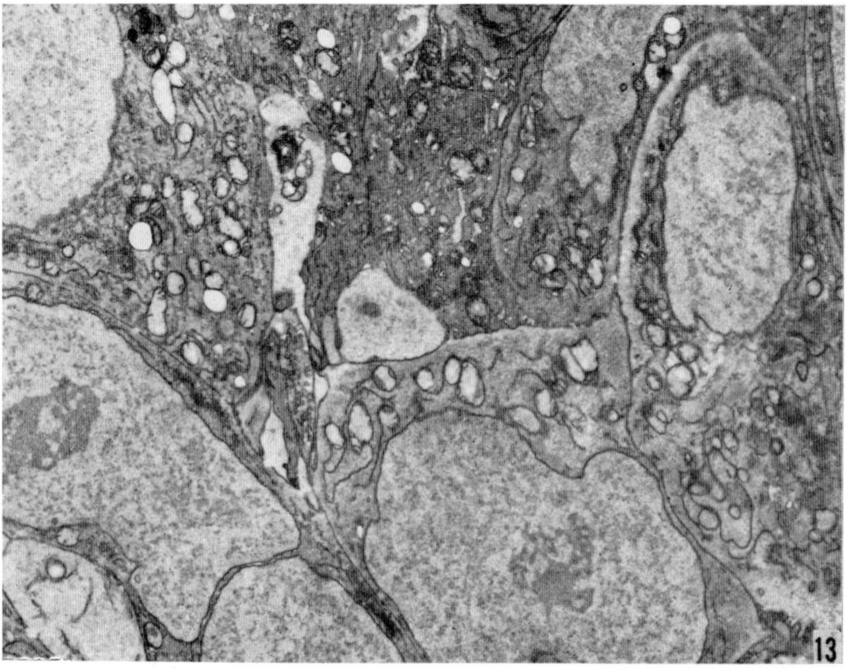

12, Syncytial trophoblast of the closing plate. Note the presence of a relatively undifferentiated cytotrophoblast cell within the syncytium in the center of the picture. ×8,200.

13, A region where invasive trophoblast (dark cells in upper left and center of the picture) is differentiating from the cytotrophoblast. ×5,000.

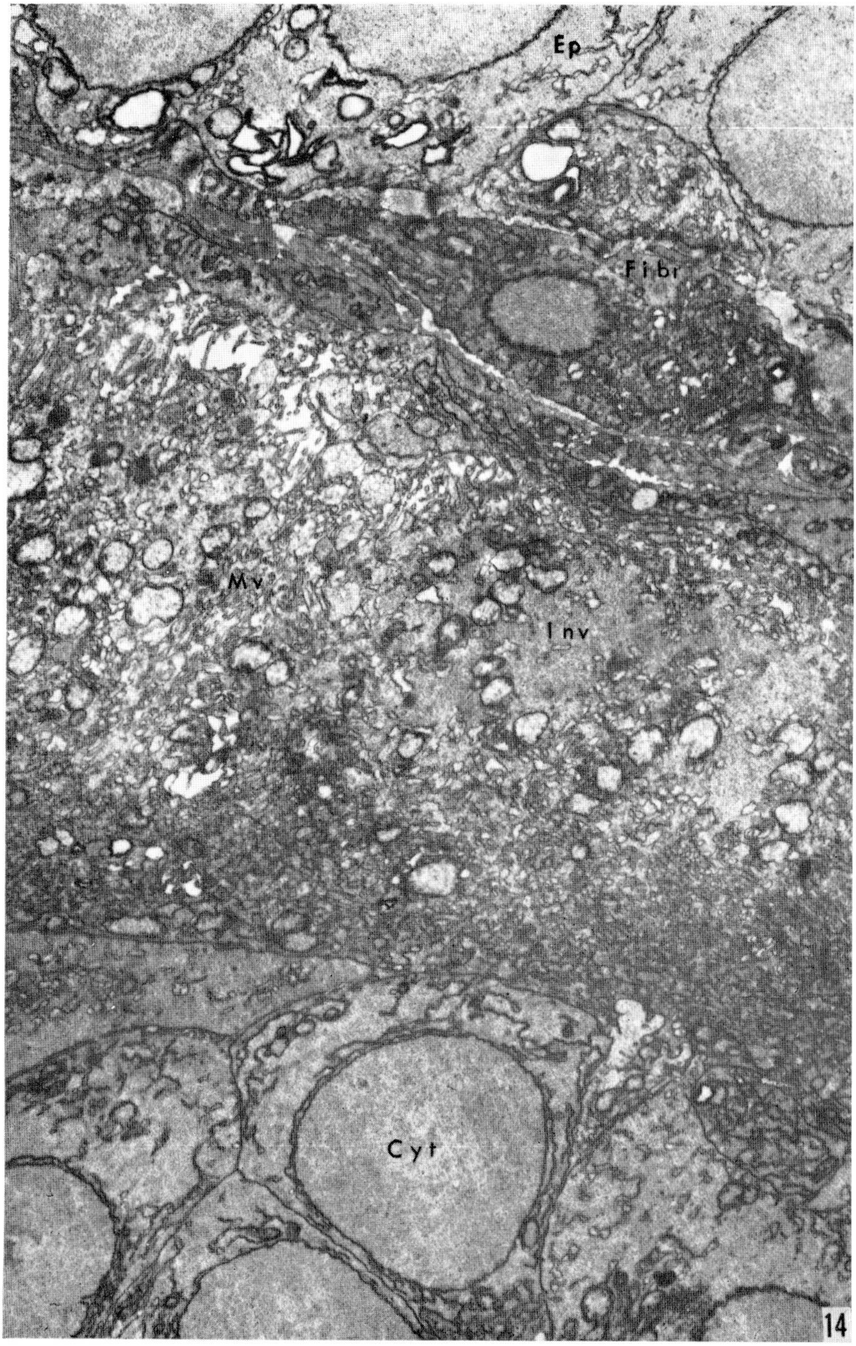

14, The glandular epithelium (*Ep*) and a fibroblast (*Fibr*) are underlaid by invasive trophoblast (*Inv*). Note that many microvilli (*Mv*) are present, especially toward the uterine tissue, but not on the border with the cytotrophoblast (*Cyt*). ×7,100.

proliferation. The cells appear embryonic in nature, undifferentiated, and with no evidence of secretory or absorptive activity. From these cells apparently arise both the trophoblast cells of the closing plate and the invasive trophoblast. In addition, the peripheral position and thickness of this ring of cell adds to the rigidity of the implantation site.

CLOSING PLATE

The cytotrophoblast thins in the center of the implantation site until a largely single layer of cells is left in the central area, constituting the limits of the extraembryonic cavity on the side toward the endometrium. This layer of cells was referred to by Patterson as the "Träger epithelium." Shortly after its formation, mesenchyme cells of the extraembryonic celom come to line the epithelium in addition to the basement membrane. As the placenta continues to expand, this epithelial layer serves to separate the exocelom from the products of cell breakdown and maternal blood and, as such, forms the closing plate.

When first formed, the cells of the closing plate are biscuit-shaped, with numerous long microvilli on their free surface and a distinct basement membrane underlying the basal surface. The endoplasmic reticulum is frequently dilated. Ribosomes are numerous, not only in association with the endoplasmic reticulum, but also free in the cytoplasm. Mitochondria are numerous and evidently swell readily during fixation. The membranes of the Golgi complex also tend to be dilated. Various types of inclusions, including granules, small lipid droplets, and numerous vesicles, are present. Later, the cell membranes separating the individual cells disappear, particularly in the basal region. However, individual, less highly differentiated cells may persist within this syncytium until the formation of cell columns (Pl. VI, *12*).

The position of the closing plate, and the abundance of surface modifications, vesicles, and inclusions in the cells, are consistent with the interpretation of the closing plate as the major absorptive surface of the implantation site.

INVASIVE TROPHOBLAST

The invasive trophoblast arises from the undersurface of the cytotrophoblast and, later, from the peripheral trophoblast (Pl. VI, *13*). It is not usually very abundant, with the greatest amount of this element being present after initial penetration of small sinuses has occurred but before broad contact with a major sinus has been established. Quite commonly, whole portions of glands will be completely surrounded by cells of the invasive trophoblast (Pl. VII, *14*). In many such glands, the epithelial cells appear quite normal. In others, both the epithelial cells and the trophoblast seem difficult to preserve. The invasive trophoblast largely disappears before the development of the cell columns and villi, although a few cells from this tissue may contribute to the area of attachment of the closing plate with the endometrium.

The invasive trophoblast forms an irregular and discontinuous penetrating face to the implantation site. During the brief existence of this element, all the maternal tissue lying between the closing plate and the basal blood sinuses of the endometrium disappears. The cells of the invasive trophoblast apparently contribute to the disintegration of the uterine tissue. There is no cytological evidence for the synthesis of digestive enzymes by these cells. Glands, when first surrounded, appear quite normal, which may indicate that disintegration by autolysis occurs only after the epithelial cells are separated from their normal vascular relationship.

Discussion

The finding of an attached blastocyst, in which the only possible evidence of invasion was the rupture of several luminal cells at the margin of the embryonic cell mass, the finding of two detached early implantation sites, the absence of any ruptured blastocysts after dipping of the implantation site, and the absence of any epithelial cells in the central region of any of the established implantation sites all suggest that the initial penetration of the endometrium is accomplished by disintegration of the luminal epithelium. No evidence for fusion of the fetal cells with the maternal cells, as suggested by Larsen (1961) for implantation in the rabbit, has been found in the armadillo.

After the initial penetration very little additional loss of luminal epithelium appears to occur. The glandular epithelium underlying the site, however, is surrounded by invasive trophoblast, after which it undergoes deterioration. In this instance, the sequence of events is consistent with the idea that the endometrial cells disintegrate when cut off from their normal vascular relationships rather than being actively digested. The subsequent enlargement of the site appears to accompany enlargement of the exocelom and the closing plate and is brought about by a distention of the uterus rather than by continued erosion.

The morphological evidence accumulated in the course of this study enables us to suggest some of the functions of the various components of the early implantation site. A great deal of additional evidence is necessary, however, before these functions can be established with certainty and the means by which they are accomplished elucidated. Because of the small size of early implantation sites in this animal and others that do not have central implantation, it is doubtful whether ordinary biochemical or physiological methods are practical. The exacting methods of Edstrom (1960) for study of nucleic acids might be modified for use in studying a larger number of substances. Another promising approach is the use of aldehydes for initial fixation, then postfixing in osmium fixatives after incubation as a method of intercellular localization of enzyme activity (see Essner and Novikoff, 1962). At the present time, however, fixation of these tissues is barely adequate for morphological investigation alone.

The rapidity of differentiation into several distinct cell types at the early implantation site is a particularly interesting phenomenon. Evidently, mesenchyme cells, symplasma, cytotrophoblast and closing plate, and invasive trophoblast are differentiated within a period of a few hours to a very few days. The relationships that determine what the direction of differentiation shall be for an individual cell are far from clear. The complexity of the relationship between the blastocyst and the endometrium is quite remarkable in this relatively primitive animal. With regard to structural sophistication, reproduction in the armadillo appears far from simple.

References

Buchanan, G. D., A. C. Enders, and R. V. Talmage. 1956. Implantation in armadillos ovariectomized during the period of delayed implantation. J. Endocrin., **14**:121–28.

Dempsey, E. W. 1953. Electron microscopy of the visceral yolk-sac epithelium of the guinea pig. Am. J. Anat., **93**:331–63.

Enders, A. C. 1960*a*. Development and structure of the villous haemochorial placenta of the nine-banded armadillo (*Dasypus novemcinctus*). J. Anat., **94**: 34–45.

———. 1960*b*. Electron microscopic observations on the villous haemochorial placenta of the nine-banded armadillo (*Dasypus novemcinctus*). *Ibid.*, pp. 205–15.

———. 1962. The structure of the armadillo blastocyst. *Ibid.*, **96**:39–48.

Enders, A. C., and G. D. Buchanan. 1959. Some effects of ovariectomy and injection of ovarian hormones in the armadillo. J. Endocrin., **19**:251–58.

Enders, A. C., G. D. Buchanan, and R. V. Talmage. 1958. Histological and histochemical observations on the armadillo uterus during the delayed and post-implantation periods. Anat. Rec., **130**:639–57.

Essner, E., and A. B. Novikoff. 1962. Cytological studies on two functional hepatomas: Interrelations of endoplasmic reticulum, Golgi apparatus, and lysosomes. J. Cell. Biol., **15**:289–312.

Larsen, J. F. 1961. Electron microscopy of the implantation site in the rabbit. Am. J. Anat., **109**:319–34.

Luse, S. A. 1957. The morphological manifestations of uptake of materials by the yolk sac of the pregnant rabbit. Macy Foundation Conf. Gestation, **4**: 115–42.

Luse, S. A., J. Davies, and M. Smith. 1959. Electron microscopy of experimental inclusions in cytoplasm and nuclei of yolk sac cells. Fed. Proc., **18**:491.

Newman, H. H., and J. T. Patterson. 1910. The development of the nine-banded armadillo from primitive streak to birth, with special references to the question of specific polyembryony. J. Morph., **21**:359–423.

Patterson, J. T. 1913. Polyembryonic development in *Tatusia novemcinctus*. J. Morph., **24**:559–684.

Wislocki, G. B., and E. W. Dempsey. 1955*a*. Electron microscopy of the human placenta. Anat. Rec., **123**:133–67.

———. 1955*b*. Electron microscopy of the placenta of the rat. *Ibid*., pp. 33–63.

Wislocki, G. B., and H. A. Padykula. 1961. Histochemistry and electron microscopy of the placenta. In W. C. Young (ed.), Sex and Internal Secretions. Baltimore: Williams & Wilkins Co.

DISCUSSION (*Chairman:* E. C. Amoroso)

Wimsatt: I have two questions. I noticed when you showed development of the fetal membranes that there was irregularity of nuclear membrane in the yolk sac epithelial cells. Is this unusual?

A. Enders: There is quite a bit of variation in the irregularity of the nuclear envelope. However, certain types of cells, such as the cytotrophoblast cells, have a less irregular nuclear envelope, while others, including the cells of invasive trophoblast and the early yolk sac, show more irregularities.

Wimsatt: What is the origin of the symplasmic masses?

A. Enders: After we found symplasmic masses associated with the trophoblast of two implantation sites that became detached during examination, I came to the conclusion that the trophoblast was a source of these masses.

Dempsey: I offer you my sympathy and admiration for having put together the identification and localization of the cells in this highly complex region. I am not sure that I am entirely convinced about the origin of the symplasma. I think it may require more material and more discussion before this question can be resolved. It is so common in so many species for the endometrium to be transformed into a symplasmic mass at about the time of implantation that one searches for evidence of this phenomenon in any new form. The mass you describe does appear to be different from the fetal type of syncytium. Thus, there are either two fetal syncytia or a fetal syncytium and a maternal symplasma.

A. Enders: On the other hand, occasional trophoblast cells contiguous with the symplasma seem to show intermediate stages (such as unusually extensive endoplasmic reticulum). However, these early stages are hard to get, and it is possible that we have missed the crucial evidence.

Dempsey: There seems to be a terminological problem also. "Symplasma" generally refers to a confluent mass of maternal cells, while "syncytium" refers to a similar configuration of fetal elements.

A. ENDERS: In that case, I should prefer to refer to this region as the "syncytial mass," at least until more evidence is accumulated.

DAVIES: Could you expand a bit on the relationship between cytotrophoblast and syncytium? How does syncytium arise from cytotrophoblast? Are there desmosomes, etc.? Is it a true syncytium or multinucleate sheets?

A. ENDERS: In later stages, where there are cell columns, the relationship between the cytotrophoblast and the syncytial trophoblast is particularly clear. In these stages, the cell columns form proliferating masses of cells at the tips of the villi. Overlying the cell columns and forming the epithelium of the vascular villi is a single layer of syncytial trophoblast (there is no Langhan's layer in the armadillo). Desmosomes form between the cells of the cell columns and the overlying syncytium. In earlier stages this type of relationship is not found.

HARRISON: I was interested in your comments on invasive trophoblast and on the histochemical investigation of the invasive characteristics. Can you expand on this? Do cells really destroy the maternal tissue?

A. ENDERS: Initial penetration of epithelium occurs. Then the two or three glands between the luminal epithelium and the larger sinuses are surrounded by invasive tissue that is clearly trophoblast. The glands look healthy at first. They then begin to appear necrotic, with fatty degeneration and membrane breakdown. We attempted to localize proteolytic activity by incubation of sections against a gelatin film. The results were equivocal, but it should be kept in mind that the finding of proteolytic activity in such sections would not mean that the enzymes were being released in the living tissue. The enzymes might be associated with the intracellular breakdown of material ingested by the trophoblast.

WIMSATT: I do not recollect that you answered explicitly Dr. Davies' question on how the syncytium arises.

DEMPSEY: I think he did answer the question, because the attachment of one cell to another cell by means of desmosomes is quite specific. The only exception, in which cells of one type are attached by desmosomes to cells of a different type, is the motor end plate. Otherwise, these structures appear to occur only between cells of related embryonic origin.

A. ENDERS: In this species it is particularly clear that the process of formation of syncytium during the period of placental expansion is from the cytotrophoblast at the tips of the villi. The villi are free in the maternal blood stream. Villi develop in the shape of flattened projections forming more aborizing projections later. After this condition is reached, all cells of the cell columns disappear and the only subsequent enlargement of villi is by increase in diameter. Since the armadillo placenta lacks a Langhans layer, anchoring villi, and a basal plate, the restriction of the cytotrophoblast to the cell columns is particularly striking. It should also be noted that there is no decidual reaction in the armadillo, in that there is neither a stromal reaction as in rodents nor an epithelial proliferation as in carnivores.

WIMSATT: Do you see former membranes "fading away"? What is the visible expression of the genesis of syncytium from cytotrophoblast?

DAVIES: The cytotrophoblastic cells divide and in some way give rise to syncytiotrophoblast. The latter may arise by fusion of daughter cells of the cytotrophoblast—the classical view—or in some obscure way nuclei may be "pumped" into the syncytial mass by repeated mitoses without the formation of cell membranes. In the rodents and the rat the syncytiotrophoblast consists of overlapping bi- or trinucleate syncytial sheets, rather than a continuous syncytial mass.

ORSINI: Could the syncytium be formed by enlargement of the cells of the cytotrophoblast? In the hamster the largest giant cells, the tertiary giant cells, may be seen to develop (in a developmental series) from smaller cells without mitoses.

AMOROSO: We cannot unravel the problem here, since it has obfuscated the minds of many workers since Strahl. It is a most confusing and difficult problem to understand, and I think there is where we must leave it.

CECILIA LUTWAK-MANN

Uterine-Blastocyst Relationships at the Time of Implantation: Biochemical Aspects

Visual inspection supported by optical methods, now increasingly involving high-power microscopy, has until recently represented the main investigational approach in the study of uterine implantation, a phenomenon that has for so long engaged the attention of naturalists, ecologists, and physiologists. Attempts to investigate chemically early mammalian development are of relatively recent origin, and, as yet, the biochemical contributions form a very small, though perhaps not entirely insignificant, sector in this field of study.

The rapidity with which analytical chemical and physical methods are being perfected augurs well for the future of this particular area of chemical embryology. One would almost say that it is not so much the technical deficiencies as the lack of interest among professional biochemists that has been responsible for the sluggish tempo of progress in this field. That, however, is not to be wondered at; it appears, and often in fact is, much more rewarding for a biochemist to work in those areas of his discipline in which there is a great deal of current interest rather than to be spending a lonely existence in what is virtually a no-man's land, trying to engage the attention and understanding of the descriptive embryologist, endocrinologist, and medical or veterinary man, a good many of whom continue to evince a distaste for biochemical intervention, perhaps because (subconsciously?) they see in it a challenge to their hitherto undisputed supremacy of thought or possibly owing to an underestimation of the intrinsic value of biochemical contribution to the problems inherent in the process of mammalian reproduction in general, and uterine implantation more specifically.

DR. CECILIA LUTWAK-MANN is Principal Scientific Officer, Agricultural Research Council Unit of Reproductive Physiology and Biochemistry, University of Cambridge, England.

By contrast with that reluctance to recognize and admit the significance of chemical findings as part and parcel of mammalian embryology, there is the attitude of those who, though not much experienced in metabolic studies, eagerly seize upon and try to invest with some deep but often farfetched meaning every minor chemical discovery, long before the original discoverer has been given time to assess properly the true significance and relevance of his own findings. Such "inspired guesses" and hypotheses cause a great deal of confusion, though undoubtedly they swell the individual scientific output! An illustrative case in point is the endometrial carbonic anhydrase. Whereas its discoverer (and present author) carefully avoided assigning to this uterine enzyme any specific function in embryonic life until more general and interspecies information was forthcoming (Lutwak-Mann, 1955), others, who contrary to usage shall remain nameless, took up the subject, spinning out rather involved theories whereby carbonic anhydrase–catalyzed alkaline carbonate was to have been the agent responsible for a peculiar "stickiness" of the surface of the implanting blastocyst. No account was taken in these theories of the fact that under physiological conditions the alkalinity of a carbonate system would be buffered by carbon dioxide. Moreover, since it has now been demonstrated that a remarkably high bicarbonate content is characteristic of the estrous uterine fluid of the rabbit (Lutwak-Mann, 1962*b;* Leone, Libonati, and Lutwak-Mann, 1963), coincident with quite low activity of endometrial carbonic anhydrase, the always improbable "carbonic anhydrase theory" of blastocyst implantation has been further weakened.

However, these reflections bear upon what is probably no more than a passing phase, soon due to come to an end, and, since more biochemically trained investigators are entering the field of mammalian reproduction, the flow of their contributions is bound to enlarge our comprehension of, among other things, that very complex set of biological events that comprises implantation and its variants. In what follows, experimental approaches rather than the experiments themselves will be described, whereby the author and her co-workers have attempted to study, in the rabbit, blastocyst-maternal relationships at stages of pregnancy immediately preceding and subsequent to implantation.

Perhaps the simplest example of the experimental procedures applied has been the study of the concentration in blastocyst fluid as compared with maternal body fluids, of sugars and other small-molecular substances, at various time intervals following parenteral administration at 6–10 days of gestation (Lutwak-Mann, 1954, 1962*a*). From the experimental results with sugars, such as, for example, glucose or fructose, it appeared that unimplanted blastocysts were almost impenetrable but that these substances increasingly gained access into the blastocyst cavity with incipient and advancing implantation. However, in the earlier experiments of this type no account has been taken of the possibility that the entry into free-lying blastocysts of even small molecules, such as glucose or fructose, may depend in the first place on whether or not such substances are capable of passing across the endometrium and into the endometrial secretion. Recently, however, some indication has been obtained that glucose or fructose, administered intravenously, does not raise materially the level of reducing sugar in the uterine estrous fluid (Lutwak-Mann, 1962*b*). The mechanism of the process whereby hexoses, and possibly other metabolites, are prevented from crossing into the uterine lumen is still under investigation. But it may explain to a large extent why maternal hyperglycemia or fructosemia fails to influence perceptibly the respective levels of these sugars in the unattached blastocysts. It is probable that the ability to resist the passage of certain metabolites and convey others readily is a property perhaps shared by the endometrium with the cells of the trophoblast, a property that may be responsible to a significant extent for observations made with respect to blastocyst permeability.

Apart from and in addition to the endometrium, there are the barriers presented to metabolite exchange by the membranes investing the blastocysts, chiefly the zona pellucida, and, ultimately, the selectivity of the trophoblast itself toward materials that reach it from the uterine secretion.

In this respect, another point deserves discussion, though so far it has scarcely been investigated, namely, that there must exist a continuous two-way exchange between the maternal environment and the young implanting embryo. It has been found repeatedly that the clearance from the blastocyst space is slow and that, for instance, glucose and salicylate (both of them substances that are easy to determine quantitatively in minute amounts of experimental material) tend to linger on in the blastocyst cavity at levels which at certain stages exceed those of the maternal fluids quite perceptibly. This is a fact of considerable biological interest, since it may explain the damaging action upon the early embryo of agents that are eliminated quite efficiently from the maternal circulation, which, however, may, so to speak, hang on, unsuspected, in the embryonic fluids for a considerable time. Thus, determinations of, say, isotopically labeled drugs or other potentially embryotropic substances in the organs or body fluids of the adult and/or pregnant animal need not necessarily reflect the conditions within the embryo or its immediate uterine environment. Here one cannot but think of the recent impressive work on the distribution of C^{14}-labeled thalidomide in orally treated laboratory animals (Faigle *et al.*, 1962). Although most instructive pharmacological and biochemical data have thus been assembled on the distribution and persistence of thalidomide following single and multiple doses in a number of organs and body fluids, no major attempt has been made, to date, to establish by the same excellent techniques the presence, continued or otherwise, of this *facultative* teratogen (if one may coin this term for it) in either the young embryo or the endometrial tissues. Yet the possibility of residual thalidomide in embryonic fluids or cells ought at least to be envisaged, in view of the extended period of its presence in the cellular elements of blood, in contrast to a much earlier clearance from the blood plasma. Nor should carrying out the requisite experiments present much technical difficulty, since the blastocyst flat-mount procedure evolved by us (Moog and Lutwak-Mann, 1958; Lutwak-Mann and Hay, 1962) lends itself extremely well to autoradiographic and similar techniques. That it would indeed be worthwhile to follow up this line of thought is indicated by our findings, whereby even preimplantation blastocysts appeared to suffer damage, largely confined to the embryonic disk, following oral treatment of pregnant rabbits with thalidomide soon after mating.

Another experimental approach that has permitted us to obtain an idea of the speed with which blastocyst permeability changes with progressing implantation has been made by studying the entry of labeled ions from the maternal circulation into the embryo and its environment (Lutwak-Mann, Boursnell, and Bennett, 1960). This enabled us to study certain comparative aspects of the incorporation of labeled ions in a variety of systems, which included (1) the free-lying blastocyst as against the enveloping endometrial secretion, (2) the preimplantation $6\frac{1}{2}$-day-old embryo as against the 12-day-old fetus, (3) the endometrial mucosa as against the secretion, on one side, and incipient placental tissue, on the other.

These experiments have corroborated what has also been inferred from other experimental approaches, namely, that even before uterine nidation the blastocyst is already a relatively highly organized entity, rich in coenzymes and vitamins (Jacobson and Lutwak-Mann, 1956; Kodicek and Lutwak-Mann, 1957), capable of a marked degree of metabolic selectivity. It was found, for instance, that, in spite of a uniformly high distribution of labeled ions in the uterine secretion, individual ions were entering the blastocysts, each at its own characteristic level, which for the ions studied was well below that of the secretion. We have taken this as an indication, even if not direct proof, of a mode of entry for labeled ions (and presumably several other metabolites as well) by "active transport" rather than by simple diffusion.

By the same approach we have been able to assess events in the uterine secretion as compared with the blastocyst fluid, both of which may be presumed to be of fundamental nutrient value to the preimplantation and implanting embryo. From the time of entry of the embryos into the uterus and during implantation, we have observed striking differences in values for labeled ions incorporated in what may be regarded as the "inner and outer aquatic medium" of the young embryos. In the endometrial secretion the uptake values registered were roughly of the same order for each ion examined; from day 5 of gestation onward (though not before then) values in the uterine secretion were devoid of major fluctuations. The blastocyst fluid, on the other hand, presented a vastly different picture of ion incorporation, in that all its uptake values were several times lower than those recorded for the secretion and, moreover, each ion was incorporated differently, some of them, like $^{32}PO_4$, ^{24}Na, and $^{35}SO_4$, presenting peak values at about $7\frac{1}{2}$–8 days, a stage at which maximum permeability of the blastocyst cavity has also been demonstrated by entirely different investigational procedures. Brambell and his co-workers (1949) showed by means of electrophoretic and ultracentrifuge studies that the blastocyst fluid of 7–8-day-old rabbit embryos, but not thereafter, contains albumin, and α-, β-, and γ-globulins, as well as fibrinogen, in similar proportions to each other as in the maternal plasma. Furthermore, agglutinins, whether actively or passively acquired, were found to pass freely from the maternal circulation into the blastocyst cavity of implanting rabbit embryos without alteration of protein structure (Brambell, Hemmings, and Rowlands, 1948). It is obvious that in the rabbit—at any rate, just before the full development of the true placenta—the blastocyst is not selective in some respects, since it was at least as permeable to foreign protein as to that of maternal origin. The retention of immunological identity by the agglutinins after their passage across the trophoblast wall constitutes, if not evidence, then certainly a strong indication that the agglutinins remained unaltered in transit. Thus, an exchange of even large-sized molecules between mother and implanting embryo (in this particular species) appears to have been proved, the trophoblast seemingly being as permeable to homologous as to heterologous protein.

The peculiarities of penetrability of the free-lying and implanting rabbit blastocyst have also been brought out by experiments in which it was demonstrated that before nidation the embryos remain impermeable to the azo-dye trypan blue, whereas from about day $7\frac{1}{2}$ onward this teratogen enters the blastocyst cavity freely (Ferm, 1956; confirmed by Lutwak-Mann, Boursnell, and Bennett, 1960).

As concerns the tissues that are in intimate contact with the implanting embryo, namely, the endometrial mucosa and incipient placental tissue, of all the labeled ions examined, $^{32}PO_4$ gave the most instructive and presumably significant results. Endometrial values for incorporation of $^{32}PO_4$ showed a progressive rise from day 6 to day 9 of gestation; this was not observed with other ions examined. Moreover, starting as early as day 7, the incorporation of $^{32}PO_4$ by the very young placental tissue exceeded several times that of the extraplacental endometrium. The placental ^{32}P-values reached a maximum on days 8–9, declining afterward. We took these observations as indicative of the special metabolic potential of the fast-developing placental tissue. When the latter has been damaged, by suitably timed estrogen pretreatment of the pregnant animal, the $^{32}PO_4$ incorporation by the placenta declined markedly.

The effect exerted by the removal of ovaries, a well-tried experimental approach in studies on implantation, has also proved enlightening as concerns events taking place during a deliberately restricted "anovarian" period (Lutwak-Mann, Hay, and Adams, 1962). First of all, we found that blastocysts did not implant on day 7 (as they do normally) if ovariectomy was done about 16–20 hours earlier. There was invariably embryonic loss, but the surviving blastocysts did not differ materially from coeval normal ones, either in over-all dimensions or those of the embryonic disks or in the extent of differentiation and development of trophoblastic knobs. The embryos' mitotic activity, ascertained in experiments with parenterally administered Colcemid, was well maintained. That such embryos were, in fact, perfectly viable was demonstrated by transferring them into suitable culture media in which they proceeded to expand and differentiate further right up to the stage of primitive groove, head process, and blood-island formation. These findings on postovariectomy blastocysts were not unexpected. We knew from other experiments in which we had administered estrogens to rabbits at 4–5 days of pregnancy that such interference with the hormonal equilibrium did not per se affect the $6\frac{1}{2}$-day-old preimplantation blastocysts but influenced them only in the subsequent stages, indirectly, owing to changes produced in the uterine environment by the estrogen treatment.

No spectacular changes were noted in the postovariectomy endometrium, at any rate as assessed either histologically or by determining carbonic anhydrase activity. It is of course probable that, because of the limited postovariectomy interval, subtle changes in the endometrium would escape all but the most exacting methods of examination.

The general impression was gained, though it was not easy to provide for it a direct proof, that the postovariectomy change chiefly responsible for failure of implantation resided in the myometrium. Presumably, because of the disturbance induced in the myometrial tonus, the blastocysts did not succeed in coming to rest at their predestined nidation "stations" sufficiently long to permit the setting-up of reciprocal vascular-trophoblastic reactions, which are essential for attachment. To what extent one could offset the deleterious effect of ovariectomy by hormonal substitution has not been adequately explored. But, in view of the brief period intervening between the removal of ovaries and autopsy, it seems most unlikely that exogenous hormones would have had a chance to counteract the loss of endogenous ovarian control.

The concentration of characteristic embryonic metabolites, namely, glucose, bicarbonate, and lactic acid, showed a significant decrease only in respect to lactate, that of the other two remaining practically unaltered. It would be most desirable to pursue further and in more detail the reasons for differences in lactic acid content between normally implanting 7-day-old blastocysts and those that fail to implant—for example, following gonadectomy or after treatment of pregnant rabbits with mercaptopurine.

In our work on embryotoxic agents (Adams, Hay, and Lutwak-Mann, 1961) we have concentrated mainly on the preimplantation blastocysts. However, we have frequently also included in these studies the period of uterine attachment so as to find out which, if any, of the numerous drugs administered maternally were capable of preventing implantation. Quite generally speaking, when the interval allowed for drug action was short, as was mostly the case in our experiments, it was seldom possible entirely to prevent blastocyst attachment, even with relatively large doses of potent agents. The situation most commonly encountered on day 7 or day 8 of gestation following drug treatment as late as day 5 or day 6 of gestation, was a partial implantation, in the sense that some blastocysts were forming apparently normal implantation domes, while others were lying free, so that one could lift them readily from the endometrial surface. Such individual differences in drug susceptibility within members of a litter, even at the blastocyst stage of embryonic development, were often observed in response to a variety of drugs given to the pregnant rabbits. In this respect it is most interesting to recall observations made by Brambell (1948), who noted variations in agglutinin titers from embryo to embryo in the same litter, at 8½ days of gestation, in rabbits immunized against *Brucella abortus*.

These as yet meager biochemical data on the blastocyst-uterine relationships at the time of implantation await extension in several directions. First, we might with profit learn more about the metabolism of the implanting embryo, in itself not an insuperable task but one worthwhile only if the metabolic measurements are accompanied by *sound* criteria of embryonic viability. Such criteria, we believe, we have at long last worked out for the rabbit blastocysts, since we can now keep them alive for up to 48 hours in readily available culture media and are, moreover, able to assess confidently the extent of their continuing growth and differentiation by means of a simple and rapid histological procedure. That should make the rabbit blastocysts an object of choice for future metabolic studies in vitro.

Next, so as to enlarge our vision and perspective, data analogous to those discussed above ought to be acquired in animal species other than the rabbit. Furthermore, much benefit would accrue from better knowledge concerning the levels at implantation time of ovarian steroids in maternal blood and their urinary excretion products, since this would give us some sort of endocrine diagnostic assessment of incipient and accomplished nidation. As a matter of fact, any approach, whether purely morphological, chemical, or physical (preferably a combination of all three), that would enable us to determine precisely the onset and termination of implantation would be invaluable. As yet, clinical determinations of ovarian hormones in blood are not really practicable. There is one reference to human implantation, sufficiently well documented to be worth mentioning, which describes a distinct rise in gonadotrophin excretion at 9 days after artificial insemination carried out on the day of the mid-cycle estrogen peak and resulting in a normal pregnancy (Brown *et al.*, 1958). The increase in gonadotrophin was followed by a rise in estrogen output and by maintenance of luteal-phase levels of pregnanediol. According to the authors, the increase in gonadotrophin was due not to pituitary but to chorionic gonadotrophin. In sows, the week of maximal excretion of estrone was observed at about 24–27 days after breeding, the levels of estradiol-17β remaining low (Lunaas, 1962). Here the time of increasing estrone excretion corresponded to the stage in which, according to Corner (1921), the fetal membranes expand and become vascularized. Since, at present, refinements in methods of hormone determination are being constantly introduced, the latter constitute the safest basis of our hopes for a satisfactory solution of the problems involved in the process of implantation and its variants.

It remains to be seen whether greater clinical and laboratory use will be made in the near future of physical methods of investigation other than recordings of basal temperature, for instance, measurements of potential across readily accessible areas of the body surface and its cavities (skin and mucous membranes), preferential fixation of some isotopes, perhaps by certain endocrine glands or the reproductive tract itself, etc. In this respect, we must keep an open and unbiased mind at all times and be receptive to any novel ideas that might helpfully present themselves to us in our quest for advancement.

REFERENCES

ADAMS, C. E., M. F. HAY, and C. LUTWAK-MANN. 1961. The action of various agents upon the rabbit embryo. J. Embryol. Exp. Morph., **9**:468–91.

BRAMBELL, F. W. R., and W. A. HEMMINGS. 1949. The passage into the embryonic yolk sac cavity of maternal plasma proteins in rabbits. J. Physiol., **108**:177–85.

BRAMBELL, F. W. R., W. A. HEMMINGS, and W. T. ROWLANDS. 1948. The passage of antibodies from the maternal circulation into the embryo in rabbits. Proc. Roy. Soc., B., **145**:390–403.

BROWN, J. B., A. KLOPPER, and J. A. LORAINE, 1958. The urinary excretion of oestrogens, pregnanediol and gonadotrophins during the menstrual cycle. J. Endocrin., **17**:401–20.

CORNER, G. W. 1921. Cyclical changes in the ovaries and uterus of the sow and their relation to the mechanism of implantation. Carnegie Inst. Wash. Contr. Embryol., **13**:119.

FAIGLE, J. W., H. KEBERLE, W. RIESS, and K. SCHMID. 1962. The metabolic fate of thalidomide. Experientia, **18**:389.

FERM, V. H. 1956. Permeability of the rabbit blastocyst to trypan blue. Anat. Rec., **125**:745–60.

JACOBSON, W., and C. LUTWAK-MANN. 1956. The vitamin B_{12} content of the early rabbit embryo. J. Endocrin., **20**:ii–iii.

KODICEK, E., and C. LUTWAK-MANN. 1957. The pattern of distribution of thiamine, riboflavin and nicotinic acid in the early rabbit embryo. J. Endocrin., **14**:xix.

LEONE, E., M. LIBONATI, and C. LUTWAK-MANN. 1963. Enzymes in the uterine and cervical fluid and certain related tissues and body fluids. J. Endocrin. **25**:551.

LUNAAS, T. 1962. Urinary oestrogen levels in the sow during oestrous cycle and early pregnancy. J. Reprod. & Fertil., **4**:13–20.

LUTWAK-MANN, C. 1954. Some properties of the rabbit blastocyst. J. Embryol. Exp. Morph. **2**:1–13.

———. 1955. Carbonic anhydrase in the female reproductive tract: Occurrence, distribution and hormonal dependence. J. Endocrin., **13**:26–38.

———. 1962*a*. Glucose, lactic acid and bicarbonate in rabbit blastocyst fluid. *Nature*, **193**:653–54.

———. 1962*b*. Some properties of uterine and cervical fluid in the rabbit. Biochim. & Biophys. Acta, **58**:637–39.

LUTWAK-MANN, C., J. C. BOURSNELL, and J. P. BENNETT. 1960. Blastocyst-uterine relationships: Uptake of radioactive ions by the early rabbit and its environment. J. Reprod. & Fertil., **1**:169–85.

LUTWAK-MANN, C., and M. F. HAY. 1962. Effect on the early embryo of

agents administered to the mother. Brit. Med. J., No. 5310 (October 13, 1962).
LUTWAK-MANN, C., M. F. HAY, and C. E. ADAMS. 1962. The effect of ovariectomy on rabbit blastocysts. J. Endocrin., **24**:185–97.
MOOG, F., and C. LUTWAK-MANN. 1958. Observations on rabbit blastocysts prepared as flat mounts. J. Embryol. Exp. Morph., **6**:57–67.

DISCUSSION (*Chairman:* E. C. AMOROSO)

DAVIES: Is the carbonic anhydrase in the blastocyst wall or in the endometrium?

LUTWAK-MANN: Only in the endometrium, so far as I know. To demonstrate its presence in the blastocyst wall would require very fine microdeterminations.

DAVIES: Do you place any significance on the relationship of the enzyme to the high bicarbonate?

LUTWAK-MANN: That possibility undoubtedly exists, though it is by no means easy to prove it directly. Inhibition, in vivo, of carbonic anhydrase in the endometrium of pregnant laboratory animals appeared to have little effect on the progress of pregnancy. On the other hand, relatively large amounts of bicarbonate are present in the uterine estrous fluid, coincident with low endometrial carbonic anhydrase activity. The interesting thing about carbonic anhydrase is its occurrence in the female reproductive tract, not only of mammals, but also of birds, fishes, and certain reptiles. One wonders whether this enzyme perhaps plays a more important role in the lower forms than in the mammal, where it may be a sort of "residual" enzyme? However, I keep a very open mind in respect to the biological significance of uterine carbonic anhydrase.

DAVIES: Do you know whether any membrane potential measurements have been made across the trophoblast wall? We made these on the allantoic membrane and got a flood of very high potassium with 50 megavolt potential.

LUTWAK-MANN: I possess no data but recognize that such measurements would be eminently desirable, provided that one could make them delicately enough not to upset the sensitive young embryo. I should be especially interested in potentials between the unimplanted blastocyst and the endometrial secretion.

GREENWALD: You have shown in previous work that antimetabolites destroy the inner cell mass without affecting the trophoblast. Have you any experiments on the uptake of ions, glucose, etc., by these altered blastocysts?

LUTWAK-MANN: Yes, indeed, we have done experiments on the uptake of labeled ions by blastocysts from mercaptopurine- or azaguaninetreated rabbits. We found very little difference, at that stage of embryonic development, as between our control values and those from the treated animals. On the other hand, the content of lactic acid was markedly diminished in 7-day-old blastocysts from mercaptopurine-treated rabbits (such blastocysts are usually incapable of implantation). When we examined the uptake of $^{32}PO_4$ in 12-day-old fetuses from mercaptopurine-injected rabbits, there was a distinct diminution in $^{32}PO_4$-uptake at that advanced stage; also, the placental tissue in these experiments showed decreased values for uptake of $^{32}PO_4$.

HARRISON: You mentioned thalidomide. Have you used it, and, if so, how did you administer it?

LUTWAK-MANN: We have used thalidomide in a limited number of experiments; it was given to rabbits orally, doses of 0.5 gm. per animal per day, having ostensibly no effects on the pregnant animal itself. The preimplantation blastocysts from these rabbits showed a peculiar "disorganization" in the area of the embryonic disk. However, it is conceivable that some of these pathological changes might be susceptible to repair in the course of further pregnancy. I certainly would not expect, in rabbits, anything more than, say, 5–10 per cent malformations from thalidomide. However, that still remains to be investigated, since hitherto this drug has always been administered after implantation.

HAFEZ: I am very much interested in the variations in the biochemical composition of the blastocyst fluid within the same litter. We have been dealing with rabbit blastocysts at day 6 postcoitum, and we have found a close relationship between the diameter of blastocyst and diameter of the inner cell mass. Would you get a correlation between the diameter of blastocyst and the biochemical composition of fluid within the same litter?

LUTWAK-MANN: We have done extensive measurements on the diameters of entire preimplantation blastocysts, as well as on the area of their embryonic disks. There are clear-cut differences between members of a litter as well as between coeval litters. I expect that we could present these differences more impressively by quantitative chemical determinations, say of nucleic acids, which is what we are now intending to do, using our blastocyst flat-mount preparations.

HAFEZ: For example, would you expect high lactic acid content in the small blastocyst?

LUTWAK-MANN: I use a very delicate micromethod to determine lactic acid, but it is not sufficiently sensitive to provide data on the differences in content between one blastocyst and another.

DE FEO: Have you studied histadine decarboxylase in the blastocyst?

LUTWAK-MANN: I have not done any experiments concerned with that enzyme.

DE FEO: If the blastocyst is a producer and releaser of histamine, would it not be reasonable to expect such an enzyme?

LUTWAK-MANN: I should have to think about that.

DE FEO: In the rat, we have found a wide range of substances to be capable of eliciting extensive deciduoma formation when injected introluminally. Among these is physiological saline. We believe that it is not necessary to postulate histamine release by the blastocyst, for, indeed, any metabolite that it might release could probably initiate the decidua.

LUTWAK-MANN: You may well be right.

E. C. AMOROSO

Summary of the Conference

THIS CONFERENCE has reached the point at which the privilege of being the chairman of this final session assumes its most onerous aspect, when, in accordance with the directives of its organizer, Dr. Enders, I must sum up the proceedings. In doing so, I shall attempt to bring into focus the many points of agreement and disagreement that have arisen during the course of our discussions and shall indicate to you to what extent my education on the biology of delayed implantation has been improved and to what extent it has not proceeded so far as it might well have done. But, if any part of this summary fails in its allusions to major points, while emphasizing minor ones unduly, you must ascribe this to my shortcomings and not to any departure from the strict neutrality that is usually associated with the chairman's function. At the outset, we can all agree that this symposium has lived up to the high expectations to which it had given rise and that it has amply justified the efforts of its organizer, Allen Enders. To him and to all the willing band of helpers, as well as to the participants, we offer our best thanks. Those who have contributed have spoken with authority, and no one present throughout these discussions can fail to have been impressed by the scope and interest of the narrative as this was unfolded in the several papers, which ranged from delayed implantation in marsupials to the fine structure of the placenta of the armadillo and ended a minute or two ago with Dr. Lutwak-Mann's analysis of uterine-blastocyst interrelationships.

The papers presented have been of a very high order of excellence, and all have provided important information, in some cases from a wholly novel point of view. The morphological descriptions of Wimsatt, of Sharman, and of Allen Enders; the experimental analyses provided by Mayer, by Deanesly, and by Shelesnyak; and the field studies undertaken by Ealey, and by Wright, Harrison, and Canivenc, all deal

DR. E. C. AMOROSO, F.R.S., is professor in the Department of Physiology, Royal Veterinary College, University of London, England.

with the same topic, but from different angles and with different instruments.

The fact that there is a community of problems has clearly emerged from our discussions, and if answers have been found to some of those that have engaged us, they will surely also provide clues to the solution of others. But the collection of all this information has, at the same time, revealed how extensive are the gaps that remain in our knowledge, and this symposium will have served a very useful purpose if, in the future, it focuses our attention on the many problems that have eluded us today and that still clamor for solution.

I turn for a moment to the individual papers and recall at the outset the introductory remarks of Dr. Hartman, who reminded us that the problem of delayed implantation has an immensely long history, having been recorded more than a century ago by Ziegler in 1843 and Bischoff in 1854. Since that time delayed implantation has been described in a variety of mammals under various conditions. Thus, it occurs spontaneously in normal gestation in the armadillo, the badger, and the roe deer, to mention the best-established instances, and was also observed by Lataste more than seventy-five years ago in mice that were pregnant and lactating at the same time.

Another type of evidence was that provided by our Australian friends, who gave us a most fascinating account of delayed implantation in marsupials. Sharman recalled that among the macropod marsupials there are several that show the phenomenon of delay. He discovered, as recently as 1954, I believe, that the period between ovulation and implantation, in a pregnancy concurrent with lactating young inside or outside the pouch, is very greatly extended, and he showed that the amount of delay corresponds in a general way to the time young are being suckled. These and other facts that Sharman presented pose fascinating problems and indicate that reproduction in these creatures is not as simple as it sometimes seems or is made out to be.

While certain instances of endocrine mechanisms in the delayed implantation of marsupials have been established, our knowledge of these processes appears rather incomplete in comparison with the elegant analyses of Canivenc and Mayer in the rat. However, when one appreciates the difficulties inherent in experimentation with the marsupials and considers that relatively few investigators devote their efforts to this aspect of biology, the investigations of Tyndale-Biscoe and of Ealey assume a new importance and inspire confidence that we are on the threshold of many exciting discoveries.

The great strength of this marsupial work, which I regard as functional morphology, lies in the fact that it has always been considered in the light of the possible course of evolution, and, without this reference, I think that morphology is likely to be barren and to fall into errors of homology. Nevertheless, one must caution our Australian friends that it would be prudent to get more of the facts and to explore them more fully before embarking on speculations that may lead us into difficulties.

A point of particular interest to me was the realization of how much of the field of delayed implantation seems to be concerned with specific histological and morphogenetic reactions, whereas the underlying physiological processes involved appear to be more generalized. This conclusion emerged, for example, from the accounts given by Wimsatt and Orsini of the morphological changes in the reproductive tracts of the black bear and the hamster, respectively. It was apparent also in the clear-cut demonstrations of Noyes and of Mayer and in those of Nutting, in which similar mechanisms were invoked to explain essentially different phenomena.

The material presented by Glenister is so new, indeed, that it should cause little surprise if many of the interpretations of the phenomena he described are modified as newer knowledge becomes available. Nevertheless, it seems to me that the in vitro cultivation of the blastocyst is so important that we must be grateful to him for his description, even in its incomplete form, and we might suggest the use of the Cartesian diver manometer for the further exploration of the biology of the blastocyst in vitro.

The analyses of Wright and Harrison, as well as those of Robert Enders, are as direct an attack on the problem of delayed implantation in the Carnivora as can at present be made. One set of problems that emerged from the investigations of these workers, and also from the work of Canivenc, concerns the question of the free life of the blastocyst. It has come as an astonishing fact, to me at least, that the blastocyst can survive as long as it does free from all hormonal influences that can be related to the ovaries. We have also seen that in the case of the badger we are dealing with the free life of a blastocyst that may be related to processes different from those in the rat and mouse, different too from those in the mink, in which pituitary influences may be involved.

In some of these species it was shown that manipulation of photoperiods was sufficient to initiate development in a blastocyst that had remained quiescent for a long time. On the other hand, our discussion not only has dealt with external factors as modulators of blastocyst development but has also shown that blastocyst development is immediately affected by the dissolution of the zona and that the latter phenomenon appears not to be dependent upon the stability of the uterine environment but to be regulated from within the egg. This was very elegantly demonstrated by Noyes, who showed that unfertilized native rat eggs that had remained in a pseudopregnant uterus for as long as fertilized donor eggs retained their zona in contrast to the donor blastocysts, in which they were lost.

This observation interests me greatly, since there are clear indications from the work of Glenister that the presence of the zona in some way precludes, or at least delays, the attachment of the blastocyst. On this account one would like to know more about the hormonal and pharmacological conditions at the time of implantation, as well as those purely mechanical factors to which Wimsatt and others have alluded. If, for example, there is a crowding of the dormant blastocysts at the cervical end of the uterine horn, the factors determining their final resting point must presumably be related to the other mechanisms that we have been considering. Hence, as Shelesnyak has suggested, we should continue to look at the problem of nidation from as many different angles as possible.

This brings me to agents and procedures that interfere with nidation, which were discussed by Warren Nelson and briefly by Shelesnyak and by Lutwak-Mann. Their analyses, though not coming strictly within the scope of the title of this symposium, must command attention, for there is no problem in human biology that clamors for a more urgent solution. In the same way, too, Shelesnyak's explorations of the cytochemical and endocrinological mechanisms in ovo-implantation constitute a field of inquiry that it is hoped will be pursued as vigorously as it can be. It is also hoped that his plea for support has not gone unnoticed. New and challenging data abound in this work, though one may not think that his interpretation is the only one possible.

I come finally to the paper by Dr. Deanesly. Her studies on the guinea pig and those of Mayer on the rat are complementary and deal with the fate of the blastocyst following oöphorectomy. Their central theme has been the endocrinological factors that underlie the patterns of behavior of the free blastocyst. How, for example, is the arousal of the dormant vesicle effected? Their contributions, together with those of Tyndale-Biscoe, stand on their own; for up to the present, at this conference at any rate, theirs have been the only ones to tackle the problem of the experimental analysis of delayed implantation.

Drawing these various lines of research together, I believe that while we have gained a great deal of information from our various contributors, and while I personally know a lot more than I did at the beginning about the possible association of endocrine factors with delayed implantation, I am still at a loss to know whether these effects are mediated through the blastocyst itself or through the endometrium. That hormones are implicated seems certain, but how they do it is still a mystery. The free blastocyst is, of course, very stubborn until the zona is denuded. Thereafter, we witness those remarkable changes in its biochemical properties which Dr. Lutwak-Mann described this morning. Her paper indicated plainly that when one considers any of the morphological problems of delayed implantation, whether they are questions of endometrial reactions, on the one hand, or embryonic development, on the other, we are dealing with the unfolding of patterns of chemical change, which become meaningful only when considered in relationship to the accompanying anatomical changes but which by themselves remain sterile. When a dozen such studies of equal amplitude have been combined with the work of the biologist, we shall have a better understanding of delayed implantation. Meanwhile, we can only salute the pioneers and hope that some years hence, when we are again wondering where we stand and what progress has been made, we may again meet under the guidance of Allen Enders and in circumstances equally congenial.

Index